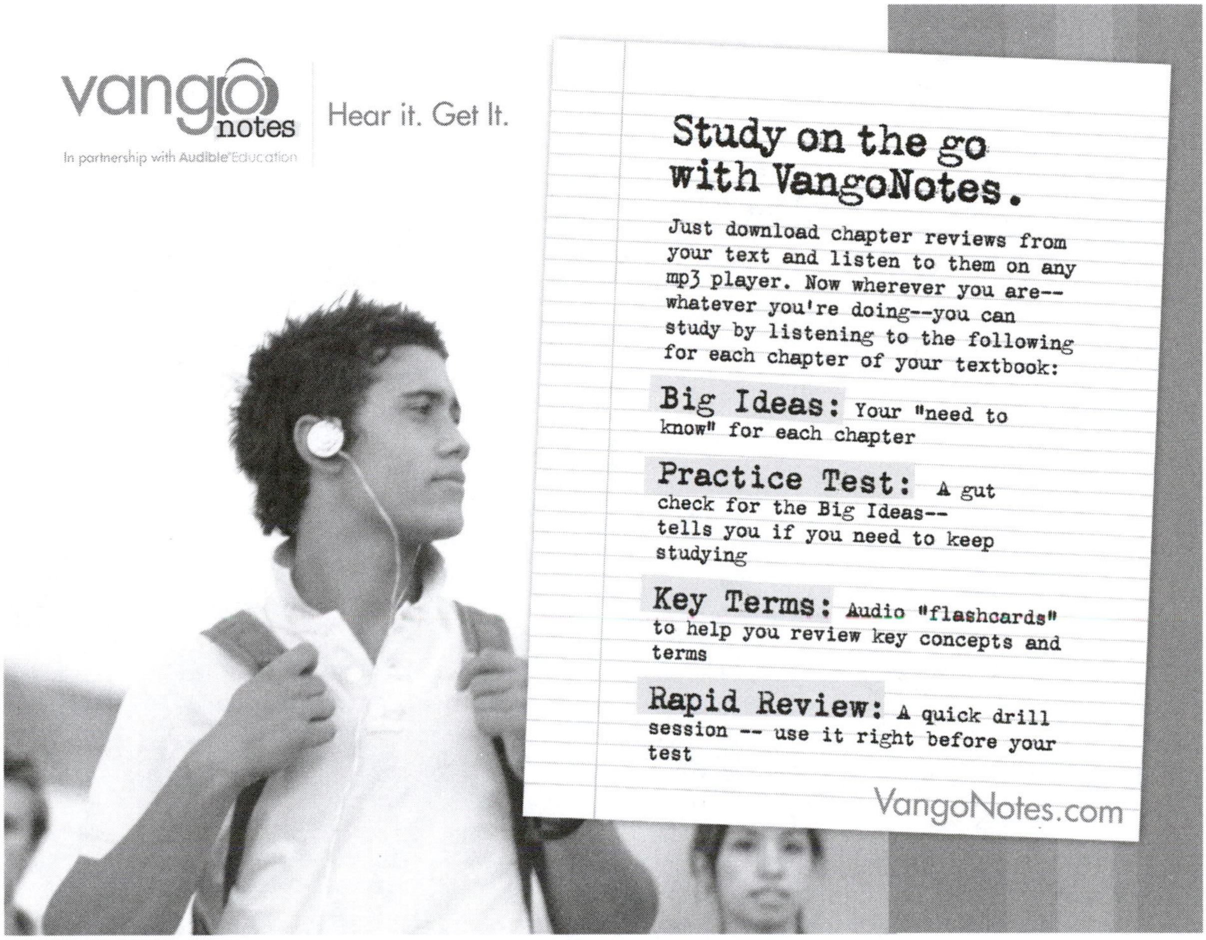
vango notes
Hear it. Get It.
In partnership with Audible Education
Study on the go with VangoNotes.
Just download chapter reviews from your text and listen to them on any mp3 player. Now wherever you are--whatever you're doing--you can study by listening to the following for each chapter of your textbook:
Big Ideas: Your "need to know" for each chapter
Practice Test: A gut check for the Big Ideas--tells you if you need to keep studying
Key Terms: Audio "flashcards" to help you review key concepts and terms
Rapid Review: A quick drill session -- use it right before your test
VangoNotes.com

Prentice Hall Nursing Reviews & Rationales

Nutrition & Diet Therapy

Second Edition

Series Editor

Mary Ann Hogan, MSN, RN

Clinical Assistant Professor
University of Massachusetts–Amherst
Amherst, Massachusetts

Consulting Editors

Evangeline DeLeon, RN

Assistant Professor
Delmar College
Corpus Christi, Texas

Margaret M. Gingrich, RN, MSN

Professor
Harrisburg Area Community College
Harrisburg, Pennsylvania

Kate Willcutts, MS, RD, CNSD

Assistant Clinical Nutrition Manager
Nutrition Services
Nursing Instructor
University of Virginia Medical Center
Charlottesville, Virginia

PEARSON
Prentice Hall

Upper Saddle River, New Jersey 07458

Cataloging-in-Publication data is on record at the Library of Congress.

Notice: Care has been taken to confirm the accuracy of the information presented in this book. The authors, editors, and the publisher, however, cannot accept any responsibility for errors or omissions or for the consequences for application of the information in this book and make no warranty, express or implied, with respect to its contents.

The authors and the publisher have exerted every effort to ensure that drug selections and dosages set forth in this text are in accord with current recommendations and practice at time of publication. However, in view of ongoing research, changes in government regulations, and the constant flow of information relating to drug therapy and drug reactions, the reader is urged to check the package inserts of all drugs for any change in indications of dosage and for added warnings and precautions. This is particularly important when the recommended agent is a new and/or infrequently employed drug.

The authors and publisher disclaim all responsibility for any liability, loss injury, or damage incurred as a consequence, directly or indirectly, of the use and application of any of the contents of this volume.

Publisher: Julie Levin Alexander
Assistant to Publisher: Regina Bruno
Editor-in-Chief: Maura Connor
Editorial Assistant: Mary Ellen Ruitenberg
Developmental Editor: Danielle Doller
Senior Managing Editor, Development: Marilyn Meserve
Managing Editor, Production: Patrick Walsh
Production Liaison: Anne Garcia
Production Editor: Jessica Balch, Pine Tree Composition
Manufacturing Manager: Ilene Sanford
Manufacturing Buyer: Pat Brown
Design Coordinator/Cover Designer: Mary Siener
Director of Marketing: Karen Allman
Senior Marketing Manager: Francisco Del Castillo
Marketing Coordinator: Michael Sirinides
Marketing Assistant: Patricia Linard
Media Product Manager: John Jordan
Manager of Media Production: Amy Peltier
New Media Project Manager: Stephen Hartner
Composition: Pine Tree Composition, Inc.
Printer/Binder: Von Hoffman, Owensville
Cover Printer: Phoenix Color Corp.

Pearson Education Ltd., *London*
Pearson Education Australia Pty. Limited, *Sydney*
Pearson Education Singapore, Pte. Ltd.
Pearson Education North Asia Ltd., *Hong Kong*
Pearson Education Canada, Ltd., *Toronto*
Pearson Educación de Mexico, S.A. de C.V.
Pearson Education—Japan, *Tokyo*
Pearson Education Malaysia, Pte. Ltd.
Pearson Education, Upper Saddle River, New Jersey

PEARSON
Prentice Hall

10 9 8 7 6 5 4 3 2 1
ISBN 0-13-243712-0

Contents

Welcome to the Prentice Hall Nursing Reviews & Rationales Series!

This series has been specifically designed to provide a clear and concentrated review of important nursing knowledge in the following content areas:

- Anatomy & Physiology
- Fundamentals & Skills
- Nutrition & Diet Therapy
- Fluids, Electrolytes, & Acid-Base Balance
- Medical-Surgical Nursing
- Pathophysiology
- Pharmacology
- Maternal-Newborn Nursing
- Child Health Nursing
- Mental Health Nursing
- Physical Assessment
- Community Health Nursing
- Leadership & Management

The books in this series are designed for use either by current nursing students as a study aid for nursing course work, for NCLEX-RN® licensing exam preparation, or by practicing nurses seeking a comprehensive yet concise review of a nursing specialty or subject area.

This series is truly unique. One of its most special features is that it has been developed and reviewed by a large team of nurse educators from across the United States and Canada to ensure that each chapter is edited by a nurse expert in the content area under study. The series editor, Mary Ann Hogan, designed the overall series in collaboration with a core Prentice Hall team to take full advantage of Prentice Hall's cutting edge technology. The consulting editors for each book, also experts in that specialty area, then reviewed all chapters and test questions submitted for comprehensiveness and accuracy. Finally, Mary Ann Hogan reviewed the chapters in each book for consistency, accuracy, and applicability to the NCLEX-RN® Test Plan.

All books in the series are identical in their overall design for your convenience. As an added value, each book comes with a comprehensive support package, including a bonus ***NCLEX-RN® Test Prep*** CD-ROM and a tear-out ***NursingNotes*** card for clinical reference and quick review.

Study Tips

Use of this book should help simplify your review. To make the most of your valuable study time, also follow these simple but important suggestions:

1. Use a weekly calendar to schedule study sessions.
   - Outline the timeframes for all of your activities (home, school, appointments, etc.) on a weekly calendar.
   - Find the "holes" in your calendar, which are the times in which you can plan to study. Add study sessions to the calendar at times when you can expect to be mentally alert and follow it!
2. Create the optimal study environment.
   - Eliminate external sources of distraction, such as television, telephone, etc.
   - Eliminate internal sources of distraction, such as hunger, thirst, or dwelling on items or problems cannot be worked on at the moment.
   - Take a break for 10 minutes or so after each hour of concentrated study both as a reward and an incentive to keep studying.
3. Use pre-reading strategies to increase comprehension of chapter material.
   - Skim read the headings in the chapter (because they identify chapter content).
   - Read the definitions of key terms, which will help you learn new words to comprehend chapter information.

- Review all graphic aids (figures, tables, boxes) because they are often used to explain important points in the chapter.

4. Read the chapter thoroughly but at a reasonable speed.
   - Comprehension and retention are actually enhanced by not reading too slowly.
   - Do take the time to reread any section that is unclear to you.
5. Summarize what you have learned.
   - Use questions supplied with this book and the ***NCLEX-RN® Test Prep*** CD-ROM to test your application of chapter content.
   - Review again any sections that correspond to questions you answered incorrectly or incompletely.

Test-Taking Strategies

We added new test-taking strategies to the rationales for every question in the series. These strategies will enable you to select the correct answer by breaking down the question, even if you don't know the correct response. Use the following strategies to increase your success on nursing tests or examinations:

- Get sufficient sleep and have something to eat before taking a test. Take deep breaths during the test as needed. Remember, the brain requires oxygen and glucose as fuel. Avoid concentrated sweets before a test, however, to avoid rapid upward and then downward surges in blood glucose levels.
- Read the question carefully, identifying the stem, the 4 options, and any critical words or phrases in either the stem or options.
  - Critical words in the stem such as "most important" indicate the need to set priorities, since more than 1 option is likely to contain a statement that is technically correct.
  - Remember that the presence of absolute words such as "never" or "only" in an answer option is more likely to make that option incorrect.
- Determine who is the client in the question; often this is the person with the health problem, but it may also be a significant other, relative, friend, or another nurse.
- Decide whether the stem is a true response stem or a false response stem. With a true response stem, the correct answer will be a true statement, and vice-versa.
- Determine what the question is really asking, sometimes referred to as the issue of the question. Evaluate all answer options in relation to this issue, and not strictly to the "correctness" of the statement in each individual option.
- Eliminate options that are obviously incorrect, then go back and reread the stem. Evaluate the remaining options against the stem once more.
- If two answers seem similar and correct, try to decide whether one of them is more global or comprehensive. If the global option includes the alternative option within it, it is likely that the more global response is the correct answer.

The NCLEX-RN® Licensing Examination

The NCLEX-RN® licensing examination is a Computer Adaptive Test (CAT) that ranges in length from 75 to 265 individual (stand-alone) test items, depending on individual performance during the examination. Upon graduation from a nursing program, successful completion of this exam is the gateway to your professional nursing practice. The blueprint for the exam is reviewed and revised every three years by the National Council of State Boards of Nursing according to the results of a job analysis study of new graduate nurses practicing within the first six months after graduation. Each question on the exam is coded to a *Client Need Category* and an *Integrated Process*.

Client Need Categories. There are 4 categories of client needs, and each exam will contain a minimum and maximum percent of questions from each category. Each major category has subcategories within it. The *Client Needs* categories according to the NCLEX-RN® Test Plan effective April 2007 are as follows:

- Safe, Effective Care Environment
  - Management of Care (13–19%)
  - Safety and Infection Control (8–14%)
- Health Promotion and Maintenance (6–12%)
- Psychosocial Integrity (6–12%)
- Physiological Integrity
  - Basic Care and Comfort (6–12%)
  - Pharmacological and Parenteral Therapies (13–19%)
  - Reduction of Risk Potential (13–19%)
  - Physiological Adaptation (11–17%)

Integrated Processes. The integrated processes identified on the NCLEX-RN® Test Plan effective April 2007, with condensed definitions, are as follows:

- Nursing Process: a scientific problem-solving approach used in nursing practice; consisting of assessment, analysis, planning, implementation, and evaluation.
- Caring: client-nurse interaction(s) characterized by mutual respect and trust and that are directed toward achieving desired client outcomes.
- Communication and Documentation: verbal and/or nonverbal interactions between nurse and others (client, family, health care team); a written or electronic recording of activities or events that occur during client care.
- Teaching and Learning: facilitating client's acquisition of knowledge, skills, and attitudes that lead to behavior change

More detailed information about this examination may be obtained by visiting the National Council of State Boards of Nursing website at http://www.ncsbn.org and viewing the *NCLEX-RN® Examination Test Plan for the National Council Licensure Examination for Registered Nurses.*[1]

[1]Reference: National Council of State Boards of Nursing, Inc. *NCLEX Examination Test Plan for National Council Licensure Examination for Registered Nurses.* Effective April, 2007. Retrieved from the World Wide Web at https://www.ncsbn.org/RN7Test_Plan_2007_Web.pdf.

HOW TO GET THE MOST OUT OF THIS BOOK

Each chapter has the following elements to guide you during review and study:

Chapter Objectives describe what you will be able to know or do after learning the material covered in the chapter.

Objectives

- ➤ Discuss legal considerations related to maternity nursing.
- ➤ Delineate ethical issues that influence maternal-newborn nursing practice.
- ➤ Identify culturally diverse health beliefs that impact the maternity cycle.
- ➤ Describe a philosophy of care that maintains maternal–newborn safety and fosters family unity.

NCLEX-RN® Test Prep

Use the CD-ROM enclosed with this book to access additional practice opportunities.

Review at a Glance contains a glossary of key terms used in the chapter, with definitions provided up-front and available at your fingertips, to help you stay focused and make the best use of your study time.

Review at a Glance

belief something accepted as true, especially as a tenet or a body of tenets accepted by an ethnocultural group

cultural competency the awareness, knowledge and skills necessary to appreciate, understand and communicate with people of diverse cultural backgrounds

family a group of individuals related by blood, marriage, or mutual goals

family-centered maternity care maternity care that is family oriented and views childbirth as a vital, natural life event rather than an illness

scope of practice legally refers to permissible boundaries of practice for nurses and is defined by statute (written law), rules and regulations, or a combination of the two

Pretest provides a 10-question quiz as a sample overview of the material covered in the chapter and helps you decide in what areas you need the most—or the least—review.

PRETEST

1 The nurse performs a vaginal examination and determines that the fetus is in a sacrum anterior position. The nurse draws which conclusion from this assessment data?

1. The fetal sacrum is toward the maternal symphysis pubis.
2. The fetal sacrum is toward the maternal sacrum.
3. The fetal face is toward the maternal sacrum.
4. The fetal face is toward the maternal symphysis pubis.

Practice to Pass questions are open-ended, stimulate critical thinking, and reinforce mastery of the chapter information.

Practice to Pass

The client scheduled for a hysterosalpingogram reports an allergy to shellfish. What should the nurse do?

NCLEX Alert identifies concepts that are likely to be tested on the NCLEX-RN® examination. Be sure to learn the information highlighted wherever you see this icon.

!

Case Study, found at the end of the chapter, provides an opportunity for you to use your critical thinking and clinical reasoning skills to "put it all together." It describes a true-to-life client case situation and asks you open-ended questions about how you would provide care for that client and/or family.

Case Study

A 14-year-old primigravida is admitted in early labor with severe preeclampsia at 42 weeks gestation. The client's blood pressure is 168/102.

1. What other assessment data would you obtain?
2. Describe the complications this client is at risk for.
3. Discuss the medications you expect to administer to this client.
4. What concerns do you have for this fetus? Why?
5. What would you teach this client and her family about her condition?

For suggested responses, see page 343.

Posttest provides an additional 10-question quiz at the end of the chapter. It provides you with feedback about mastery of the chapter material following review and study. All pretest and posttest questions contain comprehensive rationales for the correct and incorrect answers, and are coded according to cognitive level of difficulty, NCLEX-RN® Test Plan category of client need and integrated process.

POSTTEST

1 A client who is a brittle diabetic is seeking to get pregnant. The nursing working in a primary care provider's office suggests that which of the following healthcare providers would be an optimal choice?

1. A certified nurse-midwife
2. A family nurse practitioner
3. An obstetrician
4. A maternal-fetal medicine specialist

NCLEX-RN® Test Prep CD-ROM

For those who want to practice taking tests on a computer, the CD-ROM that accompanies the book contains the pretest and posttest questions found in all chapters of the book. In addition, it contains 30 NEW questions for each chapter to help you further evaluate your knowledge base and hone your test-taking skills. We included some of the newly developed alternate NCLEX Test Items, so these items will give you valuable practice with different types of questions.

Prentice Hall NursingNotes Card

This tear-out card provides a reference for frequently used facts and information related to the subject matter of the book. These are designed to be useful in the clinical setting, when quick and easy access to information is so important!

VangoNotes

Study on the go with VangoNotes. Just download chapter reviews from your text and listen to them on any mp3 player. Now wherever you are—whatever you're doing—you can study by listening to the following for each chapter of your textbook:

- **Big Ideas:** Your "need to know" for each chapter
- **Practice Test:** A gut check for the Big Ideas—tells you if you need to keep studying
- **Key Terms:** Audio "flashcards" to help you review key concepts and terms

VangoNotes are **flexible;** download all the material directly to your player, or only the chapters you need. And they're **efficient.** Use them in your car, at the gym, walking to class, wherever. So get yours today. And get studying.

About the Nutrition & Diet Therapy Book

Most nurses have limited experience in the field of nutrition, while most nutritionists have limited experience in the field of nursing. This book attempts to merge the knowledge of these two distinct disciplines into one reference source that addresses management of client nutrition in the context of the nursing practice. Chapters in this book cover "need-to-know" information about nutritional science with direct application to the nursing process. This book provides a comprehensive overview of nutritional principles and delves into building block elements (macronutrients and micronutrients) and basics of nutritional biochemistry to provide the reader with a clear, concise explanation of nutritional principles. Individual chapters focus on developmental areas of nutrition across the life span, nutritional therapeutics, nutritional support and therapeutic diets, and nutritional supplements. The last chapter examines the nutritional management of clients who experience multisystem disorders. This book is intended for use as one resource in managing a client's nutritional status and should be used in conjunction with appropriate referrals and collaboration with registered dieticians to provide client care and determine specific nutritional outcomes.

Acknowledgements

This book is a monumental effort of collaboration. Without the contributions of many individuals, this edition of *Nutrition & Diet Therapy: Reviews and Rationales* would not have been possible. Thank you to all the contributors and reviewers who devoted their time and talents to the previous edition of this book:

Contributors to First Edition
Susan E. Berkow, PhD
SEB Associates

Cindy L. Brubaker, MS, RN
Bradley University
Peoria, Illinois

Pam Hamre, RN, CNM, MS
College of St. Catherine
St. Paul, Minnesota

Mary C. Kishman, PhD (c), RN
College of Mount St. Joseph
Cincinnati, Ohio

Daryle Wane, APRN, BC, MS
Pasco-Hernando Community College
New Port Richey, Florida

Reviewers to the First Edition
Kathleen A. Hutchins-Otero, RN
San Jacinto College South
Houston, Texas

Mary Beth Kuehn, BSN, MSN
St. Olaf College
Northfield, Minnesota

Terran R. Mathers, MSN, RN
Spring Hill College
Mobile, Alabama

Kathy Watson, RN, MS, CPNP, CS
University of Arizona
Tucson, Arizona

Their work will surely assist both students and practicing nurses alike to extend their knowledge in the area of nutrition and diet therapy.

I owe a special debt of gratitude to the wonderful team at Prentice Hall Nursing for their enthusiasm for this project, as well as their good humor, expertise, and encouragement as the series developed. Maura Connor, Editor-in-Chief for Nursing, was unending in her creativity, support, encouragement, and belief in the need for this series. Danielle Doller, Developmental Editor, devoted many long hours to coordinating different facets of this project, and tirelessly and cheerfully encouraged our efforts as well. Her high standards and attention to detail contributed greatly to the final "look" of this series. Editorial Assistant, Mary Ellen Ruitenberg, helped to keep the project moving forward on a day-to-day basis, and I am grateful for her efforts as well. A very special thank you goes to the designers of the book and the production team, led by Anne Garcia, Production Editor, and Mary Siener, Designer, who brought the ideas and manuscript into final form.

Thank you to the team at Pine Tree Composition, led by Project Coordinator Jessica Balch, for the detail-oriented work of creating this book. I greatly appreciate their hard work, attention to detail, and spirit of collaboration.

Finally, I would like to acknowledge and gratefully thank my children, who sacrificed hours of time that would have been spent with them, to bring this book to publication. Their love and support kept me energized, motivated, and at times, even sane.

MaryAnn Hogan

Prentice Hall's *Nursing Notes*

NUTRITION & DIET THERAPY

Body Mass Index Table

	NORMAL						OVERWEIGHT					OBESE									
BMI	19	20	21	22	23	24	25	26	27	28	29	30	31	32	33	34	35	36	37	38	39
HGT	WEIGHT IN POUNDS																				
4-10	91	96	100	105	110	115	119	124	129	134	138	143	148	153	158	162	167	172	177	181	186
4-11	94	99	104	109	114	119	124	128	133	138	143	148	153	158	163	168	173	178	183	188	193
5-0	97	102	107	112	118	123	128	133	138	143	148	153	158	163	168	174	179	184	189	194	199
5-1	100	106	111	116	122	127	132	137	143	148	153	158	164	169	174	180	185	190	195	201	206
5-2	104	109	115	120	126	131	136	142	147	153	158	164	169	175	180	186	191	196	202	207	213
5-3	107	113	118	124	130	135	141	146	152	158	163	169	175	180	186	191	197	203	208	214	220
5-4	110	116	122	128	134	140	145	151	157	163	169	174	180	186	192	197	204	209	215	221	227
5-5	114	120	126	132	138	144	150	156	162	168	174	180	186	192	198	204	210	216	222	228	234
5-6	118	124	130	136	142	148	155	161	167	173	179	186	192	198	204	210	216	223	229	235	241
5-7	121	127	134	140	146	153	159	166	172	178	185	191	198	204	211	217	223	230	236	242	249
5-8	125	131	138	144	151	158	164	171	177	184	190	197	203	210	216	223	230	236	243	249	256
5-9	128	135	142	149	155	162	169	176	182	189	196	203	209	216	223	230	236	243	250	257	263
5-10	132	139	146	153	160	167	174	181	188	195	202	209	216	222	229	236	243	250	257	264	271
5-11	136	143	150	157	165	172	179	186	193	200	208	215	222	229	236	243	250	257	265	272	279
6-0	140	147	154	162	169	177	184	191	199	206	213	221	228	235	242	250	258	265	272	279	287
6-1	144	151	159	166	174	182	189	197	204	212	219	227	235	242	250	257	265	272	280	288	295
6-2	148	155	163	171	179	186	194	202	210	218	225	233	241	249	256	264	272	280	287	295	303
6-3	152	160	168	176	184	192	200	208	216	224	232	240	248	256	264	272	279	287	295	303	311
6-4	156	164	172	180	189	197	205	213	221	230	238	246	254	263	271	279	287	295	304	312	320

Abridged from Body Mass Index Table, National Heart, Lung, and Blood Institute, National Institute of Health

Foods High in Sodium and Potassium

High-Sodium Foods

The following foods should be limited or avoided by those with cardiovascular disease or whenever fluid retention is a problem:

- Bacon, ham, canned tuna
- Smoked meats and fish
- Pickles and other foods cured in brine
- Processed/refined foods
- Commercial bakery products
- Canned soups and vegetables
- Instant cooked cereals
- Instant potatoes or rice
- Salted snack foods
- Mineral water
- Tomato juice
- Steak/soy sauces, meat tenderizer

High-Potassium Foods

The following foods should be limited or avoided by those with renal failure or by those taking potassium-sparing diuretics:

- Bananas, citrus fruits, cantaloupe, avocados
- White and sweet potatoes
- Tomatoes
- Green leafy vegetables
- Carrots, corn, winter squash
- Fresh meat
- Whole grain products (especially bran)
- Milk, yogurt, ice cream
- Potassium-containing salt substitutes

Four-Step Method for Calculating Estimated Calorie Needs (Total Calorie Expenditure)

1. Calculate basal metabolic rate (BMR):

Multiply *healthy* weight* in lbs. by 10 (women) or 11 (men)
(Healthy weight) X (10 or 11) = A (calories for BMR)

2. Calculate calories for physical activity:

Multiply the BMR by the overall physical activity level

- 0.20 sedentary (sitting, reading, keyboarding, driving, sleeping, etc.)
- 0.30 light (light exercise not > 2 hrs/day)
- 0.40 moderate (yard work, heavy housework, relatively little sitting)
- 0.50 high (labor-intensive occupations or physical sports)

A x (physical activity factor) = B (calories used for activity)

3. Calculate calories expended in thermal effect of food (usually 10%)

Add BMR and physical activity calories together and multiply by .10
[A + B] x 0.10 = C (calories needed for thermal effect of food)

4. Calculate total daily expended calories

A + B + C = Total daily calories expended

Nutrition Facts Food Label

Nutrition Facts
Serving Size 1 cup (228g)
Servings Per Container 2

Amount per Serving	
Calories 260 Calories from Fat 120	
	% Daily Value*
Total Fat 13g	**20%**
Saturated Fat 5g	**25%**
Cholesterol 30g	**10%**
Sodium 660mg	**28%**
Total Carbohydrate 31g	**10%**
Dietary Fiber 0g	**0%**
Sugars 5g	
Protein 5g	

Clinical Manifestations Suggestive of Malnutrition

Body System	Clinical Manifestations
General findings	Apathy, listlessness, fatigue, weight not WNL
Integumentary	**Skin:** dry, flaky, pale, bruising, ↓ subcutaneous fat **Nails:** brittle, pale, ridged, spoon-shaped **Hair:** dull, dry, brittle, color loss
Gastrointestinal	**Mouth:** angular stomatitis (swollen red cracks in side of mouth) **Lips:** cheilosis (vertical fissures in lips) **Gums:** spongy, red, bleed easily, swollen, recessed **Tongue:** smooth, beefy red or magenta color, swollen, papillae hypertrophied or atrophied; anorexia, constipation, diarrhea, ↑abdomen, hepatosplenomegaly
Musculoskeletal	**Muscles:** flaccid, wasted, poor tone, difficulty walking **Skeleton:** bony deformities, prominent scapulae, poor posture **Teeth:** caries, mottling, missing
Neurosensory	Confusion, depression, sensory and motor difficulties, ↓ reflexes, burning and tingling of extremities **Eyes:** pale conjunctiva, dull or scarred cornea, xanthelasma (yellow lumps around eyes)
Cardiovascular	Cardiomegaly, hypertension, tachycardia

WNL = within normal limits

MyPyramid—www.mypyramid.gov

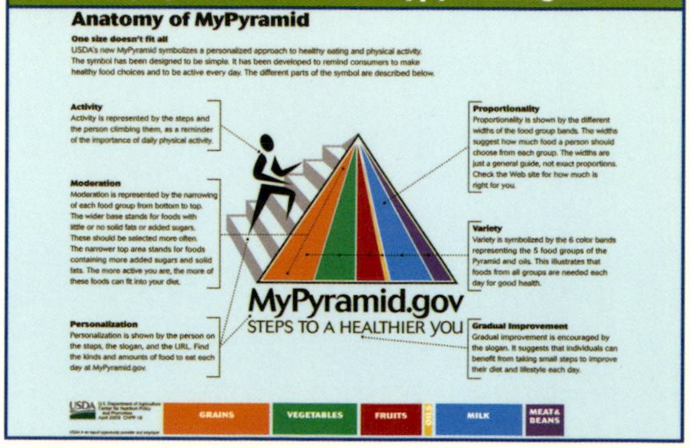

ISBN 0-13-243712-0
90000
9 780132 437127

Prentice Hall

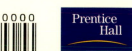

Overview of Selected Micronutrients

Micronutrient *Type* Adult RDA or AI*	**Major Functions**	**Common Food Sources**	**Signs of Deficiency**	**Signs of Excess/toxicity**
Calcium *Mineral* 1000-1300 mg*	Bone & teeth formation, blood clotting, muscle contraction Nerve transmission	Milk and milk products, cheese, yogurt, broccoli, kale, green leafy vegetables, legumes	Impaired growth (children) Osteoporosis (adults)	Renal stones, renal insufficiency Hypercalcemia Milk alkali syndrome Constipation
Iron *Mineral* 8-11 mg (men) 8-18 mg (women)	Oxygen transport via hemoglobin Acts in many enzyme systems	Red meat and poultry, beef liver, (heme sources) Clams, tofu, legumes, fortified bread & cereals (non-heme)	Weakness & fatigue Pale nailbeds or conjunctivae Impaired immunity & wound healing Intolerance to cold temperatures	GI distress & enlarged liver Hair loss, ↑ risk of infection, lethargy, joint disease Amenorrhea, impotence
Magnesium *Mineral* 310-420 mg	Bone formation Enzyme formation needed for amino acid, CHO, & cholesterol metabolism Nerve transmission Smooth muscle relaxation	Green leafy vegetables Whole grains Nuts Milk Meat & seafood Cocoa & chocolate	Usually occurs with alcohol abuse, protein malnutrition, renal disease, prolonged V/D Growth failure (children); weakness & confusion; severe: tetany, seizures, hallucinations	Rarely occurs N/V, osmotic diarrhea ↓BP & respirations Muscle weakness
Thiamine (B_1) *Water soluble vit.* 1.1-1.2 mg	Coenzyme in metabolism of CHOs and branched-chain amino acids	Whole grains, enriched breads, & cereals Liver, legumes, & nuts	Milder: A/N/V, weight loss, fatigue Severe: Beri-beri: confusion, muscle weakness/wasting, painful calf muscles, peripheral paralysis, edema, cardiomegaly, death	None reported
Riboflavin (B_2) *Water soluble vit.* 1.1-1.3 mg	Coenzyme in energy metabolism, numerous redox reactions, aids tryptophan → niacin	Organ meats Whole grains, fortified cereals Eggs, milk, & dairy products Green leafy vegetables	Dermatitis Cheilosis, glossitis Photophobia, reddening of cornea	None reported
Niacin (B_3) *Water soluble vit.* 14-16 mg	Coenzyme in energy metabolism, promotes NS functioning	Meat, fish, poultry, and other protein foods; whole grain and enriched breads & cereals	Pellagra: 4D's- dermatitis, diarrhea, dementia, and death (if untreated)	Flushing, ↓BP, & GI distress from supplements; none reported from natural foods
Vitamin B_6 *Water soluble vit.* 1.3-1.7 mg	Coenzyme in amino acid, fatty acid metabolism, Aids tryptophan → niacin Production of antibodies, hemoglobin, myelin sheaths, & insulin	Organ meats, fish, poultry, fortified soy-based meat substitutes, legumes, nuts Fruits, green leafy vegetables Fortified cereals	Dermatitis Cheilosis, glossitis Anemia Abnormal brain waves, convulsions	Supplements: Fatigue & irritability Headaches, depression, sensory neuropathy
Folate *Water soluble vit.* 400 µg	Coenzyme in DNA synthesis & amino acid metabolism	Enriched bread, grains, cereals Leafy vegetables, legumes, seeds Liver, oranges	Fatigue & fainting Depression, mental confusion Glossitis, anemia, diarrhea	Masks neurological complications of vitamin B_{12} deficiency
Vitamin B_{12} *Water soluble vit.* 2.4 µg	Coenzyme in new cell synthesis, activates folate Helps maintain nerve cells Metabolizes fatty & amino acids	Meat, fish, poultry Fortified cereals Milk, dairy products, eggs	Pallor, dyspnea, weakness, palpitations, fatigue A/C/D, indigestion, glossitis, weight loss; paresthesias (hands & feet), incoordination, irritability, poor memory, paranoia, hallucinations	None reported
Vitamin C *Water soluble vit.* 75-90 mg	Antioxidant, immune function, collagen synthesis, promotes iron absorption	Citrus fruits/juices, kiwi, cantaloupe, strawberries Potatoes, brussel sprouts, broccoli, cauliflower, spinach, cabbage, tomatoes/tomato juice	Bleeding from gums, petechiae Scurvy: delayed wound healing, anemia, softening of bones & teeth, muscle degeneration, ↑ susceptibility to infection	Abdominal cramps, nausea, diarrhea, Headache, insomnia, & fatigue Hot flashes Kidney stones, aggravation of gout
Vitamin A *Fat soluble vit.* 700-1300µg	Adaptation to dim light Gene expression Immune function Integrity of skin, mucous membranes, hair, & gums	Liver Dairy products, egg yolk Fish Ready-to-eat cereals Dark green & yellow vegetables	Night blindness, dry eyes, hardened cornea (can lead to blindness) Bone and teeth degeneration Dry, scaly, rough skin; diarrhea ↑ susceptibility to infection	Birth defects (teratological effects) Liver damage Headaches and vomiting Double vision; hair loss Bone abnormalities
Vitamin D *Fat soluble vit.* 5-15 µg	Maintain serum calcium and phosphorus levels (GI absorption, Ca^{++} release from bones, kidney reabsorption)	Sardines, salmon, fish oils, liver Eggs from hens fed Vitamin D Fortified milk, milk products, & cereals	Children: rickets: malformed or decayed teeth, retarded bone growth & bone abnormalities, weak muscles Adults: osteomalacia, osteoporosis, hypocalcemia	A/N/V/C/D, excessive thirst Headaches and fatigue Bone & muscle weakness Soft tissue calcification Liver damage (bleeding) & kidney damage or stones
Vitamin E *Fat soluble vit.* 15 mg*	Antioxidant (protects against vitamin A & PUFA destruction) Protects cell membranes	Vegetable oils, meats Unprocessed cereal grains Nuts, fruits, vegetables	↑ RBC hemolysis Anemia, edema, & skin lesions in infants	Rare Enhanced action of anticoagulant medications
Vitamin K *Fat soluble vit.* 65-80 µg	Synthesis of blood clotting proteins & bone protein that regulates serum Ca^{++}	Green leafy vegetables or those in cabbage family Liver & milk	Bleeding or hemorrhage	None reported

A = anorexia, BP = blood pressure, C = constipation, CHO = carbohydrate, D = diarrhea, GI = gastrointestinal, N = nausea, NS = nervous system, RBC = red blood cell, V = vomiting, vit = vitamin

Nutrition Basics

1

Chapter Outline

Nutritional Science Concepts
Population Guidelines
Diet Planning Guides
Food Labels and FDA Guidelines
Nutritional Status Assessment: Individual and Community
Teaching Principles

Objectives

- Review concepts of nutritional science.
- Describe Dietary Reference Intakes and diet planning guides for client populations.
- Identify measures used to analyze nutritional assessment status.
- Review food label principles and current FDA guidelines.
- Identify the importance of research and teaching principles in the area of nutrition.

NCLEX-RN® Test Prep

Use the CD-ROM enclosed with this book to access additional practice opportunities.

PRETEST

Review at a Glance

Adequate Intake (AI) guideline for intake of a nutrient when an RDA cannot be determined due to lack of scientific data on requirements

anthropometric measurements collection of specific assessment data related to physical characteristics of the body

calorie (Kcalorie) a measure of the energy content of food that translates to raising the temperature of 1 kilogram of water by 1 degree centigrade

Daily Reference Values (DRVs) established for foods that have health implications but no RDA; may be either amounts that should not be exceeded or amounts to try to consume

Daily Value (DV) reference nutrient values that appear on nutrition labels and that are based on a 2000 kcalorie diet

Dietary Reference Intakes (DRIs) comprehensive measure of nutrition and long-term health; includes updated RDAs, ULs, EAR, and AI; outlined by age and gender

Estimated Average Requirement (EAR) estimated amount of a nutrient needed to meet the requirements of half of the healthy people in a group based on gender and/or lifestyle

exchange list a diet planning tool that can be used with diabetic (and nondiabetic) clients that focuses on organizing foods by their macronutrient content; foods that are on the same exchange list are similar in macronutrient content and therefore can be "exchanged" or substituted as part of a dietary plan

health claims FDA-regulated labeling that must meet specific criteria for the claim being made

MyPyramid a graphic representation of the basic food groups illustrating number of servings that can be used in a healthy diet; they can be individualized specific to certain populations (children, adolescents, pregnant/lactating women, and the elderly) as well as to specific diets (vegetarian or Mediterranean)

nutrients groups of chemical substances that the body utilizes from the foods that are consumed (water, protein, carbohydrates, fats, minerals, and vitamins)

nutrition the foundation for life and health, based on food requirements of humans for activity, growth, maintenance, reproduction, and lactation

Recommended Daily Allowance (RDA) represents the average amount of nutrients that should be taken in on a daily basis to meet established nutrient needs

Tolerable Upper Limit (UL) highest level of a daily nutrient that is likely to create no adverse effects

vegetarian diet diet consisting only or primarily of vegetables and vegetable-based foods; some types may include eggs, dairy, and/or fish

PRETEST

1 An elderly client asks the nurse, "What's all this stuff about DRIs that I keep hearing?" Which of the following statements by the nurse provides the best explanation?

1. "They are updated nutritional guidelines that the government developed."
2. "The DRIs are guidelines for how many calories you need in a day."
3. "They refer to guidelines for weight loss for persons who are 25% overweight."
4. "Don't worry, your doctor will tell you what you need to know about nutrition."

2 The nurse is assisting the client in menu planning using MyPyramid as a standard. The nurse encourages the client to choose which of the following items on the menu to obtain an adequate daily intake of milk and dairy products?

1. 8 ounces of skim or whole milk
2. 8 ounces of milk and 2 ounces of cheese
3. One-half cup of yogurt
4. One-half cup of yogurt and one egg

3 A 34-year-old diabetic client who is receiving insulin therapy is not making healthy dietary choices to control blood glucose. The nurse would use which of the following as the most appropriate aid when reviewing diet planning with the client?

1. MyPyramid
2. Exchange list
3. Food diary
4. 24-hour recall

4 The nurse is demonstrating to a client how to read food labels. Using the label on the right, the nurse calculates the food item derives how many calories from sugars contained in the product? Provide a numerical answer.

Nutrition Facts
Serving Size 1 cup (228g)
Servings Per Container 2

Amount per Serving
Calories 260 Calories from Fat 120

	% Daily Value*
Total Fat 13g	20%
Saturated Fat 5g	25%
Cholesterol 30g	10%
Sodium 660mg	28%
Total Carbohydrate 31g	10%
Dietary Fiber 0g	0%
Sugars 5g	
Protein 5g	

5 During a client teaching session, which of the following foods would the nurse identify as belonging to the bread, cereal, rice, and pasta group of MyPyramid?

1. Peanuts
2. Coconut
3. Navy beans
4. Hot dog bun

6 The nurse is involved with a nutritional research project that involves quantifying calcium intake and osteoporosis rates of occurrence in elderly adults. The nurse concludes that this is which of the following types of studies?

1. Epidemiologic research
2. Laboratory research
3. Human studies research
4. Qualitative research

7 The nurse has taught a client to read nutrition labels. Which of the following statements by the client indicates to the nurse that the teaching has been effective?

1. "Those nutrition labels are misleading. Companies can put whatever they want on the labels."
2. "When a label says a food product helps reduce the risk of cancer, you can believe it."
3. "Food label health claims are exaggerated and based on eating abnormally large amounts."
4. "The health claims on food product labels are individually determined by each state."

8 A nurse conducting a nutrition class tells the class that the energy contained in a specific amount of a food product is measured in:

1. Joules
2. Calories.
3. Grams.
4. Pounds.

9 The school nurse is assigned to collect anthropometric data from preschool children regarding nutrition. From which of the following methods can the nurse choose to collect this type of data? Select all that apply.

1. Complete blood count (CBC)
2. Hemoglobin
3. Body mass index (BMI)
4. Triceps skin folds
5. Albumin

10 When assessing a client's nutritional status, the nurse uses the client's Body Mass Index (BMI) to determine:

1. Apple- versus pear-shaped body type.
2. Metabolic rate of the individual.
3. Hypercholesterolemia.
4. Relative fatness or weight to height.

➤ *See pages 17–18 for Answers and Rationales.*

I. NUTRITIONAL SCIENCE CONCEPTS

A. Definitions

1. **Nutrition** refers to the science studying the relationship of humans to food; the foundation for life and health based on food requirements needed by humans for activity, growth, maintenance, reproduction, and lactation; and the intake, digestion, and utilization of nutrients for tissue maintenance and provision of energy
2. **Nutrients** are substances that the human body utilizes from foods that are consumed; include six categories: water, proteins, carbohydrates (CHOs), fats (or lipids), minerals, and vitamins
   - ! **a.** Essential: nutrients required for human life that the body cannot manufacture
   - **b.** Nonessential: nutrients that the body needs but that the body can manufacture
   - **c.** Macronutrients: organic nutrients that provide energy and are classified as proteins, fats, and carbohydrates; also referred to as energy-yielding nutrients
   - ! **d.** Micronutrients: nutrients that the body needs in small amounts; serve to regulate and control the functions of the body; all micronutrients are either vitamins or minerals
3. ! **Calorie (Kcalorie)** represents the energy measurement of nutrients that foods provide
   - **a.** Proteins and carbohydrates (CHOs) each provide 4 kcalories per gram
   - **b.** Fats provide 9 kcalories (kcal) per gram
   - **c.** Alcohol provides 7 kcal per gram and is considered a source of empty calories because it provides no nutritional value
4. Nutrient density refers to the concentration of nutrients in a given amount of a food source relative to its caloric content; considers calories, carbohydrates, fats, proteins, vitamins, and minerals and water; the higher the nutrient density, the greater the nutritional value in a small amount of food
   - **a.** High nutrient density refers to greater nutritional content value in a specified amount of food
   - **b.** Foods that are high in nutrient density provide more nutrients per kcal and are used to improve the diet for clients at risk for nutritional deficiencies; these can add weight gain if taken in sufficient quantities
   - **c.** Foods that are low in nutrient density provide fewer nutrients per kcal and thus a higher calorie intake is needed to obtain needed nutrients; these can lead to weight loss if they are eaten and calorie intake is reduced

B. Nutritional research methods

1. Epidemiological research methods utilized in nutrition reflect examination of nutrition as a factor in the frequency and distribution of disease and other health-related events in a given population and provide information relative to patterns or correlations

2. Laboratory studies utilized in nutrition reflect examination of clinical hypotheses in a controlled clinical setting whereby chemical composition of foods, nutritional requirements/function, and determinants at cellular levels are assessed; these studies can utilize animal models as part of their clinical research methods
3. Human studies utilized in nutrition reflect examination of human subjects through deliberate manipulation of nutritional intake (depletion–repletion or balance studies)
4. Reliability and validity are measures of the accuracy of research
   a. Reliability refers to the accuracy (consistency) of a study and is often measured by the ability to replicate a study to obtain the same results
   b. Validity refers to the extent to which the study really examines/measures or determines what it purports
   c. Clinical research studies utilize statistical evaluation methods to determine both reliability and validity; appropriate interpretation of results provide a credible body of scientific evidence
5. ! It is critical that nutritional research be based on sound scientific principles, incorporating reliability and validity; clinical evidence can then be obtained and interpreted for use
   a. Utilize peer review and scientific journals to obtain accurate information
   b. Examine clinical research methods and clinical data to verify reliability and validity of methodology
   c. Accurately interpret clinical data for utilization with specific populations

II. POPULATION GUIDELINES

A. **Dietary Reference Intakes (DRIs)** represent a set of four standards used to provide a comprehensive measure of nutrition and long-term guidelines that are utilized to both assess and plan diets for healthy individuals in both the United States and Canada; they include updated RDAs, upper limits for safe intake (Tolerable Upper Limits or UL), Estimated Average Requirements (EAR), and Adequate Intake (AI); DRIs are outlined by age and gender

1. ! DRIs are standards used to support both group and individual diet planning for healthy individuals
   a. Determination of age, gender, and life-stage groups help to prioritize nutritional concerns
   b. Recognition of children, adolescents, adults, the elderly, and pregnant/lactating women is critical in determining nutritional requirements for these groups
2. **Estimated Average Requirement (EAR)** is the estimated amount of a nutrient needed to meet the requirements of half of the healthy people in a group based on gender, age, and life-stage groups; it is based on bioavailability, reducing risk of disease, and prevention of nutrient deficiency
3. ! **Recommended Dietary Allowances (RDAs)** represent calculated nutrient needs for healthy individuals based on gender, age, and life-stage groups; they are calculated using the EAR as a baseline and then increasing amounts to satisfy requirements of the majority of healthy individuals
4. **Adequate Intake (AI)** represents an estimate guideline for intake of a nutrient in an individual when an RDA cannot be determined due to lack of scientific data on requirements

Table 1-1 Healthy People 2010 Goals, Objectives, and Nutritional Target Areas

Goals	Objectives	Nutritional Target Areas
An increase in the span of healthy life for Americans. A reduction of health disparities among Americans.	Establishment and promotion of healthy behaviors. Establishment and promotion of healthy food communities. Access to preventive healthcare services for all Americans. Prevention of disease and clinical disorders.	Weight control issues (obesity, overweight, underweight) Dietary intake issues (fat—saturated, trans fat, fruit and vegetables, grains, sodium and iron) School nutrition issues (meals and snacks) and anemia in pregnancy Nutrition education, assessment, planning, and security issues

Practice to Pass

The nurse is providing nutrition education to a community group on the Healthy People 2010 Initiative. What information should be included?

5. **Tolerable Upper Limits (UL)** represents the highest (maximum) level of a daily nutrient that is likely to result in no adverse effects in an individual

B. **Healthy People 2010 Initiative:** developed by U.S. Department of Health and Human Services, the initiative focuses on health promotion and disease prevention through healthy choices in diet, weight control, and prevention of other nutritional risk factors (Refer to Table 1-1 and visit the Healthy People 2010 Web site at *http://www.health.gov/healthypeople/*)

III. DIET PLANNING GUIDES

! A. **The *MyPyramid* food guidance system** is a visual representation of five basic food groups (bread, cereal, rice, and pasta group; vegetable group; fruit group; milk, yogurt, and cheese group; meat, poultry, fish, dry beans, eggs, and nuts group; fats, oils, and sweets group) that provide a basis for nutrition education, general meal planning, and evaluation of overall food intake patterns (refer to Figure 1-1)

! 1. MyPyramid establishes recommendations for amount of food per group based on age, gender, and activity level

! 2. Fats, oils, and sweets are located in the yellow section of the pyramid and are to be used sparingly

! 3. MyPyramid can be adapted to various groups according to cultural and religious preferences and needs in pregnancy/lactation

! B. **The Exchange List System** represents a diet planning system that divides food into three groups based on their macronutrient content: carbohydrates, meat and meat substitutes (proteins), and fats; each group is further divided into subgroups so that each constituent in the subgroup contains the same exchange value when eaten in a clearly defined by portion size (see Table 1-2, p.8); published by the American Diabetes Association and the American Dietetic Association; it is a tool utilized for weight reduction programs and nutritional therapy planning, including diabetic meal planning

! 1. Using the exchange list system of diet planning is a more accurate method to ensure specific energy and macronutrient composition

! 2. It is critical to have a complete understanding of how the exchange system works in order to accurately use this diet planning guide; collaboration with a dietitian/nutritionist is essential in promoting compliance and providing nutritional education (refer to Box 1-1 for Exchange List Guidelines, p. 8)

C. **Carbohydrate counting:** a dietitian determines a client's dietary needs, the carbohydrate allowance given, divides food intake into meals and snacks

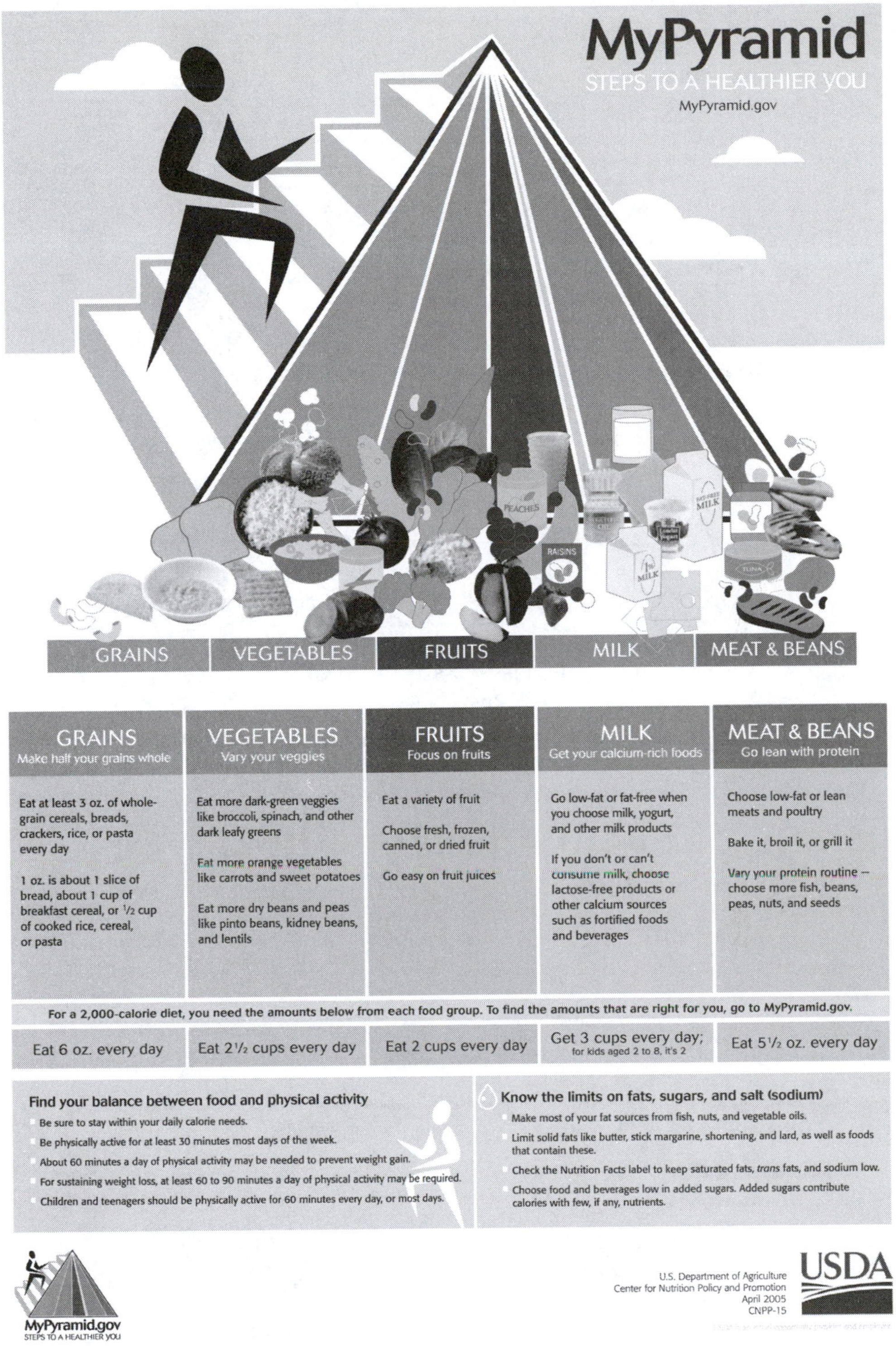

Figure 1-1

MyPyramid food guidance system (http:www.mypyramid.gov)

D. **Vegetarian diets** represent diet planning guides whereby an individual restricts products that are derived from animal sources

1. There are different degrees of vegetarianism that reflect the extent of this dietary restriction
    a. Vegan: the client eats only vegetable products and avoids all animal products

Table 1-2

Exchange List System

Group	Subgroups
Carbohydrate group	Starch, fruit, milk, vegetables, and other carbohydrates
Meat and meat substitute group	Very lean, lean, medium-fat, and high-fat
Fat group	Monounsaturated, polyunsaturated, and saturated

Practice to Pass

The adolescent client states that she has become a vegetarian. What additional information does the nurse need?

b. Lacto-vegetarian: the client eats dairy products (milk, cheese, yogurt) and vegetable products

c. Lacto-ovo-vegetarian: the client eats dairy products (milk, cheese, yogurt), eggs, and vegetable products

d. Pesco-vegetarian: the client eats fish and vegetable products; most pesco-vegetarians also eat dairy and eggs

e. Pollo-vegetarian: the client eats chicken and vegetable products; may also eat eggs and dairy products

! 2. The use of vegetarianism as a diet planning guideline and lifestyle choice has both defined health benefits and potential health risks

a. Health benefits: decrease in cholesterol levels, blood pressure, diabetes, cardiac disease, certain types of cancer, and obesity

b. Health risks: protein, mineral, and vitamin deficiencies due to inadequate intake

! 3. Clients who follow a vegetarian diet must be knowledgeable regarding the use of complementary proteins in order to prevent nutritional deficiencies

IV. FOOD LABELS AND FDA GUIDELINES

A. **FDA food labeling laws** ensure that food product labels include accurate information and identify nutrients contained in the product

B. **USDA labeling laws** ensure that meat and poultry products are safe, wholesome, and accurately labeled; pertain to fresh, frozen, and processed meat, poultry, and egg products; include information on the amount of added water and fat content

Box 1-1

Exchange List Guidelines

- Determine adequate weight based on body frame size and correlate with calories needed to maintain the metabolic rate to obtain the caloric intake.
- Determine the macronutrients (protein, CHOs, and fats) based on dietary standard recommendations of 10–35% protein, 45–65% CHOs, and 35% or less fats, which will provide a caloric measurement.
- Calculate the distribution of kcalories to grams to provide a weight measurement of dietary intake that will enable the individual to start making dietary choices.
- Recognize that the client's overall health status may influence other nutrient needs; conditions such as elevated lipids, disease processes, and/or vitamin or mineral deficiencies could affect dietary planning.
- Once caloric intake and grams of macronutrients have been determined, use standardized energy nutrient per servings information to start the dietary selection process.

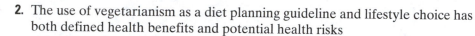

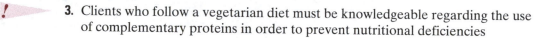

Figure 1-2

Nutrition Facts Food Label

Nutrition Facts

Serving Size 1 cup (228g)
Servings Per Container 2

Amount Per Serving	
Calories 250	Calories from Fat 110
	% Daily Value*
Total Fat 12g	**18%**
Saturated Fat 3g	**15%**
Trans Fat 3g	
Cholesterol 30mg	**10%**
Sodium 470mg	**20%**
Total Carbohydrate 31g	**10%**
Dietary Fiber 0g	**0%**
Sugars 5g	
Protein 5g	
Vitamin A	**4%**
Vitamin C	**2%**
Calcium	**20%**
Iron	**4%**

* Percent Daily Values are based on a 2,000 calorie diet. Your Daily Values may be higher or lower depending on your calorie needs.

	Calories:	2,000	2,500
Total Fat	Less than	65g	80g
Sat Fat	Less than	20g	25g
Cholesterol	Less than	300mg	300mg
Sodium	Less than	2,400mg	2,400mg
Total Carbohydrate		300g	375g
Dietary Fiber		25g	30g

Practice to Pass

The nurse is providing nutrition education to a client who desires to lose weight. What should the nurse say to explain the health claims on food product labels and what they mean?

C. Required elements of labeling from the Nutrition Labeling and Education Act of 1990

1. List of ingredients is presented in descending order by weight
2. Nutrition Facts (see Figure 1-2) represent a grouping of information relative to standard serving size, the amount of servings per product, listing of calories with percent of calories from fat, list of important nutrients (total and saturated fat, trans fat, cholesterol, sodium, total CHOs, dietary fibers and sugars, and protein), percent daily values, and calories per gram standards for macronutrients
   - a. **Daily Values (DV)** are reference nutrient values (amount of nutrient in food) based on a 2000 kcalorie diet using the Reference Daily Intake or Daily Reference Value with regard to nutrition labeling
   - b. Reference Daily Intakes (RDIs) reflect reference values for vitamins and minerals based on the highest amounts previously suggested by the RDAs
   - c. **Daily Reference Values (DRVs)** are established for foods that have health implications (total fat, saturated fat, cholesterol, total CHO, dietary fiber, sodium, potassium, and protein) but no RDA; recommended use assists with disease prevention and health promotion

D. Description of labeling terms and *health claims*

1. Defined terms (Refer to Table 1-3)
   - a. FDA labeling laws require that the manufacturer comply with specific terminology and use of descriptors in labeling food products

Table 1-3

Defined Labeling Terms

Term	Definition
Free	Contains virtually none of the nutrient (< 0.5 gram per serving); can refer to calories, sugar, sodium, salt, fat, saturated fat, and cholesterol
Low	Contains a small enough amount of a nutrient in the product (contains ≤ 3 grams per serving of fat or < 20 mg of cholesterol); can be used without concern for exceeding dietary recommendations; can refer to sodium, calories, fat, saturated fat, and cholesterol
Very Low	Refers to sodium only < 35 mg
Reduced or Less*	Contains a 25% reduction in a nutrient compared to the regular product in a food product that has been altered
Light or Lite	1/3 fewer calories in an altered food product or 50% less fat than a comparable regular product
Good Source	Provides 10–19% of the Daily Value for a nutrient per serving
High, Rich in, or Excellent Source	Provides > 20% of the Daily Value for a nutrient
More	Provides > 10% of a desirable nutrient than a comparable product
Lean	Meat or poultry product containing < 10 grams fat, < 4.5 grams saturated fat, and < 95 mg cholesterol per 100 grams and standard sized serving
Extra Lean	Meat or poultry product containing < 5 grams fat, < 2 grams saturated fat, and < 95 mg cholesterol per 100 grams and standard sized serving
Healthy	"Healthy" levels of total fat, saturated fat, cholesterol, and sodium

*Products that are labeled as "less" do not have to be altered but still reflect a 25% reduction.

!

b. It is important that clients are aware of exactly what each term refers to regarding the use of "free," "low," and "light" with regard to food products because this can affect dietary planning and food selections

2. Allowable health claims (Refer to Table 1-4)

!

a. The FDA allows for food products to list health claims for nutrients that have established health–disease relationships for cancer, heart disease, hypertension,

Table 1-4

Health Claims Approved for Use

Nutrient	Health Claim
Calcium	Osteoporosis
Fat; fruits and vegetables	Cancer ↑ or ↓, respectively
Sodium	High blood pressure
Folic acid	Neural tube defects
Sugars	Dental decay
Saturated fat and cholesterol; soluble fiber from psyllium seed husk or whole oats; fiber-containing grain products, fruits, and vegetables; soy protein	Risk of coronary heart disease ↑ or ↓, respectively

stroke, neural tube defects, osteoporosis, and dental decay, provided that they meet specific criteria

! **b.** Foods that carry health claims should not exceed 20% of DV for total fat, saturated fat, cholesterol, or sodium; provide a good source (≥ 10%) of DV for protein, dietary fiber, vitamins A and C, calcium, and iron; and reflect established scientific evidence for disease relationships

c. Structure-function claims, such as "slows aging," can be made without FDA approval

! **3.** Collaboration with a dietitian/nutritionist will help the client obtain information relative to nutrition labeling and establish the client's knowledge base

a. Sample nutrition labels can be utilized as part of a teaching program to illustrate the specific components of food labels and allow the client to identify and discuss diet choices

! **b.** Clients should be encouraged to read nutrition labels as part of their regular shopping routine in order to make informed dietary choices

V. NUTRITIONAL STATUS ASSESSMENT: INDIVIDUAL AND COMMUNITY

! **A. Documented history**

1. Dietary intake record: the client records every food and beverage consumed during a set time (often a one-week period); this record is then analyzed for nutrient content

2. 24-hour recall: dietary intake recording tool in which every food and beverage consumed in the last 24 hours is recalled either verbally or in writing; will be most accurate if the client starts with the most recent meal and works backwards; is greatly affected by changes in usual eating patterns and routines

3. Food diary: intake recording tool, similar to dietary intake record, but also includes emotions and reasons for eating; especially helpful for persons desiring to lose weight and those with anorexia and/or bulimia

4. Review of systems (ROS): asking the client about each body system for symptoms of nutrition problems related to excess or deficiency (example: constipation as a result of low fiber and water intake)

5. Nutritional screening initiatives (NSIs): funding is provided to public health and similar agencies for performing nutritional screening of special populations, such as pregnant women or the elderly

a. NSIs provide a 3-step approach to determine nutritional health of the individual, to assess those at increased nutritional risk, and then to provide a more comprehensive examination of the identified individual with poor nutrition

b. An initial screening is done using a checklist approach; self-evaluation by the individual identifies "warning" signs of poor nutrition with self-scoring (0–2: recheck in 6 months; 3–5: moderate risk, examine changes and recheck in 3 months; and 6 or more: high nutritional risk and referral to next level of screening)

c. A level I Screen involves calculating the body mass index or BMI (see next section), evaluating eating habits, and assessing environment to determine risk level with appropriate referral to next screening if needed

Practice to Pass

The nurse is performing nutritional screening for overnutrition and undernutrition using anthropometric data. What measurements does the nurse collect on each client? How does the nurse use the data?

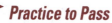

Practice to Pass

The client wants to know if he is obese or overweight. He is 6′ tall and weighs 275 lbs. What is this client's Body Mass Index (BMI)?

d. A level II Screen involves incorporating anthropometric data (see next section), laboratory data, and clinical evidence with detailed assessment of eating habits, environment, functional status, and mental/cognitive status

6. After a diet history is completed, nutrient content can be determined through a comparison of the data collected with food composition tables or through a computerized diet analysis program

B. ***Anthropometric measurements***

1. Height, weight, and body size are obtained and compared to a table of norms for reference; Metropolitan Life Insurance Table is most commonly used; the client is categorized as underweight, at ideal weight, or overweight; does not take % of body fat or lean muscle into account

2. Body Mass Index (BMI): assesses relative weight for height; calculated by dividing the weight in kilograms (2.2 pounds = 1 kg) by the square of the height in meters (2.54 cm = 1 inch)—Weight ÷ $(\text{Height})^2$ = BMI; charts or nomograms may be used to calculate BMI (see Figure 1-3)

a. BMI provides a range with which to evaluate a healthy body weight ("healthy" range is between 18.5 and 24.9)

b. A BMI < 17 reflects underweight status while a BMI of 25 or higher reflects overweight/obesity

Figure 1-3

Body Mass Index Nomogram

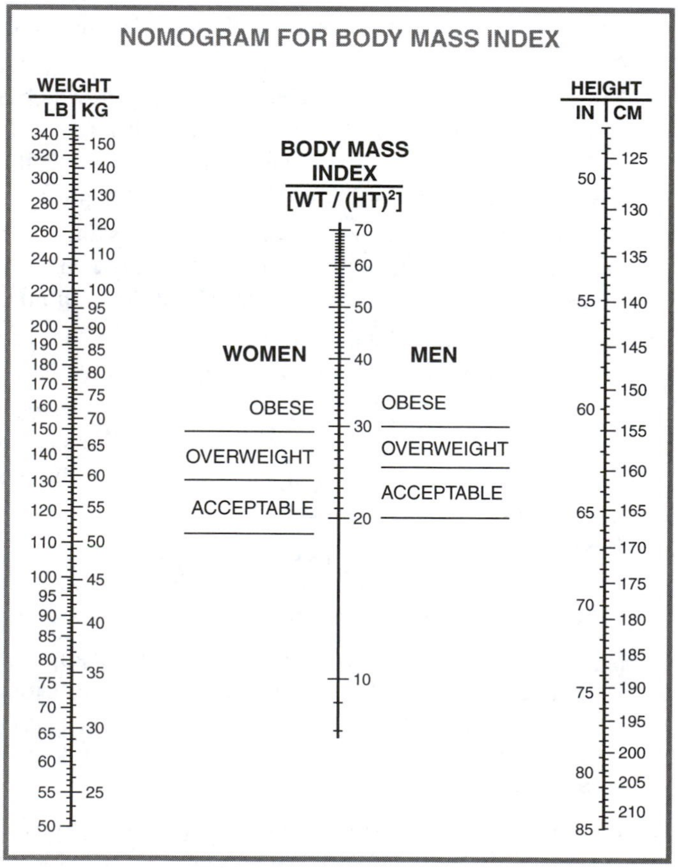

c. BMI silhouettes can be used as a visual tool with a client to determine both body image perception and recognition of body weight

d. BMI does not reflect body composition; individuals with greater muscle mass development may appear to be to be overweight and yet not have increased body fat

e. High or low BMIs do correlate with clinical pathology and disease pathology in population studies

! 3. The Basal Metabolic Rate (BMR) measures the body's consumption of oxygen and therefore the rate of calories burned when the body maintains basic metabolic activities—the higher the BMR, the more calories the client can take in without weight gain; lean muscle tissue mass most directly affects the BMR; the BMR decreases about 2% during each decade after the maximum at age 30

! a. Activities and clinical conditions can affect the BMR; it is increased with activity, stress, temperature, pregnancy, smoking, caffeine, stress; BMR changes during growth spurts and is decreased with sleep, fasting, or starvation states, and undernutrition

! b. Calculation of BMR in accordance with type of activity/lifestyle is necessary in order to determine exact caloric requirements

! 4. The distribution of body fat is important in assessing health risk potential because central (truncal) obesity (increased intra-abdominal fat in the individual) is associated with increased risk of disease

a. Determination of waist circumference and/or hip–waist ratio correlates with the "apple" versus "pear" body type and reflects risk pattern for disease ("apple" types are at greater risk than "pear" types)

b. The use of fat fold measurements as part of anthropometric data can help to determine the distribution of body fat in the individual

Practice to Pass

The client has an albumin level of 3.0 grams/dL. What does this indicate about the client's nutrition?

5. Skin fold measurements using calipers provide an objective measurement of body fat stores and nutritional status

a. The triceps skin fold (TSF) is the most commonly used measurement performed using the subscapular and suprailiac skin folds

b. The mid-arm circumference (MAC) provides information relative to muscle and fat stores and is used to calculate the mid-arm muscle circumference (MAMC)

c. The MAMC provides information about skeletal muscle mass and distinguishes differences in muscle and body fat

C. Laboratory and diagnostic measurements

! 1. There is no single laboratory value that accurately measures nutritional status

a. Albumin is decreased in stress and illness, during bedrest, and after trauma or surgery; it is normal in chronic malnutrition (marasmus); however, it is still used in many settings for nutritional screening (see Table 1-5)

! b. Prealbumin levels are a more sensitive indicator of nutritional status due to shorter half-life and because they respond to short-term changes in protein stores; however, they are low in infection/inflammation, and high in renal failure and use of steroids

! c. Transferrin levels are poor measures of visceral protein stores because of their changes related to iron stores

Table 1-5

Serum Albumin Levels

Category	Serum Albumin Level
Normal	3.5 grams/dL
Mild depletion	2.8–3.4 grams/dL
Moderate depletion	2.1–2.7 grams/dL
Severe depletion	<2.1 grams/dL

! **d.** Albumin, prealbumin, and transferrin levels may be used to evaluate clinical response in clients receiving total parenteral nutrition (TPN) and overall nutritional status in other clients as part of the global assessment

2. Total lymphocyte count (TLC) decreases as protein stores become depleted, which has implications for immune system function

! **3.** Screening for specific nutrient deficiencies: hemoglobin levels reflect iron intake; transferrin carries iron from the intestine through the serum and drops more rapidly than albumin

VI. TEACHING PRINCIPLES

A. Individual client teaching concerns

1. Use established nutritional standards such as MyPyramid, BMR silhouette profile, anthropometric data, biochemical data, and food history assessment to identify nutritional problems and identify knowledge deficit

! **2.** Use visualization of serving sizes to help clients identify accurate serving sizes and use "real" food diagrams or pictures to assess client's level of knowledge (refer to Table 1-6)

! **3.** Assess client for cultural dietary preferences and incorporate culturally based food intake patterns or restrictions into dietary teaching

4. Include client and family members in nutritional teaching to provide a more comprehensive focus to managing a dietary pattern, especially when the client is a child, adolescent, or and elderly person

! **5.** Collaborate with a dietitian and other members of the healthcare team in order to provide education, monitor compliance, and evaluate response to treatment

B. Group and community client teaching concerns

1. Provide broad-based information on topics that are relevant to group and community needs

Table 1-6

Visualization of Serving Sizes—Selected Examples

Serving Size	Visual Cue
2–3 ounces meat	Deck of playing cards or cassette tape
1/2 cup cooked pasta	One ice cream scoop
1 medium fruit	Tennis ball or average fist

2. Provide factual information through a variety of methods (handouts, display of materials, audiovisuals, etc.) to groups/community so that information will be aimed at many different types of learners
3. Provide a method for evaluation; validate effectiveness of teaching through formative (ongoing) and summative (final) evaluations
4. Make referrals to dietitian and healthcare provider for further information, assessments, and followup care

C. Client population teaching concerns

1. Provide information based on specific population needs related to geographic location, environmental and lifestyle factors, and age-related topics
2. Use multimedia approach including books, Internet, and pamphlets to provide continuous access to information and refer to appropriate dietitian or healthcare provider for followup
3. ! Understand the demographics of the population being taught, paying attention to specific cultural/religious concerns, age appropriateness, lifestyle issues, and geographic issues in order to focus on what clients need to know and what information must be conveyed with regard to public health issues

Case Study

You are a nurse in the community. You are planning the content for a 1-hour community class on Healthy People 2010.

1. What information will you include?
2. How will you restate the first goal—an increase in the span of healthy life for Americans—in plain words?
3. How will you explain the second goal—reduction of health disparities among Americans?
4. What are the nutritional target areas identified in Healthy People 2010?
5. How will you present the MyPyramid as it relates to Healthy People 2010?

For suggested responses, see page 317.

POSTTEST

1 What consistent statement in the *Dietary Guidelines for Americans 2005* should the nurse include in teaching the client to stay healthy?

1. Restrict almost all fat and cholesterol.
2. Balance the intake of food with physical activity.
3. Include higher amounts of milk and meats.
4. Increase portions to ensure adequate amounts of nutrients.

2 A client has received teaching of basic nutritional principles. The nurse determines the client needs additional teaching when he states:

1. "Alcohol is the chemical basis of one of the essential nutrients."
2. "Protein and carbohydrates are examples of macronutrients."
3. "Water is necessary for human life."
4. "Calcium is a micronutrient."

3 The nutrition consult done on a client indicates the body mass index (BMI) is 17. Based on this information the nurse identifies which of the following nursing diagnoses as being most appropriate?

1. Impaired growth
2. Deficient knowledge: nutrition
3. Imbalanced nutrition: less than body requirements
4. Risk for injury: dehydration

4 Which of the following data choices would the nurse utilize as anthropometric measurements in determining a client's nutritional status?

1. Height and weight
2. Hemoglobin and albumin
3. Total lymphocyte count (TLC)
4. 24-hour dietary recall

5 The nurse teaching a client about food product labeling explains that a label that reads "Light Salad Dressing" contains:

1. 50% less fat than comparable regular product.
2. 35% less sodium than comparable regular product.
3. 20% more protein than comparable regular product.
4. At least 50% fewer calories than a comparable regular product.

6 The nurse caring for a client with a low basal metabolic rate (BMR) recognizes the client would be most likely to experience which of the following nutritional problems?

1. Undernutrition
2. Obesity
3. Low serum albumin
4. Low hemoglobin

7 The nurse is instructing a client on how to maintain a food diary. The nurse explains the diary should include:

1. Every type of food and beverage consumed in the past week.
2. Exact amounts of foods and beverages consumed in the past twenty-four hours.
3. Exact amounts of food consumed along with feelings and reasons for eating.
4. When and where food is consumed during the last week.

8 The nurse is instructing a client who wants to begin following a vegetarian diet about foods that provide protein. The nurse explains that which of the following choices would be appropriate for this client? Select all that apply.

1. Soy
2. Beans
3. Nuts
4. Turkey
5. Wheat germ

9 The nurse is reviewing the laboratory test results on an assigned client that indicate a decreased transferrin level. The nurse interprets that this finding would be associated with which of the following in the client?

1. Low dietary iron intake
2. Recent episode of blood loss
3. Malnutrition, especially lack of protein
4. Recent bacterial infection

10 The nurse is writing a care plan for a client at risk for a nutritional deficit. An appropriate goal would be:

1. Client will wear prescribed oxygen at 2 liters/minute.
2. Client will verbalize two healthy nutritional practices.
3. Client will maintain current weight.
4. Client will monitor weight twice daily at the same times each day.

See pages 18–20 for Answers and Rationales.

POSTTEST

ANSWERS & RATIONALES

Pretest

1 **Answer: 1** A Daily Recommended Intake (DRI) is a nutritional guideline that goes beyond the RDAs. It includes Tolerable Upper Limits and Adequate Intake amounts and is established by the government to provide a more comprehensive approach to nutrition. Option 2 is incorrect because DRIs do not merely relate to caloric intake. Option 3 is incorrect because DRIs are not based solely on weight variables but reflect a recommended intake of nutrient factors. Option 4 is incorrect—even though the physician is knowledgeable, any one healthcare provider does not have complete knowledge of nutritional therapies. A collaborative approach is necessary to provide information to the client.
Cognitive Level: Application **Client Need:** Health Promotion and Maintenance **Integrated Process:** Teaching and Learning **Content Area:** Foundational Sciences: Nutrition **Strategy:** Note the critical word *best,* indicating some options may be partially correct. Eliminate option 4 because it does not offer an explanation to the client. Eliminate options 2 and 3 since they do not completely address DRIs. **Reference:** Nix, S. (2005). *Williams' basic nutrition and diet therapy* (12th ed.). St. Louis, MO: Elsevier Mosby, pp. 8, 196.

2 **Answer: 2** MyPyramid recommends three servings a day from milk, cheese, and dairy products. One serving is equal to 8 ounces of milk or ¾ ounces of cheese. Option 1 does is equal to one serving, but not a day's supply. Option 3 is an insufficient amount. Option 4 is also insufficient, and eggs are not part of the milk category.
Cognitive Level: Application **Client Need:** Health Promotion and Maintenance **Integrated Process:** Nursing Process: Implementation **Content Area:** Foundational Sciences: Nutrition **Strategy:** Note that question asks for adequate *daily* intake, not just a single serving size. Options 1 and 3 are similar and can be eliminated. Eliminate option 4 since eggs are not part of the milk and dairy group. **Reference:** www.mypyramid.gov.

3 **Answer: 2** The use of an exchange list is recommended by the American Dietetic Association for use by diabetic clients for meal planning. Option 1 is incorrect: Even though the MyPyramid is developed by the USDA to illustrate healthy diet choices, the use of an exchange system is geared specifically to equivalent carbohydrate contents that are critical for a diabetic client. Options 3 and 4 are incorrect because they are not diet planning guides but rather examples of tools that can be used to evaluate nutritional status.
Cognitive Level: Application **Client Need:** Health Promotion and Maintenance **Integrated Process:** Nursing Process: Planning **Content Area:** Foundational Sciences: Nutrition **Strategy:** Note the question asks for a method or guide to diet planning. Eliminate options 3 and 4 since they involve record keeping of a diet, but do not involve planning. Recall knowledge of diabetic diets to choose exchange lists. **Reference:** Nix, S. (2005). *Williams' basic nutrition & diet therapy* (12th ed.). St. Louis, MO: Elsevier Mosby, pp. 380–381.

4 **Answer: 20** Sugars are a carbohydrate (CHO), and each gram of CHO or sugar contains 4 kcal. Multiply 5 grams $\times$ 4 = 20 calories.
Cognitive Level: Application **Integrated Process:** Teaching and Learning **Client Need:** Health Promotion and Maintenance **Content Area:** Foundational Sciences: Nutrition **Strategy:** Identify how many grams of sugar are listed on the label. Be sure to select just sugar, not total CHOs. Use simple mathematics to multiply and arrive at calories/gram. **Reference:** Grodner, M., Long, S., & DeYoung, S. (2004). *Foundations and clinical applications of nutrition* (3rd ed.). St. Louis, MO: Elsevier Mosby, pp. 43, 45.

5 **Answer: 4** A hot dog bun is found in the bread, cereal, rice, and pasta group. Option 1 is incorrect—peanuts are found in the meat, poultry, and fish group because they are considered to be legumes. Options 2 and 3 are incorrect—coconut is found in the vegetable group; navy beans are in the meat, poultry, and dried beans group.
Cognitive Level: Application **Client Need:** Health Promotion and Maintenance **Integrated Process:** Nursing Process: Implementation **Content Area:** Foundational Sciences: Nutrition **Strategy:** Recall knowledge of the food groups to eliminate options 1, 2, and 3, which are protein and vegetable groups. **Reference:** Rolfes, S., Pinna, K. & Whitney, E. (2006). *Understanding normal and clinical nutrition* (7th ed.). Belmont CA: Wadsworth & Thomson Learning, pp. 44–45.

6 **Answer: 1** Epidemiologic nutritional research studies nutritional factors that influence the cause, frequency, and distribution of disease, injury, or other health-related events in a defined human population. Option 2 is incorrect because laboratory research is used to test scientific hypothesis in a controlled setting. Option 3 is incorrect because the use of human studies research

involves manipulation of variables affecting nutrient intake. The stated example above relates to an intake study that is attempting to correlate rates of disease occurrence. Option 4 is incorrect because qualitative research looks at the quality of a given variable. The nutritional research study proposed does not provide enough information relative to type and amount of calcium intake, so one cannot categorize this research as either qualitative or quantitative.
Cognitive Level: Comprehension **Client Need:** Health Promotion and Maintenance **Integrated Process:** Nursing Process: Analysis **Content Area:** Foundational Sciences: Nutrition **Strategy:** Note the critical word *quantifying* and that a specific population, the elderly, is being studied. Recall knowledge of types of research to choose option 1. **Reference:** Grodner, M., Long, S., & DeYoung, S. (2004). *Foundations and clinical applications of nutrition* (3rd ed.). St. Louis, MO: Elsevier Mosby, p. 39.

7 **Answer: 2** Health claims on food products are regulated by the FDA, are trustworthy, and are based on scientific evidence. The food products making the claims must meet specific rigid criteria. Options 1 and 3 are incorrect because FDA regulations are strictly enforced, and companies must comply with federal guidelines or risk penalty. Option 4 is incorrect—food product labels are regulated by the FDA and not by individual states.
Cognitive Level: Application **Client Need:** Health Promotion and Maintenance **Integrated Process:** Nursing Process: Evaluation **Content Area:** Foundational Sciences: Nutrition **Strategy:** The question is asking to assess effectiveness of teaching. Recall specific knowledge of labeling standards and laws to choose option 2. **Reference:** Nix, S. (2005) *Williams' basic nutrition & diet therapy* (12th ed.). St. Louis, MO: Elsevier Mosby, pp. 233–235.

8 **Answer: 2** Calories or kilocalories are the most commonly used measurement of a food product's energy. Grams and pounds reflect weight measurements. Joules represent electrical energy.
Cognitive Level: Application **Client Need:** Health Promotion and Maintenance **Integrated Process:** Teaching and Learning **Content Area:** Foundational Sciences: Nutrition **Strategy:** Critical words are *energy* and *measurement.* Recognize that options 1, 3, and 4 are measures of weight and quantity and thus they can be eliminated. **Reference:** Nix, S. (2005). *Williams' basic nutrition & diet therapy* (12th ed.). St. Louis, MO: Elsevier Mosby, p. 5

9 **Answer: 3, 4** Height, weight, and skin fold thickness are common anthropometric data (measurement of body parts) obtained by the nurse, as well as the body mass index. Options 1 and 2 are incorrect: CBC (and hemoglobin, which is a test included in the CBC) reflect laboratory parameters. Option 5 is incorrect because albumin is a type of serum protein and is another laboratory measurement.
Cognitive Level: Application **Client Need:** Health Promotion and Maintenance **Integrated Process:** Nursing Process: Planning **Content Area:** Foundational Sciences: Nutrition **Strategy:** Critical words are *anthropometric data* and *measurement.* Eliminate option 2 since it does not involve an actual measurement. Note also that options 1, 2, and 5 are distracters relating to diagnostic studies and not anthropometric data. **Reference:** Nix, S. (2005). *Williams' basic nutrition & diet therapy* (12th ed.). St. Louis, MO: Elsevier Mosby, p. 311.

10 **Answer: 4** The Body Mass Index (BMI) is calculated by taking the weight in kilograms and dividing by the height in meters squared. It assesses weight compared to height, or fatness. Option 1 is incorrect—these are merely descriptive terms that relate to body frame variables and overall distribution of weight. Option 2 is incorrect because the metabolic rate of an individual relates to basal metabolic rate (BMR). Option 3 is incorrect, because BMI does not detect hypercholesterolemia. Elevated cholesterol levels can be found in individuals with differing BMI values because both genetic and metabolic factors influence its development.
Cognitive Level: Analysis **Client Need:** Physiological Integrity: Physiological Adaptation **Integrated Process:** Nursing Process: Assessment **Content Area:** Foundational Sciences: Nutrition **Strategy:** The focus of the question is the purpose or applicability of BMI. Recall BMI involves measurement of height and weight. Eliminate options 2 and 3 since they are refer to metabolism and blood chemistries. Eliminate option 1 since it is a shape, not related to height and weight. **Reference:** Nix, S. (2005). *Williams' basic nutrition & diet therapy* (12th ed.). St. Louis, MO: Elsevier Mosby, p. 193.

Posttest

1 **Answer: 2** The 2005 Dietary Guidelines apply the principles of scientific evidence in promoting health and reducing risk of chronic disease through diet and physical activity. Option 2 is correct because it includes the two key components found in more than one guideline topics, option 1 is incorrect because guidelines to recommend a total fat intake of 20–35% and less than 300 mg of cholesterol per day. Options 3 and 4 are incorrect because under the topic "Food Groups to Encourage" milk is mentioned but only sufficient amounts while staying within energy needs.
Cognitive Level: Application **Client Need:** Health Promotion and Maintenance **Integrated Process:** Teaching and Learn-

ing **Content Area:** Foundational Sciences: Nutrition **Strategy:** Note the critical word in the stem of the question "consistent" option 1 is the only choice mentioned more than once. **Reference:** Rolfes, S., Pinna, K. & Whitney, E. (2006). *Understanding normal and clinical nutrition* (7th ed.). Belmont CA: Wadsworth & Thomson Learning, pp. 41–42.

2 **Answer: 1** Alcohol provides calories but is not an essential nutrient. All of the other choices reflect statements that are consistent with basic nutritional knowledge.
Cognitive Level: Application **Client Need:** Health Promotion and Maintenance **Integrated Process:** Teaching and Learning **Content Area:** Foundational Sciences: Nutrition **Strategy:** Note the question asks to identify the need for further teaching, indicating a false response question. Thus, you need to look for an option that indicates an incorrect statement. Identify options 2, 3, and 4 as being correct statements, leading to option 1 as the answer to the question. **Reference:** Nix, S. (2005). *Williams' basic nutrition & diet therapy* (12th ed.). St. Louis, MO: Elsevier Mosby, pp. 11–15.

3 **Answer: 3** A BMI of less than 18.5 is classified as underweight. The most important nursing diagnosis is Imbalanced nutrition: less than body requirements because the client's intake is not sufficient to maintain a normal BMI. A low BMI places client as risk for respiratory diseases, TB, digestive diseases, and some cancers, but does not create risk for dehydration (option 4). The client could also be at risk for impaired growth, depending on age and specific nutritional deficits existing, but this information is not provided. The client could also have a knowledge deficit, but this is also not evident from the question, so would not be the most appropriate diagnosis.
Cognitive Level: Analysis **Client Need:** Health Promotion and Maintenance **Integrated Process:** Nursing Process: Planning **Content Area:** Foundational Sciences: Nutrition **Strategy:** Critical words are *most appropriate,* indicating some or all options may be indicated, but one is more correct. Eliminate options 1 and 2 since insufficient information is given in question to support their choice. Recall knowledge of BMI norms to choose option 3. **Reference:** Grodner, M., Long, S., & DeYoung, S. (2004). *Foundations and clinical applications of nutrition* (3rd ed.). St. Louis, MO: Elsevier Mosby, pp. 24, 405–407.

4 **Answer: 1** Height and weight are physical parameters that are considered to be anthropometric measurements. Options 2 and 3 are incorrect because they represent laboratory/diagnostic test results. Option 4 is incorrect because a 24-hour dietary recall is part of a documented history.
Cognitive Level: Application **Client Need:** Health Promotion and Maintenance **Integrated Process:** Nursing Process: Assessment **Content Area:** Foundational Sciences: Nutrition **Strategy:** The critical words are *anthropometric measurement.* Recall knowledge of them to eliminate options 2 and 3, since they are laboratory measurements. Eliminate option 4 because it is not a measurement. **Reference:** Grodner, M., Long, S., & DeYoung, S. (2004). *Foundations and clinical applications of nutrition* (3rd ed.). St. Louis, MO: Elsevier Mosby, pp. 401–403.

5 **Answer: 1** The terms "light" or "lite" can only be used if the product has greater than or equal to 1/3 fewer calories or greater than or equal to 50% less fat than a comparable regular product. Option 2 is incorrect—it refers to sodium levels, and the term "light" is related to specific caloric levels and/or fat. Option 3 is incorrect because it refers to an increased protein level. Option 4 is incorrect because the caloric decrease stated is much higher than the identified level.
Cognitive Level: Application **Client Need:** Health Promotion and Maintenance **Integrated Process:** Teaching and Learning **Content Area:** Foundational Sciences: Nutrition **Strategy:** Note that the question describes a food as "light," which refers to the fat content. Eliminate options 2 and 3 since they refer to sodium and protein content. Choose option 1 over 4 as it specifically addresses fat content. Recall knowledge of food labeling requirements. **Reference:** Grodner, M., Long, S., & DeYoung, S. (2004). *Foundations and clinical applications of nutrition* (3rd ed.). St. Louis, MO: Elsevier Mosby, pp. 42–44.

6 **Answer: 2** A low BMR occurs when calories are being burned at a slower than normal rate; therefore, weight gain may occur. Option 1 is incorrect because a low BMR would correlate with increased weight gain due to possible endocrine disturbances. Options 3 and 4 are incorrect because they reflect poor nutritional status, fatigue, and decreased oxygen-carrying capacity, which can occur because a variety of other metabolic factors, not only nutrition.
Cognitive Level: Analysis **Client Need:** Physiological Integrity: Physiological Adaptation **Integrated Process:** Nursing Process: Analysis **Content Area:** Foundational Sciences: Nutrition **Strategy:** Critical words are *most likely,* indicating there is a tendency for it to occur. Eliminate options 3 and 4 because they do not reflect metabolism. Choose option 2 since weight gain correlates with a slowed metabolism. **Reference:** Grodner, M., Long, S., & DeYoung, S. (2004). *Foundations and clinical applications of nutrition* (3rd ed.). St. Louis, MO: Elsevier Mosby, pp. 248–249.

7 **Answer: 3** A food diary involves recording intake of foods and beverages over a specific period of time and also includes emotions and rationales for eating. It can

be used to help clients identify unhealthy patterns, and it can also be used for weight loss and bulimia/anorexia. Option describes a dietary intake record, which does not include emotions and reasons. Option 2 describes a 24-hour recall. Option 4 might or might not be part of a food diary.
Cognitive Level: Application **Client Need:** Health Promotion and Maintenance **Integrated Process:** Teaching and Learning **Content Area:** Foundational Sciences: Nutrition **Strategy:** Note the word *diary* is part of the plan, indicating more than just listing of food items will be involved. Eliminate options 1 and 2 since they just include food quantities. Eliminate option 4 because it is very general and less specific than option 3. **Reference:** Grodner, M., Long, S., & DeYoung, S. (2004). *Foundations and clinical applications of nutrition* (3rd ed.). St. Louis, MO: Elsevier Mosby, pp. 408–411.

8 **Answers: 1, 2, 3** Soy, beans, and nuts are part of the protein group and would be appropriate for a vegetarian. Vegetarians do not eat animals that must be killed prior to consumption; most vegetarians (other than vegans) will consume eggs, legumes, and dairy products.
Cognitive Level: Application **Client Need:** Health Promotion and Maintenance **Integrated Process:** Teaching and learning **Content Area:** Foundational Sciences: Nutrition **Strategy:** Notice that the client is vegetarian; eliminate option 4 since it is of animal origin. Recall knowledge of protein-containing foods. Eliminate option 5 since it is a grain. **Reference:** Grodner, M., Long, S., & DeYoung, S. (2004). *Foundations and clinical applications of nutrition* (3rd ed.). St. Louis, MO: Elsevier Mosby, pp. 154–156.

9 **Answer: 3** Transferrin levels provide information relative to iron stores and visceral protein. Option 1 is incorrect—transferrin does not specifically relate to a low dietary intake level. Option 2 is incorrect because transferrin levels do not relate to blood loss through hemorrhage, they relate to body stores. Option 4 is incorrect because transferrin levels are not affected by bacterial infections.
Cognitive Level: Application **Client Need:** Physiological Integrity: Reduction of Risk Potential **Integrated Process:** Nursing Process: Analysis **Content Area:** Foundational Sciences: Nutrition **Strategy:** The question requires knowledge of transferrin. A key word is *decreased* level. Recall transferrin reflects stored iron to eliminate option 1. Eliminate options 2 and 4 since transferrin is not related to blood loss or infection. **Reference:** Grodner, M., Long, S., & DeYoung, S. (2004). *Foundations and clinical applications of nutrition* (3rd ed.). St. Louis, MO: Elsevier Mosby, p. 223.

10 **Answer: 2** Promoting healthy nutritional practices incorporates both the categories of undernutrition and overnutrition. The correct option provides a goal that is global and relevant to nutrition. Option 1 and 4 are incorrect because they reflect an intervention, not a goal. Option 3 is incorrect because weight maintenance would only be an appropriate goal if the client is underweight and there is insufficient information to determine this.
Cognitive Level: Application **Client Need:** Health Promotion and Maintenance **Integrated Process:** Nursing Process: Planning **Content Area:** Foundational Sciences: Nutrition **Strategy:** Question requires identifying a goal that is realistic and relevant. Eliminate options 1 and 4 since they are nursing intervention, not goals. Eliminate option 3 since the question did not identify a weight problem. **Reference:** Grodner, M., Long, S., & DeYoung, S. (2004). *Foundations and clinical applications of nutrition* (3rd ed.). St. Louis, MO: Elsevier Mosby, pp. 19–24.

References

Cataldo, C., DeBruyne, L., & Whitney, E. (2006). *Nutrition and diet therapy* (7th ed.). Belmont, CA: Wadsworth & Thomson Learning, pp. 3–28.

Dudek, S. (2006). *Nutrition essentials for nursing practice* (5th ed.). Philadelphia: Lippincott, pp. 1–20.

Grodner, M., Long, S., & DeYoung, S. (2004). *Foundations and clinical applications of nutrition: A nursing approach* (3rd ed.) St. Louis, MO: Mosby, pp. 19–45, 223–249, 401–436.

Kozier, B., Erb, G., Berman, A., & Burke, K. (2004). *Fundamentals of nursing: Concepts, process and practice* (6th ed.). Upper Saddle River, NJ: Prentice Hall, pp. 1126–1143.

Lutz, C. & Przytulski, K. (2006). *Nutrition and diet therapy* (4th ed.). Philadelphia: F. A. Davis, pp. 3–34.

Nix, S. (2005). *Basic nutrition and diet therapy* (12th ed.). St. Louis: Mosby, pp. 4–13.

Rolfes, S., Pinna, K., & Whitney, E. (2006). *Understanding normal and clinical nutrition* (7th ed.). Belmont, CA: Wadsworth & Thomson Learning.

USDA Food Safety and Inspection Service website: http://www.fsis.usda.gov/OPPDE/larc/; accessed 10/1/05.

USDA. MyPyramid website: http://www.mypyramid.gov; accessed 10/1/05.

Macronutrients

2

Chapter Outline

Macronutrients
Protein
Lipids
Carbohydrates

Objectives

- ➤ Identify the physiological functions of protein, lipids, and carbohydrates.
- ➤ Describe the importance of each group of macronutrients in maintaining homeostasis.
- ➤ Review food sources for each group of macronutrients.
- ➤ Identify intake recommendations for each group of macronutrients.
- ➤ Describe the potential impact of macronutrient excess or deficiency on clients.

NCLEX-RN® Test Prep

Use the CD-ROM enclosed with this book to access additional practice opportunities.

PRETEST

Review at a Glance

amino acids building block components of protein that have a specific chemical configuration

Atwater's physiological factors represent energy per weight calculation of protein, lipids, and carbohydrates in the diet: 4 kcal/gram for carbohydrates and protein and 9 kcal/gram for lipids

biological value indicator of protein quality that looks at the amount of nitrogen that the body retains

branched chain amino acids (BCAA) amino acids—isoleucine, leucine, and valine—that are found in the body in skeletal muscle and can be used in TPN solutions for clinical treatment of clients with liver and renal disease

carbohydrate chemical compound that includes carbon, hydrogen, and oxygen with hydrogen/oxygen ratio similar to that found in water (H_2O)

complementary protein two incomplete proteins added together in the diet to form a complete protein that has all essential amino acids

conditionally essential amino acids amino acids that become essential to the body due to certain metabolic conditions

eicosanoids fatty acid derivatives that have been found to regulate blood pressure, blood clotting, and immune activity in the body (leukotrienes, prostaglandins, and thromboxane)

essential amino acids protein building blocks that are needed for life and must be supplied to the body because the body cannot directly synthesize them

fiber structural component of plants

glycemic index a grading system in which a number is assigned for each food's potential to affect serum blood glucose; the higher the glycemic index, the higher the elevation response of the blood glucose to that food substance; similarly, the lower the glycemic index, the lower the response level

hydrogenated fat result of a chemical process whereby hydrogen is added to fats (increasing saturation), resulting in altered physical characteristics that enhance shelf life, resist oxidative changes, and cause trans fatty acids to be produced due to chemical transformation

lipid chemical compound that includes triglycerides, phospholipids, and sterols

nitrogen balance the balance between nitrogen consumed and nitrogen excreted in the body as a result of overall metabolic function; can be classified as positive, negative, or neutral, depending on body's metabolic needs and demands

nonessential amino acids protein building blocks needed for life that can be synthesized by the body from the breakdown or combination of other chemical structures

omega-3 fatty acid PUFA-linolenic (essential) that is identified by chemical structure (omega-3 indicates position of carbon double bond in the molecule) and that provides health benefits in the body

omega-6 fatty acid PUFA-linoleic (essential) that is identified by chemical structure (omega-6 indicates position of carbon double bond in the molecule) and that provides health benefits in the body

protein chemical structure containing carbon, hydrogen, and oxygen with nitrogen as the distinguishing chemical feature

protein energy malnutrition (PEM) clinical deficiency state in which energy, protein, or both occur that leads to malnutrition

saturation chemical term indicating the absence of double bonds whereby a molecule is holding onto the maximum of hydrogen ions

PRETEST

1 Which information should the nurse provide to a client who is planning to begin a low-carbohydrate (CHO) diet to lose weight?

1. A minimum level (50–100 grams/day) of CHOs is needed in the body in order to prevent protein breakdown.
2. Lowering of CHOs is the only way to effect sustained weight loss.
3. A decrease of CHOs in the diet will not affect other nutrient proportions in the body.
4. The client should increase dietary fiber level to compensate for decreased CHOs.

2 The nurse has instructed a vegetarian client regarding the use of complementary proteins in the diet. Which of the following statements by the client indicates that client teaching has been adequate?

1. "I will eat gelatin for dessert."
2. "I will eat more complete protein food sources."
3. "I will increase my intake of fruits and eat a wide variety of them."
4. "I will eat different plant food products together to provide complementary proteins."

3 A client asks the nurse, "How can I best reduce cholesterol in my diet?" Which of the following is the nurse's best response?

1. "No more than 30% of your diet should come from saturated fats."
2. "Check the labels on foods to identify cholesterol content."
3. "Limit intake of cholesterol to 300 mg a day."
4. "Do not eat any eggs or products containing eggs."

4 When assessing a client's nutritional status, the nurse concludes that which of the following conditions is most likely to affect the action of protein in the body?

1. Serum potassium level of 4.0 mEq/L
2. Serum sodium level of 145 mEq/L
3. A state of slight fluid overload
4. A state of positive nitrogen balance

5 The nurse is teaching a client ways to reduce total fat intake in the diet. The nurse instructs the client to increase intake of which of the following to achieve this result?

1. Trans-fatty acids
2. Omega-3 fatty acids via fish oil supplements
3. Hydrogenated food products
4. Vegetables, fruits, and grains

6 When caring for a client with a diet history of high animal protein intake, the nurse interprets that the client is at risk for developing which of the following?

1. Marasmus
2. Diarrhea
3. Cardiac disease
4. Diabetes

7 A client has received teaching about the function of lipids in the body. The nurse determines further information is required when the client states that fats:

1. Are an integral part of cell membranes.
2. Act as the primary source of energy in the body.
3. Support and cushion internal organs.
4. Maintain temperature by providing insulation.

8 Which of the following artificial sweeteners would the nurse recommend for a client who has phenylketonuria (PKU)?

1. Equal™
2. Sweet 'n' Low™
3. Nutrasweet™
4. Aspartame

9 A food diary indicates that a client is taking in an average of 35 grams of fat per day. The nurse calculates that the client is obtaining how many kilocalories from fat in the daily diet? Provide a numerical response.

Answer: ________________________

10 The nurse is preparing to teach a group of 16-year-olds in a health class about essential nutrients. Which of the following statements would the nurse use to best describe the concept of an essential nutrient?

1. "An essential nutrient provides all the necessary energy requirements for the body."
2. "Nutrients that are essential are supplied to the body in their active form, as the body cannot synthesize them from other sources."
3. "An essential nutrient provides the same amount of fat, protein, and carbohydrates."
4. "An essential nutrient can be synthesized in the body from precursor forms."

See pages 37–40 for Answers and Rationales.

I. MACRONUTRIENTS

A. Definition

1. Are large molecule groupings that are needed by the body to maintain normal physiologic functioning
2. Consist of **protein, lipids,** and **carbohydrates** (CHOs)

! B. Atwater's physiological factors (Kcalories per gram)

1. Protein and CHO provide 4 kcal/gram
2. Lipids (fats) provide 9 kcal/gram
3. Correlation of kcalories (energy) per weight (composition)

II. PROTEIN

A. Function

1. Structural component
   - **a.** Collagen provides structural integrity and is found in tendons, ligaments, and fascia
   - **b.** All body cells contain some form of protein (found in bones, muscles, skin, hair, nails, and blood vessels)
   - **c.** Nitrogen is the distinguishing element that identifies the composition of protein
2. Enzyme component
   - **a.** Participates in chemical reactions throughout the body in the form of nucleoproteins (DNA/RNA)
   - **b.** Participates in digestive enzymes
   - **c.** Participates in contraction of muscles (actin/myosin)
3. Transport component
   - **a.** Albumin is a major protein in plasma that helps to transport free fatty acids and binds with certain medications in the body
   - **b.** Hemoglobin is a protein that has oxygen-carrying capacity
   - **c.** Ferritin and transferrin are protein carriers that are connected with iron storage and transfer in the body
   - **d.** Myoglobin is a protein carrier found in muscle cells
   - **e.** Lipoproteins (protein + fat) help to carry cholesterol and fat-soluble vitamins in the body
   - **f.** Protein binding in the body can affect serum concentrations of calcium as well as certain medications
4. Defense component
   - **a.** Antibodies are large proteins found in the blood that respond to a specific antigen (foreign substance)
   - **b.** Immunoglobulins are a group of five structurally distinct humoral antibodies that are secreted in response to specific antigens (IgA, IgE, IgD, IgG, and IgM)
5. Fluid and acid-base component
   - **a.** Circulating proteins help to maintain osmotic pressure balance throughout the body

Table 2-1

Essential, Nonessential, and Conditionally Essential Amino Acids

Essential Amino Acids	Nonessential Amino Acids	Conditionally Essential Amino Acids
Histidine	Alanine	Arginine
Isoleucine	Asparagine	Carnitine
Leucine	Aspartic Acid	Cysteine
Lysine	Glutamic Acid	Citrulline
Methionine	Glutamine	Taurine
Phenylalanine	Glycine	Tyrosine
Threonine	Proline	
Tryptophan	Serine	
Valine		

Practice to Pass

How does the amount of protein in the body affect fluid dynamics?

Practice to Pass

What nutritional benefits do the use of branched chain amino acid formulations provide in TPN solutions?

b. Low albumin levels (hypoalbuminemia) lead to edema formation and fluid shifting

c. Proteins act as a buffer system in the body to maintain normal acid-base balance

B. Building block units

1. Amino acids

   a. **Essential amino acids:** a group of nine amino acids that the body cannot produce that must be obtained from food sources or other means (refer to Table 2-1)

   b. **Nonessential amino acids:** a group of eight amino acids that the body can synthesize from other substrates already in the body (refer again to Table 2-1)

   c. **Conditionally essential amino acids:** a group of six nonessential amino acids that are needed by the body in special situations when the body has undergone stress, trauma, or illness (refer again to Table 2-1)

2. Genetic sequencing and chemical arrangements

   a. Peptides are a series of chemical bonds that join amino acids (building block units) together to form a protein molecule

   b. Transamination involves a chemical process whereby one amino group is removed from an amino acid and combined with carbon fragments to form another amino acid

   c. Deamination involves a chemical process whereby the amino group (NH_2) is removed from an amino acid

   d. Denaturation involves a chemical process whereby a protein undergoes structural changes due to heating, acid/base imbalances, or alcohol

   e. **Branched chain amino acids (BCAA)** represent valine, leucine, and isoleucine (three of the essential acids)

      1) Decreased levels are seen in clients with extensive trauma, leading to catabolism, which increases their need for replacement

      2) Total parenteral nutrition (TPN) solutions made up of BCAA may be used in the treatment of liver disease or kidney failure because decreased levels are also found with these disorders; however, studies show no improvement in client outcomes; therefore, the use of BCAA in TPN has decreased

C. Recommendations for protein intake in the diet (see Box 2-1)

1. Percent in the diet (10–35% recommended)

a. A healthy adult requires 0.8 grams/kg of body weight

b. Special group concerns are noted for clients with developmental considerations (such as infants, children, and pregnant and lactating women), clients with new tissue/repair concerns (trauma, stress, and burns) and clients with increased metabolic requirements (athletes and disease states); vegetarian clients may fall into a special group concern depending on whether they get adequate protein sources in their diet from alternate foods

2. Protein quality

a. **Biological value** is a measurement of protein in terms of how usable it is by the body (or how easily it converts from being a food protein to a body protein)

!

1) Proteins with high biologic value have essential amino acids present in adequate proportions to meet minimum body needs (eggs, fish, poultry, lean meat, and dairy products)

2) Proteins with low biologic value do not have adequate amounts of essential amino acids to meet minimum body needs (grains, nuts, seeds, and legumes)

b. Complete proteins are foods high in biologic value that provide all essential amino acids and are usually of animal origin and soy protein (exception is gelatin)

c. Incomplete proteins are foods low in biologic value and are usually of plant origin (exception is soybean)

d. A **complementary protein** results from when two incomplete protein sources are combined to form a protein that now has essential amino acids in adequate amounts (e.g., macaroni and cheese, cereal and milk, and peanut butter sandwich)

e. Other methods that can be used to determine protein quality are amino acid scoring, Net Protein Utilization (NPU), and Protein Efficiency Ratio (PER)

1) Amino acid scoring looks at evaluating amino acid composition in reference to a standard protein source

2) NPU looks at the amount of nitrogen that is eaten in food products rather than absorbed levels of nitrogen

3) PER looks at weight gain as a measure of the effectiveness of protein quality in an individual client

Practice to Pass

What instructions would you give to an adult client to meet adequate protein levels in his diet?

Box 2-1

Recommendations for Protein in the Diet

- The adult RDA is 0.8 grams/kg/day, which correlates to roughly 10% of total calories.
- Depending on the client's developmental age and growth pattern, additional protein may be required (infants, children, pregnant and lactating women).
- Additional factors such as environment, stress, activity, and overall health status will influence dietary protein needs.
- Clients with health problems related to liver and renal dysfunction will have their protein intake closely monitored so as to avoid complications from the body's inability to handle protein load.
- A dietary pattern of choosing proteins by combining complementary proteins is adequate in meeting nutritional needs.
- Clients with genetic disorders such as sickle cell disease and phenylketonuria (PKU) will have their protein intake closely monitored so as to avoid complications due to enzyme deficiencies.

D. Food sources

1. Animal sources and eggs: most protein sources are of high biologic value and are of animal origin
2. Soy proteins constitute a high biologic value protein source, and soy products can be substituted in the diet to meet protein needs (e.g., vegetarian diet)
3. Added proteins to processed foods
   a. Casein: protein in cow's milk that provides taste and texture
   b. Gelatin: dietary protein added for stabilization and thickening (not high in biologic value even though of animal origin)
4. Amino acids added to foods
   a. Aspartame: artificial sweetener composed of amino acids (phenylalanine and aspartic acid); the active ingredient in Equal™ and Nutra Sweet™
   b. Monosodium glutamate (MSG): spice/preservative composed of amino acid (glutamate); an additional source of sodium in the diet
   c. Genetic engineering: protein research development is looking at establishing genetic coding information for use in disease treatment and prevention
   d. Anabolic products: sold to athletes to supposedly maximize muscle growth

E. Health concerns

1. **Protein energy malnutrition (PEM)**
   a. Kwashiorkor is an acute deficiency state of protein due to inadequate intake leading to edematous presentation (hepatomegaly); often seen in response to illness or infection
   b. Marasmus is a chronic deficiency state of protein or energy or both in combination that leads to poor absorption and a thin, matchstick appearance; serum albumin levels can be normal in marasmus
   c. Protein deficiencies can result in anemia, weight loss due to tissue wasting, and edema formation due to decreased colloid osmotic pressure
2. High protein diets
   a. Increased protein in the diet may lead to exclusion of other needed nutrients and cause other deficiencies
   b. Increased protein in the diet can place more stress on the kidneys and may lead to renal deterioration (urea cycle helping to get rid of extra protein)
   c. There is a correlation between increased dietary protein and increased incidence of heart disease (high protein and high in fat), obesity, and osteoporosis (due to loss of calcium)
   d. Protein and amino acid supplements offer no benefit to body and may be harmful
3. **Nitrogen balance** (intake = amount excreted)
   a. Negative: client consumes less than excreted indicating protein and/or calorie deficiency and tissue breakdown (stress, trauma, or illness); net catabolism occurs
   b. Positive: client consumes more than excreted indicating building up of tissue (growth periods); net anabolism occurs
4. Amino acid relationships in metabolism
   a. Sickle cell: an autosomal recessive genetic disorder in which amino acid glutamine is replaced by valine on the hemoglobin molecule, causing chronic mutations to occur, resulting in pain and infection

b. Phenylketonuria (PKU): an autosomal recessive genetic disorder in which the phenylalanine hydroxylase enzyme (that converts phenylalanine to tyrosine) is missing or defective, leading to increased levels of the amino acid phenylalanine that can lead to mental retardation; PKU diet excludes high-protein/nutrient-dense foods and limits the amount of phenylalanine consumed in the diet

c. Tryptophan conversion to niacin: 60 mg of dietary tryptophan = 1 mg niacin; the amino acid precursor tryptophan is converted to nicotinic acid in the body (vitamin B_3–niacin)

d. Homocysteine levels (an amino acid produced as the essential amino acid methionine is broken down) and cardiovascular disease: increased levels of homocysteine are associated with cardiovascular disease, platelet adhesions and subsequent thrombus formation, and decreased levels of B complex vitamins

III. LIPIDS

A. Function

1. Structural component

a. Found in all cell membranes and participates in cell metabolism, absorption, and transport

b. Is stored as adipose tissue in the body (body has an endless capacity to store fat)

c. Provides cushioning and protection for vital organs

d. Provides skin lubrication in the form of secretions of sebaceous glands

e. Provides insulation (subcutaneous fat) to regulate body temperature and aids in nerve impulse transmission

2. Transport component: lipoproteins (protein + lipid component)

a. Chylomicrons carry triglycerides in the bloodstream after meals (largest and lightest, constitute 80–90% of triglycerides)

b. Very-low-density lipoproteins (VLDLs) transport triglycerides from liver to tissue (constitute 55–65% of triglycerides); normal serum range is 51–197 mg/dL

! c. Low-density lipoproteins (LDLs) are plasma proteins with triglyceride components that carry cholesterol to cells; increased levels are associated with incidence of heart disease ("bad" cholesterol); optimal serum range is $<$100 mg/dL

! d. High-density lipoproteins (HDLs) are plasma proteins that carry fat in the bloodstream to tissue or to the liver to be excreted; cardioprotective in that increased levels are associated with decreased incidence of heart disease ("good" cholesterol); optimal serum range is $\geq$ 60 mg/dL based on age

B. Building blocks

1. Fatty acids

a. Essential fatty acids (FAs) consist of linoleic (**omega–6 FA**), arachidonic, and linolenic acids (**omega–3FA**) that must be supplied in the diet because the body cannot manufacture them

b. Nonessential fatty acids are those that can be manufactured in the body and do not require dietary ingestion

2. Fatty acid configuration

a. Saturated versus unsaturated

1) **Saturation** refers to the maximum amount of hydrogen ions that fat can hold

Practice to Pass

A client does not understand how any form of cholesterol could be considered "good." How would you explain the concept of HDL as being the "good" cholesterol?

2) The presence of double bonds differentiates lipids as to whether they are saturated or unsaturated and defines physical characteristic properties

! 3) A saturated fat contains no double bonds, is usually of animal origin, and is solid at room temperature

! 4) An unsaturated fat contains double bonds, is usually of plant origin, and is liquid at room temperature

b. Monounsaturated versus polyunsaturated

1) An FA with one carbon-to-carbon double bond is considered to be monounsaturated

2) An FA with more than one carbon-to-carbon double bond is considered to be polyunsaturated (polyunsaturated fatty acids—PUFA)

c. Omega-3 and omega-6 fatty acids

1) Omega-3: linolenic (essential FA) has been shown to have preventive effects on heart disease (decreased blood clotting tendency, decreased blood pressure, and decreased cardiac mortality); found in fatty fish, salad, cooking oil, margarine, and fish oils

2) Omega-6: linoleic (essential FA) has been shown to lower serum cholesterol levels, prolong clotting time, help prevent cardiovascular disease, and aid in brain development; found in vegetable oils, peanuts, and eggs

3) Trans-fatty acids (change from cis to trans configuration in chemical structure) are associated with increased incidence of cardiovascular disease by increasing LDL levels and decreasing HDL levels

3. Glycerides

a. Mono- and diglycerides represent fatty acids joined to a glycerol backbone structure

1) 1 FA + glycerol = monoglyceride

2) 2 FA + glycerol = diglyceride

b. Triglycerides represent 3 FAs joined to a glycerol component; they represent most of the dietary fat and are stored as adipose tissue in the body

4. Phospholipids and sterols

a. Lecithin is a phospholipid that acts as an emulsifier in the body and can be used as an additive to food products to stabilize consistency; found in plant and animal foods

b. Cholesterol is a sterol compound that is produced by the liver and is also found in dietary sources

1) Functions include: component of bile salts that aids digestion, essential component of cell membranes (brain, nerve, and blood), required for production of hormones (cortisone, adrenaline, estrogen, and testosterone) and vitamin D

2) Increased levels are associated with coronary artery disease

3) Lipoprotein carriers recognize cholesterol

C. Recommendations for lipid intake in the diet (see Box 2-2)

1. Percent in the diet (< 35% total, < 10% saturated recommended)

a. Healthy adult

1) Not to exceed 35% of total calories but not less than 10% of daily total kcalories

2) Dietary cholesterol intake of < 300 mg per day

Box 2-2

Recommendations for Lipids in the Diet

- ➤ Maintain acceptable range of no less than 20% and no more than 35% in the daily diet.
- ➤ Keep percentage of saturated fats to a maximum of 10% in the daily diet.
- ➤ Limit daily cholesterol intake to 300 mg daily. Remember, the body makes cholesterol as well, so there is no need to add additional dietary sources.
- ➤ Read labels on food products used for hidden sources of fat content in foods. Evaluate the percentage of calories derived from fat in the food product and consider the 30% limit.
- ➤ Trim excess fat on food items prior to eating and use a minimum of fat/oils in cooking processes. Do not let the cooking method used be the source of dietary fat.
- ➤ Limit the amount of organ meats and eggs to prevent excess dietary cholesterol levels. Use alternative food items such as egg substitutes or egg whites as egg sources in the diet.
- ➤ Limit the amount of processed hydrogenated food items in the diet as they have been shown to have high levels of trans fatty acids, which have been correlated with cardiovascular disease and other health problems.
- ➤ Eat more sources of omega-3 fatty acids in the diet for their health benefits.
- ➤ Replace saturated fats and trans fats with monounsaturated and polyunsaturated fats.

b. Special population groups

1) Clients with diabetes, cardiovascular disease, cancers, and who are obese should limit their fat intake because documented evidence has shown higher incidence of health problems

2) Elderly clients, children, and pregnant clients should monitor their fat intake and maintain recommended dietary levels in order to prevent health problems

! **2.** Types of fat (see Box 2-3)

a. Saturated /unsaturated fats: it is recommended that a decreased proportion of saturated fats and increased proportion of unsaturated fats in the diet will help maximize health benefits

b. Cholesterol and triglyceride (fat) concerns: dietary cholesterol should be < 300 mg per day; triglyceride (fat) restriction should be in keeping within 35% guideline

c. Serum cholesterol level (total) should be < 200 mg/dL; serum triglyceride level should be < 150 mg/dL

d. **Hydrogenated fats** represent a chemical process whereby hydrogen is added to fat, thereby increasing saturation (adding double bonds)

1) This process causes formation of trans-fatty acids

2) This process is done to extend the shelf life of a food product

3) Process can be partial or complete (partially hydrogenated or completely hydrogenated)

e. **Eicosanoids** (leukotrienes, prostaglandins, and thromboxanes) are derivatives of long-chain PUFA fatty acids made by the body that regulate blood pressure, clotting, and other body functions by variations of hormone effects

Practice to Pass

What effect will an increase in the use of hydrogenated food products in the diet have on a client's fat intake?

D. Food sources

1. Natural fat sources are found in many dietary food sources since most animal and plant foods contain some percentage of fat

Box 2-3

Saturated versus Unsaturated Fats

- Saturated fats include butter, chocolate, coconut, egg yolks, ice cream, milk and milk products, meats, and palm oil.
- Saturated fats are usually solid at room temperature and are of animal origin.
- Saturated fats imply that the fat molecules are holding the maximum number of hydrogen ions (saturated = full).
- Unsaturated fats can be categorized as mono- or polyunsaturated fats.
- Monounsaturated fats are found in avocados, canola and olive oil, nuts, sardines, and peanut oil.
- Polyunsaturated fats (PUFA) are found in oily fish, soybeans, safflower oil, soybean oil, sunflower oil, and tofu. Omega-3 and omega-6 are examples of PUFA.
- Unsaturated fats are usually liquid at room temperature and are of plant origin.
- Unsaturated fats imply that the fat molecules contain less than the maximum number of hydrogen ions (unsaturated = not full).

2. Added fats found in processed foods are usually due to the hydrogenation process
3. Artificial fat products include alternative items that are specifically produced to replace fat content in the diet
   - **a.** CHO fat replacements are used to flavor, thicken, and stabilize certain foods
   - **b.** Protein fat replacements are used to add textural changes to the food item so that it tastes and feels more like fat
   - **c.** Fat replacements have similar properties to traditional fats but offer fewer kcalories per serving
   - **d.** Olestra is FDA-approved for use as an additive fat substitute in the diet that cannot be absorbed by the body and is found in certain snack foods; a label indicating possible symptoms (abdominal cramping and loose stools) and altered absorption of fat-soluble vitamins is put on the food product label; this factor may be of concern in clients who have altered metabolism and fat-soluble vitamin deficiencies
4. Labeling used to denote fat content in food items has been defined under FDA guidelines because there are many different descriptive terms used on food products that refer to fat content ranging from *fat free, low, reduced,* or *lean;* refer to specific FDA labeling guidelines for a complete description of terms
   - **a.** *Fat-free* items must contain less than 0.5 gram of fat per serving size
   - **b.** *Low* fat items must contain 3 grams or less of fat per serving size
   - **c.** *Reduced* can be further categorized as being reduced in fat, saturated fat, or cholesterol content
   - **d.** *Lean* refers to specific totals of fat, saturated fat, and cholesterol per 100 grams of food item

E. Health concerns

1. Essential fatty acid (EFA) deficiency is very rare, but can cause significant nutritional problems and is usually seen in clients with PEM or clients taking parenteral nutrition without recognition/replacement of EFA; associated with skin abnormalities (dermatitis, poor healing), growth failure, or reproductive failure

2. Lipids and cardiovascular disease
   a. Lipids increase plaque formation that contributes to the development of atherosclerosis
   b. HDL and LDL levels
      1) HDL is cardioprotective
      2) Increased LDL levels are associated with heart disease
   c. Dietary risk factors include excess saturated fat, increased cholesterol levels, and intake of trans fatty acids in the diet
   d. Cardioprotective effects of lipids are seen with omega-3 and omega-6 fatty acids, increased monounsaturated fats in the diet, increased fiber and antioxidants, and moderate alcohol consumption
3. Lipids and cancer
   a. There are beneficial effects of omega-3, omega-6, and monounsaturated fats in the diet
   b. Colon cancer has been associated with increased fat and low fiber levels in the diet
   c. Breast cancer may be related to increased levels of saturated fats in the diet

IV. CARBOHYDRATES

A. Function

1. Structural component
   a. Carbohydrate (CHO) contains carbon, hydrogen, and oxygen in proportions similar to H_2O
   b. Is a component of cell membranes and cell walls
2. Energy component: CHOs are the major source of energy in the diet
3. Cellular component: CHOs function to spare body protein, prevent ketosis, and regulate blood glucose levels in order to maintain normal function of the brain

B. Building block units

1. Monosaccharides (basic unit)
   a. Glucose
      1) Also known as blood sugar or dextrose
      2) Component of all three dietary dissacharides
   b. Fructose
      1) Most concentrated form of sugar
      2) High fructose corn syrup (HFCS) is often used as an additive, sweetener
   c. Galactose: breakdown of milk sugar (lactose)
2. Disaccharides (two monosaccharides joined together)
   a. Maltose = glucose + glucose
   b. Sucrose = glucose + fructose (table sugar, sugar beets, and sugar cane)
   c. Lactose = glucose + galactose (milk sugar)
3. Complex polysaccharides
   a. Glycogen is the storage form (animal starch) that is found in the liver and muscle tissue and helps to sustain glucose levels

Practice to Pass

Why is dietary fiber necessary in the human diet?

b. Starches provide the major source of CHOs in the diet (grains, cereals, breads, pasta, starchy vegetables, and legumes)

4. **Fibers** (roughage, bulk, adds volume not fuel)
   a. Cellulose (plant starch) is found as a primary constituent of plant cells and cannot be digested by human enzymes
   b. Hemicellulose is the primary constituent of cereal fibers
   c. Pectins represent nonstructural polysaccharides that are soluble fibers and provide thickening and consistency
   d. Gums and mucilages are nonstructural polysaccharides that are extracted from plants and used as additives/stabilizers
   e. Lignin is a nonpolysaccharide that is considered a "wood" portion of the plant
   f. Soluble versus insoluble fiber
      ! **1)** Insoluble fiber is derived from structural parts of plants that promote regularity and decreased risk of cancer and diverticular disease (e.g., wheat bran and nuts)
      2) Soluble fiber is derived from inside plant cells and decreases cholesterol, regulates blood glucose levels, and increases satiety (e.g., oatmeal and broccoli)

C. Recommendations for carbohydrate intake in the diet (see Box 2-4)

1. Percentage of simple carbohydrates
   a. Healthy adult
      ! **1)** Minimum of 50–100 grams CHO daily to spare protein and prevent ketosis
      2) Encourage use of whole foods, fresh fruits, and fiber

Box 2-4

Recommendations for Carbohydrates in the Diet

- A minimum amount of CHO is needed in the diet to spare protein and prevent ketosis (50–100 grams/day).
- A 45–65% CHO content is recommended in the daily diet along with 25–38 grams of fiber per day.
- Most U.S. diet patterns include sufficient CHO sources; often the client is not aware of the CHOs found in most food choices. It is important to read labels so as to become familiar with natural versus added sugars and the sugar content that is already in the food item.
- Clients with defined health risks such as diabetes should closely monitor their CHO intake in order to maintain consistency of blood glucose levels.
- The inclusion of adequate fiber and complex CHOs in the diet helps to regulate elimination patterns and can be cardioprotective as well as offer cancer protection and provide weight control.
- Use sugar substitutes within appropriate guidelines because the body does not distinguish between regular and synthetic sugars when they are broken down to constituent parts. It may prove beneficial to use regular sugar and include the amount in dietary CHO calculations.
- Monitor intake of foods with HFCS on the label because client may not be aware of hidden CHO sources in the diet that are adding to daily CHO levels.
- Hidden CHO sources in the diet may contribute to empty calories that can promote weight gain.

b. There are special group concerns for the young and for elderly clients due to potential alterations in blood glucose levels and elimination patterns

2. Percentage of complex carbohydrates
   a. Healthy adult
      1) 45–65% calories in the daily diet
      2) Encourage use of whole grains, legumes, vegetables, and other foods that are high in nutrient density and fiber and low in fat
   b. There are special group concerns for the young and for elderly clients due to potential effects on blood glucose levels and elimination patterns
3. Percentage of fiber
   a. Healthy adult: recommended 25–38 grams of dietary fiber per day
   b. There are special group concerns for clients with altered elimination patterns because natural use of fibers can help to normalize function
   c. Dietary fiber should be increased on a gradual basis to decrease the incidence of GI symptoms such as bloating, flatulence, and diarrhea
   d. Increased fluid intake (water) should accompany increased levels of fiber in the diet to prevent potential imbalances
   e. Increased amounts of insoluble fiber can reduce the absorption of certain minerals (Ca, Fe, Zn, and Mg)
   f. Adequate fiber is found in food products; it is recommended that food sources be used to increase dietary levels rather than fiber supplements

D. Food sources

1. Natural sugars include honey, molasses, brown sugar, and maple syrup
2. Refined sugars are simple CHOs that have low nutrient density (white sugar, white bread, candy bars, and cola) and have been altered or processed
3. Added carbohydrates to processed foods include modified starch thickeners (pectins, gums), HFCS (fructose), and sugar substitutes (saccharin)

E. Health concerns

1. Blood glucose regulation
   a. Hormonal response
      1) Regulating hormones between the blood and the cell include insulin, glucagon, and epinephrine
      2) Insulin release by beta cells of the pancreas occurs in response to blood glucose elevations
      3) Glucagon is released after meals in response to decreased blood glucose levels
      4) Epinephrine (adrenal gland stress hormone) acts to release glucose from storage in the liver

   ! b. **Glycemic index** (see Table 2-2)
      1) Provides an estimate of how foods affect serum blood glucose level
      2) Foods with a high glycemic index (potatoes and bread) raise the blood glucose level rapidly
      3) Foods with a low glycemic index (dairy products and pasta) do not cause the blood glucose level to rise as rapidly

Table 2-2

Glycemic Index of Selected Food Products

Low Glycemic Index	Moderate Glycemic Index	High Glycemic Index
Apple	Banana	Bagel
Apricot	Corn	Carrots
Bran cereals	Ice Cream	Graham crackers
Chocolate	Popcorn	Honey
Milk	Rice	Soft drinks
Yogurt	Sweet Potato	White bread

2. Nursing bottle syndrome
   a. Development of dental caries can occur due to prolonged contact of infant with bottle if infant/child is put to sleep with a bottle as a pacifier
   b. Periodontal disease is also promoted due to bacterial interaction with dietary proteins and production of acids
3. Proportional amount of carbohydrates in the diet
   a. Clients who experience changes in CHO metabolism are prone to developing diabetes
   b. Excess CHO is converted to and stored as glycogen and stored as fat
   c. Increased dietary fiber has significant health benefits with regard to lowering risk of bowel disorders, cardiovascular disease, and colon cancer
   d. Excess fiber can cause altered elimination patterns such as constipation if fluid intake is not adequate
   e. Increased intake of sugars in the diet can lead to obesity, elevated triglycerides, and dental caries
   f. Decreased levels of CHOs in the diet can lead to tissue breakdown (as protein sparing effect of CHO is not available) leading to ketosis and metabolic acidosis

Case Study

A 58-year-old male client has recently been diagnosed with coronary artery disease and hypertension. The physical examination reveals BP of 150/90, pulse of 80, respiratory rate of 22, and oral temperature of 99.2°F. The client is coming in to the clinic for a followup visit (one month into the treatment plan) for additional nutritional instruction regarding hypercholesterolemia because his lipid profile indicates HDL of 28, LDL of 280, and triglyceride level of 150.

1. What information does the lipid profile reveal?
2. What impact does hypercholesterolemia have on the client's overall health status?
3. What dietary instructions can you provide to the client that will help reduce dietary fat intake and lower serum cholesterol levels?
4. What other tests might be needed to determine the client's overall nutritional status?
5. What other treatment methods might be included in this client's plan of care that might affect nutritional outcomes?

For suggested responses, see page 317.

POSTTEST

1 The nurse is providing dietary counseling to a client with coronary artery disease (CAD). The nurse encourages intake of foods high in omega-3 fatty acids, such as those found in which of the following?

1. Fish oils
2. Whole grains
3. Grapefruit
4. Poultry

2 Laboratory results indicate a client has elevated homocysteine levels. The nurse explains to the client that this can contribute to which of the following?

1. Decreased utilization of essential amino acids
2. Increased metabolic production of B vitamins
3. Increased risk of atherosclerotic disease
4. Decreased absorption of lipids

3 The nurse explains to a client who is following a low protein diet that which consequence could possibly occur?

1. Increased risk of coronary artery disease
2. Frequent episodes of steatorrhea
3. Development of pyelonephritis
4. Impaired immune function

4 The nurse has conducted dietary teaching with a client who has heart disease. In evaluating the effectiveness of the session, the nurse concludes that the best outcome is obtained when the client selects which of the following food items from a sample restaurant menu?

1. Turkey casserole in a cream sauce
2. Barbecued beef ribs
3. Baked chicken breast with skin
4. Baked fish coated in bread crumbs

5 The nurse would include which strategy as most appropriate in the care plan of a client who needs to limit intake of trans-fatty acids?

1. Teach client to read nutrition labels checking for hydrogenated fats.
2. Have client select low-cholesterol foods from a dietary plan.
3. Assist client to choose non-dairy foods when filling out the menu.
4. Ask client to name three foods high in saturated fats.

6 Which of the following consequences would the nurse anticipate in a client who has had prolonged carbohydrate (CHO) deficiency?

1. Ketosis and metabolic acidosis
2. Anemia and edema
3. Skin lesions and weight loss
4. Dental caries and obesity

7 The nurse has instructed a client on complementary proteins. Which diet selection by the client illustrates that the client has understood the material presented?

1. Eggs and bacon
2. Pinto beans and rice
3. Fish and chips
4. Hamburger and fries

8 Which of the following dietary methods could the nurse best utilize in a plan of care for a client to minimize the risk of dental caries?

1. Use hard candies to prevent dryness of the oral cavity.
2. Eat air-popped popcorn when eating a snack food.
3. Limit intake of soft drinks to one or two a day.
4. Rinse mouth after eating candy or anything sweet.

9 Which of the following signs should the nurse check for in a client who admits to eating a lot of snack foods containing Olestra?

1. Numbness in fingers
2. Headaches
3. Abdominal cramping
4. Dizziness

10 A client needs to follow a low-fat diet. Which of the following products would the nurse instruct the client to avoid using when cooking? Select all that apply.

1. Solid margarine
2. Shortening
3. Coconut oil
4. Corn oil
5. Canola oil

ANSWERS & RATIONALES

Pretest

1 **Answer: 1** CHOs are the primary energy source used to maintain the body and a minimum level of CHOs (50–100 grams/day) is needed in order to avoid protein breakdown. Option 2 is incorrect because there are other methods (besides lowering CHO intake) to establish sustained weight loss. Option 3 is incorrect—a balanced intake of all three macronutrients is needed in order to maximize function, prevent breakdown of constituent products, and maintain energy. Option 4 is incorrect because an increase in dietary fiber will not compensate for a decrease in total CHOs. Although dietary fiber provides health benefits related to elimination and cholesterol levels, an increase in fiber above current recommendations (20–35 grams/day) may cause an increase in GI symptoms and lead to constipation. **Cognitive Level:** Application **Client Need:** Health Promotion and Maintenance **Integrated Process:** Nursing Process: Planning **Content Area:** Foundational Sciences: Nutrition **Strategy:** Critical words are *low CHO* and *lose weight.* Recognize there are many ways to approach weight reduction and eliminate option 2. Eliminate options 3 and 4 since they are incorrect statements. **Reference:** Rolfes, S., Pinna, K. & Whitney, E. (2006). *Understanding normal and clinical nutrition* (7th ed.). Belmont, CA: Wadsworth & Thomson Learning, pp. 47–49.

2 **Answer: 4** The use of complementary proteins in a diet pattern refers to the combining of different plant proteins in a day to form a complete protein that is of high biologic value. Vegetarians should receive instruction on this method in order to maintain required essential amino acid requirements in the body and prevent clinical deficiencies that could arise due to their choice of vegetarianism. Option 1 is incorrect: Gelatin is an animal protein of low biologic value and would not be included in a vegetarian diet. Option 2 is incorrect because the idea of complementary proteins is to combine food choices and not merely to increase the amount of complete protein sources. Option 3 is incorrect because an increase in fruits will not provide complete protein. **Cognitive Level:** Analysis **Client Need:** Health Promotion and Maintenance **Integrated Process:** Nursing Process: Evaluation **Content Area:** Foundational Sciences: Nutrition **Strategy:** Note that the critical word in the question is *complementary* and this word is repeated in option 4. Recall knowledge of complete versus complementary proteins to eliminate options 1 and 2. Eliminate option 3 because fruits are not adequate protein sources. **Reference:** Nix, S. (2005) *Williams' basic nutrition & diet therapy* (12th ed.) St. Louis: Elsevier Mosby, p. 47.

3 **Answer: 3** It is recommended that cholesterol intake be limited to 300 mg a day. No more than 10% of fats should be saturated. Checking labels is advisable but does not provide the client with specific guidelines. Eggs can be eaten but should be limited to 2–3/week. **Cognitive Level:** Analysis **Client Need:** Health Promotion and Maintenance **Integrated Process:** Communication and Documentation **Content Area:** Foundational Sciences: Nutrition **Strategy:** The question addresses reduction of cholesterol. Eliminate option 2 since it does not answer the client's question. Eliminate options 1 and 4 because they are incorrect. **Reference:** Rolfes, S., Pinna, K. & Whitney, E. (2006). *Understanding normal and clinical nutrition* (7th ed.). Belmont, CA: Wadsworth & Thomson Learning, pp. 66–67.

4 **Answer: 4** Nitrogen balance refers to the concept of a balanced protein state in the body to support metabolism. A client who is in positive nitrogen balance is taking more nitrogen in and excreting less nitrogen in order to meet metabolic needs (growth state with increased demands). Options 1 and 2 are incorrect because they represent normal range findings for sodium and potassium levels in the body. It is important to note that protein function does depend on the interaction of acid/base and serum electrolytes in order to function effectively, and the nurse must be alert to look at pertinent laboratory findings. A slight state of fluid overload (option 3) is less significant than a state of positive protein balance, which correlates directly with the question. **Cognitive Level:** Analysis **Client Need:** Health Promotion and Maintenance **Integrated Process:** Nursing Process:

Analysis **Content Area:** Foundational Sciences: Nutrition **Strategy:** Note that options 1 and 2 are normal lab values and can be eliminated. Recall nitrogen is the core molecule of protein to choose option 4. **Reference:** Dudek, S. (2006) *Nutritional essentials for nursing practice* (5th ed.). Philadelphia: Lippincott Williams & Wilkins, p. 49.

5 **Answer: 4** Vegetables, fruits, and grains in the diet are low in fat and are rich in nutrients and phytochemicals. Option 1 is incorrect because trans-fatty acids are associated with increased cardiovascular risks. Option 2 is incorrect because the use of fish oil supplements can interfere with bleeding times, diabetic state, immune status, and wound healing. A balanced level of omega-3 and omega-6 fatty acids is recommended in the diet using natural sources. Option 3 is incorrect because the process of hydrogenation increases the amount of trans-fatty acid and would not be a prudent choice.
Cognitive Level: Application **Client Need:** Health Promotion and Maintenance **Integrated Process:** Teaching and Learning **Content Area:** Foundational Sciences: Nutrition **Strategy:** Note question addresses reduction of fats. Eliminate options 1 and 3 because they suggest increasing fats. Eliminate option 2 since it does not address fat intake. **Reference:** Rolfes, S., Pinna, K. & Whitney, E. (2006). *Understanding normal and clinical nutrition* (7th ed.). Belmont, CA: Wadsworth & Thomson Learning, pp. 64–67.

6 **Answer: 3** Increased intake of animal protein may be associated with cardiac disease because animal food protein sources are also high in saturated fat content. Options 1 and 2 reflect clinical conditions in which there are protein losses due to either intake or cell breakdown. Diabetes (option 4) is associated with excessive caloric intake or an autoimmune origin.
Cognitive Level: Analysis **Client Need:** Health Promotion and Maintenance **Integrated Process:** Nursing Process: Analysis **Content Area:** Foundational Sciences: Nutrition **Strategy:** Critical words are history of *high animal protein intake* and *increased risk.* Eliminate options 1 and 2 since they are associated with protein losses or deficits. Recall correlation of animal protein sources with fat to choose option 3. **Reference:** Rolfes, S., Pinna, K. & Whitney, E. (2006) *Understanding normal and clinical nutrition* (7th ed.) Belmont, CA: Wadsworth & Thomson Learning, p. 84.

7 **Answer: 2** Lipids are not a primary energy source but rather serve as an energy reserve in the body. CHOs are the primary energy source of the body. Options 1, 3, and 4 are incorrect as they all represent functions of lipids in the body (part of cell membranes, support of internal organs, and insulation).
Cognitive Level: Analysis **Client Need:** Health Promotion and Maintenance **Integrated Process:** Nursing Process: Evaluation **Content Area:** Foundational Sciences: Nutrition **Strategy:** This question requires identifying one incorrect answer, as 3 options are correct. Recall options 1, 3, and 4 are normal functions of fat and eliminate them. **Reference:** Rolfes, S., Pinna, K. & Whitney, E. (2006). *Understanding normal and clinical nutrition* (7th ed.). Belmont, CA: Wadsworth & Thomson Learning, pp. 56–57.

8 **Answer: 2** A client with PKU has a genetic condition that prevents the utilization and conversion of the amino acid phenylalanine, leading to increased levels with toxic clinical manifestations. The product Sweet 'n' Low contains saccharin as the sweetening agent, which will not cause problems for the PKU client. All of the other options are incorrect, because both Equal and Nutrasweet (options 1 and 3) contain aspartame (option 4) as their active ingredient. Aspartame contains aspartic acid, a methyl group, and phenylalanine. Intake of these products can be dangerous for a client who has a clinical diagnosis of PKU; warning labels are found on packages of these food products denoting this fact.
Cognitive Level: Analysis **Client Need:** Health Promotion and Maintenance **Integrated Process:** Nursing Process: Implementation **Content Area:** Foundational Sciences: Nutrition **Strategy:** The question requires specific recall of PKU and the content of artificial sweeteners. If you had difficulty answering the question, review this content. **Reference:** Rolfes, S., Pinna, K. & Whitney, E. (2006). *Understanding normal and clinical nutrition* (7th ed.). Belmont, CA: Wadsworth & Thomson Learning, pp. 41–42.

9 **Answer: 315** Each gram of fat supplies 9 kcal. Multiply the 9 kcal by 35 (the number of daily grams of fat in the diet) to obtain a result of 315 kcal. ($9 \times 35 = 315$)
Cognitive Level: Analysis **Client Need:** Health Promotion and Maintenance **Integrated Process:** Nursing Process: Implementation **Content Area:** Foundational Sciences: Nutrition **Strategy:** The core issue of the question is knowledge that each gram of fat contains 9 kilocalories. Take time to become familiar with these basic nutritional facts if this question was difficult. **Reference:** Rolfes, S., Pinna, K. & Whitney, E. (2006). *Understanding normal and clinical nutrition* (7th ed.). Belmont, CA: Wadsworth & Thomson Learning, p. 56.

10 **Answer: 2** Essential nutrients are needed by the body in their original form, as the body cannot synthesize them from other materials in the body. Option 1 is incorrect—an essential nutrient does not provide all the necessary energy requirements for the body. Option 3 is incorrect—essential nutrients differ in their amounts of fat, protein, and carbohydrates. Option 4 is incorrect because this statement describes a nonessential nutrient.

Cognitive Level: Analysis **Client Need:** Health Promotion and Maintenance **Integrated Process:** Teaching and Learning **Content Area:** Foundational Sciences: Nutrition **Strategy:** Note the word *best,* indicating all or some options may be correct, but one provides a more thorough answer. Options 2 and contain similar concepts, but recall essential nutrients cannot be synthesized to choose option 2. **Reference:** Rolfes, S., Pinna, K. & Whitney, E. (2006). *Understanding normal and clinical nutrition* (7th ed.). Belmont, CA: Wadsworth & Thomson Learning, p. 7.

Posttest

1 **Answer: 1** Omega-3 fatty acids have been shown to reduce risk factors associated with heart disease. They are found in fatty fish, fish and flaxseed oils, and cooking oils. **Cognitive Level:** Application **Client Need:** Health Promotion and Maintenance **Integrated Process:** Nursing Process: Implementation **Content Area:** Foundational Sciences: Nutrition **Strategy:** The question requires recall of knowledge of foods high in omega 3 fatty acids. Since fatty acids are the product of fat breakdown, eliminate options 2 and 3 since they do not contain or have very little fat. Eliminate poultry (option 4) since it contains saturated fat in the skin. **Reference:** Dudek, S. (2006). *Nutritional essentials for nursing practice* (5th ed.). Philadelphia: Lippincott Williams & Wilkins, p. 38.

2 **Answer: 3** Clinical evidence has supported that elevated homocysteine levels correlate with increased risk for the development of atherosclerotic heart disease and deficiencies of certain B complex vitamins. Option 1 is incorrect—homocysteine is an amino acid that is produced by the breakdown of the amino acid methionine. Option 2 is incorrect because elevated homocysteine levels are associated with vitamin B deficiencies. Option 4 is incorrect because homocysteine metabolism is not related to lipid absorption.
Cognitive Level: Application **Client Need:** Health Promotion and Maintenance **Integrated Process:** Teaching and Learning **Content Area:** Foundational Sciences: Nutrition **Strategy:** A critical word is *increased.* Recall homocysteine is associated with cardiovascular disease to choose option 2. **Reference:** Rolfes, S., Pinna, K. & Whitney, E. (2006). *Understanding normal and clinical nutrition* (7th ed.). Belmont, CA: Wadsworth & Thomson Learning, p. 186.

3 **Answer: 4** Clients with deficient protein intake are at risk for immune dysfunction and fatigue. High protein intake may put clients at risk of coronary heart disease, not low protein. Steatorrhea is usually associated with altered fat metabolism. Pyelonephritis is an infection and is not caused by low protein diets.
Cognitive Level: Application **Client Need:** Health Promotion and Maintenance **Integrated Process:** Teaching and Learning **Content Area:** Foundational Sciences: Nutrition **Strategy:** Critical words are *low protein diet.* Eliminate option 1 because it is related to high protein intake. Option 2 is associated with fat metabolism. Recall protein is needed for adequate cellular metabolism to choose option 4. **Reference:** Rolfes, S., Pinna, K., & Whitney, E. (2006). *Understanding normal and clinical nutrition* (7th ed.). Belmont, CA: Wadsworth & Thomson Learning, pp. 81–83.

4 **Answer: 4** Clients with heart disease benefit from foods that are low in fat and, if hypertensive, low in salt. Baked fish without added sources of fat represent the best choice on the sample menu. The turkey would be a good choice if it did not have a cream sauce, which is high in fat. Beef is high in fat because it is an animal product and contains more fat than poultry. The baked chicken would be a better choice if the skin were removed, because skin is high in fat also.
Cognitive Level: Application **Client Need:** Health Promotion and Maintenance **Integrated Process:** Nursing Process: Evaluation **Content Area:** Foundational Sciences: Nutrition **Strategy:** Note animal foods provide richest sources of fat, so the beef can be eliminated first followed by the poultry. This leaves fish as the best choice, especially since there are no added sauces or coatings that contain fat. **Reference:** Rolfes, S., Pinna, K. & Whitney, E. (2006). *Understanding normal and clinical nutrition* (7th ed.). Belmont, CA: Wadsworth & Thomson Learning, pp. 66–67.

5 **Answer: 1** Trans-fatty acids are found in processed hydrogenated foods. The other options address reduction of cholesterol and saturated fats in the diet, but do not address trans-fatty acids specifically. Some foods high in cholesterol and fat, although they should be reduced, may not be high in trans-fatty acids.
Cognitive Level: Application **Client Need:** Health Promotion and Maintenance **Integrated Process:** Nursing Process: Planning **Content Area:** Foundational Sciences: Nutrition **Strategy:** A critical concept in the question is trans fatty acids. Options 2 and 4 can be eliminated since they address cholesterol and saturated fats. Recall hydrogenated fats are a common source of trans fatty acids to choose option 1. **Reference:** Rolfes, S., Pinna, K., & Whitney, E. (2006). *Understanding normal and clinical nutrition* (7th ed.). Belmont, CA: Wadsworth & Thomson Learning, pp. 59, 63.

6 **Answer: 1** A state of prolonged CHO deficiency can lead to protein breakdown that results in formation of ketone bodies and altered acid-base balance (metabolic acidosis). Options 2 and 3 are incorrect because they are associated with protein deficiency and lipid deficiency, respectively. Option 4 is incorrect—these are associated with an increased amount of CHOs in the diet.

Cognitive Level: Analysis **Client Need:** Health Promotion and Maintenance **Integrated Process:** Nursing Process: Analysis **Content Area:** Foundational Sciences: Nutrition **Strategy:** Critical words are *prolonged deficiency* and *CHOs.* Eliminate option 4 as it is associated with excessive CHO intake. Recognize options 2 and 3 are associated with protein and fats to eliminate them. **Reference:** Rolfes, S., Pinna, K. & Whitney, E. (2006). *Understanding normal and clinical nutrition* (7th ed.) Belmont, CA: Wadsworth & Thomson Learning, pp. 47–49.

7 **Answer: 2** Pinto beans and rice are examples of the use of complementary protein because this combines two different food items to yield a complete protein source. All of the other options do not combine to make a complete protein source. A complete protein source provides all of the essential amino acids and is of high biologic quality and value.

Cognitive Level: Analysis **Client Need:** Health Promotion and Maintenance **Integrated Process:** Nursing Process: Evaluation **Content Area:** Foundational Sciences: Nutrition **Strategy:** Recall knowledge of combining plant proteins to attain a complete protein. Eliminate options 1, 3, and 4 since they include meat proteins. **Reference:** Rolfes, S., Pinna, K. & Whitney, E. (2006). *Understanding normal and clinical nutrition* (7th ed.). Belmont, CA: Wadsworth & Thomson Learning, pp. 85, 91–93.

8 **Answer: 3** High intake of sugars (CHOs) is associated with dental caries and progression of dental disease. By limiting the intake of soft drinks in the diet, one is reducing the daily CHO content. Hard candies are mainly composed of sugar and will contribute to dental disease, because they increase the sugar medium in the oral cavity (option 1). Even air-popped popcorn can easily become lodged between the teeth, leading to food's remaining in the oral cavity and bacterial progression (option 2). Option 4 is incorrect because rinsing of the mouth after eating candy will not effectively remove the extra sugar that the candy provided. Brushing and flossing the teeth would prove to be a better option because this would remove food remnants.

Cognitive Level: Application **Client Need:** Health Promotion and Maintenance **Integrated Process:** Nursing Process: Planning **Content Area:** Foundational Sciences: Nutrition **Strategy:** Note the critical word *best,* indicating one option is a better choice. Consider the residual effect of candy, soda and popcorn residue on teeth to eliminate options 1, 2, and 4. **Reference:** Rolfes, S., Pinna, K. & Whitney, E. (2006). *Understanding normal and clinical nutrition* (7th ed.). Belmont, CA: Wadsworth & Thomson Learning, pp. 38–39.

9 **Answer: 3** Olestra blocks absorption of fat in the diet, sometimes causing abdominal cramping and loose stools. It is not associated with the symptoms in options 1, 2, and 4.

Cognitive Level: Application **Client Need:** Physiological Integrity: Physiological Adaptation **Integrated Process:** Nursing Process: Assessment **Content Area:** Foundational Sciences: Nutrition **Strategy:** Recall knowledge of the function of Olestra to block fat. Note options 1, 2, and 4 all are similar in relating to the neurovascular status. Blockage of fat would occur in the intestines, providing a clue to the abdominal cramping. **Reference:** Rolfes, S., Pinna, K. & Whitney, E. (2006). *Understanding normal and clinical nutrition* (7th ed.). Belmont, CA: Wadsworth & Thomson Learning, pp. 71–73.

10 **Answers: 1, 2, 3** The degree of unsaturation is in the firmness of fats at room temperature. The polyunsaturated vegetable oils are liquid; therefore the more saturated animal fats are solid. Options 1 and 2 are solid and should be avoided. Option 3 should also be avoided because even though coconut oil is oil, not all oils of vegetable origin are polyunsaturated.

Cognitive Level: Application **Client Need:** Health Promotion and Maintenance **Integrated Process:** Teaching and Learning **Strategy:** The critical word "avoid" in the question stem tells you that the correct answer(s) will be items that are incorrect to use when trying to lower fat content in the diet. **Content Area:** Foundational Sciences: Nutrition **Reference:** Rolfes, S., Pinna, K. & Whitney, E. (2006). *Understanding normal and clinical nutrition* (7th ed.). Belmont, CA: Wadsworth & Thomson Learning, pp. 38–39.

References

Cataldo, C., DeBruyne, L. K., & Whitney, E. (2006). *Nutrition and diet therapy* (7th ed.). Belmont, CA: Wadsworth, pp. 31–89.

Dudek, S. G. (2006). *Nutrition essentials for nursing practice* (5th ed.). Philadelphia: Lippincott, pp. 20–91.

Kozier, B., Erb, G., Berman, A. J., & Burke, K. (2004). *Fundamentals of nursing: Concepts, process, and practice* (7th ed.). Upper Saddle River, NJ: Prentice Hall, pp. 1116–1118.

LeMone, P., & Burke, K. (2004). *Medical-surgical nursing: Critical thinking in client care* (3rd ed.). Upper Saddle River, NJ: Prentice Hall, pp. 427–429.

Lutz, C., & Przytulski, K. (2006). *Nutrition and diet therapy* (4th ed.). Philadelphia: F. A. Davis, pp. 35–73.

National Heart, Lung, & Blood Institute Web site. National Cholesterol Education Program, http://www.nhlbi.nih.gov/guidelines/cholesterol/index.htm, accessed 10/1/05.

Nix, S. (2005). *Williams' basic nutrition & diet therapy* (12th ed.). St. Louis, MO: Elsevier, pp. 15–53.

Rolfes, S., Pinna, K., & Whitney, E. (2006). *Understanding normal and clinical nutrition* (7th ed.). Belmont, CA: Wadsworth & Thomson Learning, pp. 108–213.

Micronutrients

3

Chapter Outline

Micronutrients
Water-Soluble Vitamins
Fat-Soluble Vitamins
Water
Major Minerals
Trace Elements

Objectives

- Identify the physiological functions of micronutrients (vitamins, minerals, and trace elements).
- Describe the importance of each group of micronutrients in maintaining homeostasis.
- Identify food sources for each group of micronutrients.
- Identify intake recommendations for each group of micronutrients.
- Describe the potential impact of micronutrient excess or deficiency and the effect on clients.
- Explain therapeutic treatments to correct deficiency states.

NCLEX-RN® Test Prep

Use the CD-ROM enclosed with this book to access additional practice opportunities.

PRETEST

Review at a Glance

alpha fetoprotein (AFP) a protein substance produced by the body that is used as a biochemical marker to denote possible malignancies and neural tube defects

antioxidant a chemical substance that prevents the attachment of oxygen molecules that can cause damage to cell membranes

bioavailability a term that denotes the usable portion of a nutrient or substance that can be absorbed and/or utilized in the body

deficiency state a state in which an essential nutrient (or nutrients) is lacking or diminished as a result of altered metabolism or increased requirements that lead to attributable clinical manifestations

enriched a term that indicates nutrients are added to a food product in amounts that may be even higher than original levels to compensate for nutrient loss during processing

excess state a state in which increased levels of essential nutrient (or nutrients) are found in the body due to altered metabolism or increased usage that leads to attributable clinical manifestations

fat-soluble vitamins vitamins A, D, E, and K that can be dissolved in fat substances

fortification the addition of nutrients to a food product that are not otherwise seen in the original food item

heme absorbable form of iron found in animal products

megaloblastic anemia an anemia that presents with large (macrocytic) red blood cells circulating in the body, leading to decreased hemoglobin capacity and specific clinical manifestations

micronutrient a vitamin or mineral that is needed by the body in small amounts

nonheme a form of iron that is poorly absorbed in the body and is found in plant and animal products

nutritional anemia a term for a group of anemias that are characterized by clinical nutritional deficiencies that result in specific symptoms; correction with the proper nutrient leads to resolution of symptoms; treatment may be short-term (acute) or long-term (chronic) depending on etiology of deficiency

overload syndromes a group of clinical states that are characterized by overproduction, underexcretion, or overuse of various nutrients that lead to profound metabolic disturbances with attributable symptoms

oxalates a group of compounds found in certain food products such as spinach and other green leafy vegetables that act as binders in the body and affect absorption of certain nutrients, leading to decreased bioavailability

pernicious anemia a type of nutritional anemia that is due to a clinical deficiency of vitamin B_{12} as a result of the loss of intrinsic factor; gastric surgery can lead to development of this anemia state that may then require life-long therapy to treat clinical symptoms

phytates a group of compounds found in certain food products such as grains and seeds that act as binders in the body and affect absorption of certain nutrients, leading to decreased bioavailability

pica the craving and ingestion of nonfood substances such as ice, clay, and dirt, often the first indicator that an iron deficiency anemia is present

precursor a substance that is in an inactive form that requires modification to change into the active form

trace elements minerals (elements) that are required by the body in very small amounts and are also found in the body in very small amounts

water-soluble vitamins vitamin C and B-complex vitamins that can be dissolved in water solutions

PRETEST

1 The nurse encourages a client with macrocytic nutritional anemia to increase intake of which of the following micronutrients?

1. Calcium
2. Vitamin B_{12}
3. Iron
4. Vitamin B_1

2 The nurse tells the mother of a newborn infant who received an injection of phytonadione (AquaMephyton) in the delivery room that this injection is the same as vitamin K, which will prevent development of which clinical condition?

1. Hemorrhagic disease of the newborn
2. Hepatitis B
3. Skin infections in the newborn
4. Dehydration

3 While obtaining a stool specimen for a guaiac test, the nurse discovers that the client has been taking large doses of vitamin C for the past several days. The nurse considers which of the following information when deciding what action to take?

1. There will be no effect on the test results.
2. The test may show in a false positive result.
3. The test may show in a false negative result.
4. The test results will be open to interpretation.

4 A child presents with bowed legs and a pigeon breast on physical examination. The nurse suspects these deformities to be caused by a deficiency of which of the following nutrients?

1. Vitamin A
2. Vitamin D
3. Folic acid
4. Phosphorus

5 The nurse concludes that a client has an adequate understanding of potassium-rich foods when the client makes which of the following selections from a luncheon menu?

1. Baked potato topped with broccoli and cheese
2. Grilled cheese sandwich and pretzels
3. Pasta salad and roll
4. A bagel with cream cheese and dill pickle

6 Which nutrient deficiencies might the nurse expect to see in the client who reports eating a large number of whole grain products in the diet?

1. Calcium, zinc, iron, and magnesium
2. Calcium and phosphorus
3. Calcium, vitamin D, and phosphorus
4. Sodium and chloride

7 A client diagnosed with anemia who is being treated with iron replacement therapy is not responding to clinical treatment and reports tingling and paresthesias of the extremities. The nurse questions the client to determine if the client:

1. Is compliant with iron replacement therapy.
2. Has an underlying medical condition of diabetes that is complicating the course of treatment.
3. May also have a vitamin B_{12} deficiency that may account for presentation of neuropathy symptoms.
4. May be taking vitamin C supplements that may account for presentation of neuropathy symptoms.

8 Which of the following symptoms, if seen in a client who takes large doses of over-the-counter niacin to treat high cholesterol, would be of most concern to the nurse?

1. Warmth and flushing of the skin
2. Heartburn and abdominal fullness
3. Dryness of the mouth
4. Occasional diarrhea

9 The nurse is assessing the dietary intake of a client with a biotin deficiency. The nurse identifies that the frequent intake of which of the following foods may have contributed to the deficiency?

1. Raw eggs
2. Liver
3. Dark green vegetables
4. Citrus fruits

10 The nurse is instructing a client who has been started on iron supplements. In order to increase absorption of the iron, the nurse suggests the client take them with which of the following?

1. Milk
2. Orange juice
3. Green leafy vegetables
4. A full glass of water

See pages 79–81 for Answers and Rationales.

I. MICRONUTRIENTS

A. Definition

1. Small molecule groups that are needed by the body to maintain normal physiologic functioning
2. Micronutrients can be further subdivided into major minerals and minor minerals (or **trace elements**)

3. Vitamins are also included in this category and can be further subdivided into **water-soluble** and **fat-soluble vitamins**

B. **Concept properties**

! 1. **Bioavailability** refers to the amount of a nutrient that the body can use that is of good quality
   a. Factors leading to increased bioavailability are efficiency of digestion, adequate nutrition status, and quality of nutrient absorbed
   b. Factors leading to decreased availability are source of nutrient, method of food preparation, and whether other foods that interfere with absorption (binders) are taken at the same time
   c. Refer to Table 3-1 for a listing of factors that influence the bioavailability of vitamins and minerals in the body

Table 3-1

Factors That Influence the Bioavailability of Vitamins and Minerals in the Body

Vitamin/Mineral	Increased Availability	Decreased Availability
Thiamin	Enrichment/fortification	ETOH, antithiamin factors, heat and oxygen
Riboflavin		Light sensitive, medications*
Niacin	Tryptophan, enrichment	Corn, medications*
Biotin	Cooking of eggs denatures the protein avidin	Avidin (protein found in raw eggs), PCM, TPN, tube feedings, heat, acid-base
Panthothenic acid		ETOH, heat, acid/base
Vitamin B_6	Fortification	Processing, heat and light, medications* (act as vitamin antagonists)
Folic acid	Enrichment/fortification, synthetic form	Natural form, heat, light, air, and medications*
Vitamin B_{12}	Fortification	Absence of intrinsic factor, heat, light, air, microwave, medications, low stomach acid, and lack of or diseased ileum
Vitamin C		Oxygen, light, heat, and medications*
Vitamin A	Fortification, active form (provitamin A activity)	Heat and malabsorption states
Vitamin D	Fortification, active form (metabolite), increased Ca	Heat, malabsorption states, and medications*
Vitamin E		Oxygen, metal, light, cooking process, storage, heat, malabsorption states, and medications*
Vitamin K	Active forms (phylloquinones and menaquinones)	Malabsorption states and medications*
Sodium		FEAB imbalance and medications*
Potassium	Medications*	Licorice (glyceric acid), medications* and cooking in water
Calcium	Fortification, lactose, acid, and antacids	Oxalates, phytates, high fiber, milk-alkali syndrome, and medications*

Table 3-1 (*cont.*)

Vitamin/Mineral	Increased Availability	Decreased Availability
Magnesium	Active form of vitamin D	Increased calcium, fat, phosphorus, and medications*
Phosphorus	Food additives, vitamin D, and medications*	
Iron	MFP, vitamin C, ferrous form, heme sources, ETOH, increased calcium, and hemochromatosis	Increased consumption of dairy products, oxalates, phytates, tannins, and increased Cu, Zn, and Mn
Iodine	Fortification	Goitrogens
Copper		Increased Zn, Fe, Ca, Mn, phytates, alkaline, and medications*
Zinc		Increased Fe, Ca, folate, phytates, oxalates, and fiber act as chelating agents, and caffeine

*Medications—Refer to specific nutrients in text for a partial listing of medications.

2. **Precursors** refer to "inactive forms" or starting points from which other substances develop
3. Organic nature and inorganic nature are descriptions about whether micronutrients can be altered or destroyed during the handling or preparation process as a result of their chemical composition
4. ! Solubility refers to the degree to which a substance can dissolve in a water or fat medium
   a. ! Fat-soluble vitamins—A, D, E, and K
   b. Water-soluble vitamins—B complex and C
   c. Carbohydrate (CHO) and protein molecules are water soluble
   d. Lipids are insoluble in water
5. Toxicity refers to an excess of a substance that can cause harm or damage due to accumulation in the body
   a. Serum levels of minerals and vitamins may or may not reflect body stores of the nutrient
   b. Dietary Reference Intake (DRI) has set Tolerable Upper Intake Levels on certain micronutrients
6. Genetic errors in metabolism are processes whereby there is insufficient production, absorption, or excretion of substances resulting in clinical **deficiency states** (too little) or **excess states** (too much)
7. See Box 3-1 for concerns about meeting micronutrient needs

Practice to Pass

Explain how the concept of bioavailability affects the utilization of micronutrients in the body.

II. WATER-SOLUBLE VITAMINS

A. B vitamin complex

1. Functions as coenzymes throughout the body in a series of chemical reactions and binding sites
2. Involved in metabolism of all macronutrients (CHO, lipids, and protein)

Box 3-1

Concerns for Clients' Meeting Micronutrient Needs

- Focus should be on eating a healthy, balanced diet that includes adequate food sources of all micronutrients.
- Referral to a dietitian may be needed if clinical deficiency occurs or if client has contributory disease processes that may interfere with absorption and metabolism of nutrients.
- Client education may be required to advise of dietary factors and medication profiles that may lead to altered absorption states.
- Accurate history and review of systems may yield data about nutritional alterations that may be corrected with adequate sources of micronutrients in the diet.
- It is important to note that many B vitamin deficiencies occur together and the client should be assessed for multiple deficiencies and treated accordingly to restore balance.
- Focus on client education to maintain homeostasis in the body by meeting nutritional needs and staying within RDA guidelines to prevent both deficiency and toxicity states.
- Focus on client education so that client is aware of nutritional terms such as enrichment and fortification of food sources so that dietary choices are logically supported.

! **3.** See Table 3-2 for a summary of the role, food sources, and deficiency or excess states of B vitamins

B. Vitamin B_1–thiamin

1. Role and function in the body

a. Coenzyme in CHO metabolism

b. Vitamin part of coenzyme TPP (thiamin pyrophosphate—pyruvate) to acetyl-coA in TCA cycle

2. Dietary sources

a. Pork, wheat germ, and black-eyed peas

b. Fortified (**fortification**—adding nutrients to a food item) cereals and **enriched** (replacing nutrients lost during processing) grains

c. Handling and preparation losses can occur during grain processing or during heating process

d. Ingestion of foods containing antithiamin factors (certain fish, tea, coffee, blueberries, and cabbage) in large quantities can decrease absorption and lead to deficiency symptoms

3. Recommendations in the diet

a. RDA for adult male is 1.2 mg/day

b. RDA for adult female is 1.1 mg/day

c. There are increased needs in growth states (pregnancy and lactation) and for athletes

! **4.** Deficiency states

a. Beriberi is a clinical deficiency state that presents with neurological deficits (disorientation, short-term memory loss, jerky eye movements, staggered gait, and weakness) that can lead to cardiac failure; it can be further subdivided in to dry and wet types

b. Dry beriberi causes CNS presentations (paralysis and muscle wasting)

Table 3-2
B Complex Vitamins

Vitamin	Role/function	Food Sources	Deficiency	Excess
Thiamin (B_1)	Coenzyme	Pork, wheat germ, and fortified cereals	Beriberi Wernicke-Korsakoff syndrome	
Riboflavin (B_2)	Coenzyme	Milk and enriched grains	Ariboflavinosis Cheilosis Magenta tongue	
Niacin (B_3)	Coenzyme	Peanuts, legumes, and enriched grains	Pellagra (3 Ds = dermatitis, diarrhea, and dementia)	Flushing Abnormalities in blood glucose level and liver function
Pantothenic acid (B_5)	Coenzyme	Meat and whole grains	Rash and fatigue	
Pyridoxine (B_6)	Coenzyme	Pork, organ meats, whole grains, and wheat germ	Nutritional anemia Dermatitis Altered nerve function	Sensory neuropathy
Cobalamin (B_{12})	Coenzyme	Animal protein	Pernicious anemia, dementia	Masks vitamin B deficiency
Folic Acid	Coenzyme	Orange juice, meat, and leafy green vegetables	Nutritional anemia Neural tube defects Hyperhomo-cysteinemia	
Biotin	Coenzyme	Egg yolks and liver	Dermatitis Hair loss Loss of appetite Depression Glossitis	

The importance of B complex vitamins in the body is that they participate in a large number of reactions as co-enzymes that are necessary for metabolism of essential and nonessential nutrients and production of energy.

   c. Wet beriberi affects cardiac function (tachycardia and edema)
   d. Wernicke-Korsakoff syndrome is a clinical state of encephalopathy seen in clients with alcoholism, noted by the presence of mental changes, psychosis, and coma

5. Excess is excreted in urine, so nontoxic

6. Therapeutic treatment

   a. In reported clinical deficiency states, the addition of thiamin in the diet or in a supplement form is beneficial
   b. With an at-risk population group such as those with alcoholism, it is important to resolve the underlying nutritional problems in order to maintain adequate absorption of nutrients
   c. Thiamin preparations are available for use in PO (enteric coated), IM, and IV routes
   d. Dosages vary depending on use as a dietary supplement, to replace deficiency, or to provide clinical treatment of beriberi; refer to drug text for specific dosing requirements based on clinical indication and client age groups

C. Vitamin B_2–riboflavin

1. Roles and function in the body
   a. Coenzyme in protein and energy metabolism, and conversion of other vitamins into active forms (B_6, niacin, folate, and K) by direct or indirect methods
   b. Coenzyme forms are FMN (flavin mononucleotide) and FAD (flavin adenine dinucleotide)
   c. Thyroid adrenal hormone controls the conversion to the coenzyme forms
2. Dietary sources
   a. Organ meats, milk, legumes, and vegetables
   b. Found in whole or enriched grain products
   c. Handling and preparation losses occur because of light sensitivity; most products are packaged in cardboard or other opaque containers to minimize losses
3. Recommendations in the diet
   a. RDA for adult male is 1.3 mg/day
   b. RDA for adult female is 1.1 mg/day
   c. Increased needs are seen in growth states (pregnancy and lactation) and major body healing that coincide with increased protein needs of the body
4. Deficiency states (!)
   a. Ariboflavinosis (can occur with loss of other B vitamins—B_1 and B_3) refers to a clinical deficiency state that affects the skin, eyes, mouth, and tongue and results in the development of a normocytic anemia
   b. Oral lesions such as cheilosis (cracks at the corners of the mouth) and eye problems (such as photophobia, tearing, and burning) are seen with this deficiency state
   c. Drug interactions are seen with chlorpromazine (Thorazine), imipramine (Tofranil), and amitriptyline (Elavil); these drugs can interfere with conversion of this vitamin to its active coenzyme form
5. (!) Excess is excreted in urine, so it is nontoxic; may see yellow-orange urine
6. Therapeutic treatment
   a. Can be given PO
   b. Usually there are also other B vitamin deficiencies and therefore additional or combination vitamin therapy may be warranted by the oral or parenteral route
   c. The dosage needed to treat clinical deficiency is 5–10 mg/day orally

D. Vitamin B_3–niacin

1. Roles and function in the body
   a. Functions as part of respiratory enzymes and is involved in energy expenditure
   b. Nicotinic acid (major form in the body) and nicotinamide help make the active coenzymes NAD (nicotinamine adenine dinucleotide) and NADP (nicotinamine adenine dinucleotide phosphate)
   c. (!) Precursor to niacin is the amino acid tryptophan (60 mg of dietary tryptophan = 1 mg of niacin)
   d. Niacin has cholesterol-lowering properties and causes peripheral vasodilation
2. Dietary sources
   a. Found in meat, peanuts, legumes, and coffee

b. The inclusion of large amounts of corn in the diet interferes with the dietary conversion of tryptophan to niacin (corn is high in the amino acid leucine, which interferes with tryptophan conversion)

3. Recommendations in the diet
   a. Male daily requirement is 16 NE (niacin equivalents)
   b. Female daily requirement is 14 NE (niacin equivalents)
   c. There are increased requirements in growth states (pregnancy and lactation)

! 4. Deficiency states
   a. Pellagra is the clinical deficiency state that is characterized by the three Ds: dermatitis, diarrhea, and dementia
   b. Drug interactions are seen with isoniazid (INH) and hydralazine (Apresoline) that can lead to clinical deficiency states
   c. Carcinoid syndrome can exist when serum blood tryptophan levels are low due to increased serotonin synthesis from tumors; this leads to symptoms similar to pellagra
   d. Hartnup disease is a rare genetic disorder that is characterized by decreased absorption of tryptophan that causes symptoms similar to those of pellagra

! 5. Excess states
   a. Increased histamine levels are associated with increased doses of nicotinic acid (leads to skin flushing)
   b. Increased uric acid levels can occur as excess niacin competes for renal excretion
   c. Peptic ulcer disease (PUD) can be aggravated from large doses of niacin due to gastrointestinal distress
   d. Large doses may cause liver damage and gout

6. Therapeutic treatment
   a. Medication is available in PO (extended release, capsules, and elixir), IM, and IV forms
   ! b. Initial cholesterol lowering dose is 1 gram TID and maintenance dose ranges from 1–2 grams TID
   c. Vitamin dosage ranges from up to 300 mg/day for pediatric clients to up to 500 mg/day for adults
   d. Refer to drug text for specific dosages related to treatment of pellagra
   e. Dosages in the range of 100–300 mg/day can be used to treat neuropathies by increasing peripheral vasodilation
   ! f. Clients who have diabetes mellitus should be monitored closely when taking niacin products for potential hyperglycemic reactions

E. Biotin

1. Roles and function in the body
   a. Coenzyme in metabolism that functions in the tricarboxylic (TCA) cycle for release of energy
   b. Involved in gluconeogenesis (synthesis of fatty acids, amino acids, and purines)

2. Dietary sources
   a. Found in liver, kidney, meat, tomatoes, and egg yolk
   b. Avidin is a protein found in raw egg whites that binds biotin and prevents it from being absorbed

c. Handling and preparation losses are seen with heat

3. Recommendations in the diet
   a. AI (allowable intake) of 30 mcg/day for both male and female clients
   b. No RDA has been established for this vitamin
4. Deficiency states
   a. Typically rare in humans unless large number of raw egg whites are consumed in the diet
   b. Phenylketonuria (PKU) leads to a functional biotin deficiency because high phenylalanine levels inhibit enzyme activity
   c. Complications of long-term total parenteral nutrition (TPN) therapy can result in a deficiency if biotin is not included in the TPN solution
   d. Deficiency can occur in clients with protein-energy malnutrition (PEM)
   e. Clinical signs of biotin deficiency are nausea, thinning hair, hair loss, and depression
   f. Biotindase deficiency is a genetic disorder (autosomal recessive) that leads to a clinical deficiency state resulting in delayed development, seizures, and rashes; it can prove fatal without biotin correction
5. Excess states
   a. No toxic effects have been reported in the clinical setting
   b. No UL (upper limit) has been indicated
6. Therapeutic treatment
   a. 200–1,000 mcg can be given daily to reverse clinical symptoms of deficiency
   b. ! Cook eggs and limit the number of raw eggs in the diet to minimize risk exposure to avidin
   c. Make sure biotin is included in tube feedings and total parenteral nutrition (TPN) solutions

F. Vitamin B_5–panthothenic acid

1. Roles and function in the body
   a. Coenzyme in the formation of coenzyme A (important factor in the TCA cycle)
   b. Involved in fat, cholesterol, and **heme** (iron-containing portion of hemoglobin molecule) formation and amino acid activation
2. Dietary sources
   a. Found in whole grain cereals and legumes
   b. Widely found in animal tissues
   c. Handling and preparation losses are seen with heat and acid conditions
3. Recommendations in the diet
   a. There is no established RDA for this vitamin
   b. AI (allowable intake) is 5 mg/day for both male and female clients
4. Deficiency states
   a. Fatigue, paresthesias, weakness, and leg cramps can occur with clinical deficiency
   b. Neurological manifestations, such as restlessness and irritability, along with endocrine manifestations such as hypoglycemia can occur

c. "Burning feet syndrome" seen in malnourished clients may be a result of clinical deficiency

5. Excess states

a. Diarrhea can occur with excess levels of this vitamin

b. Fluid retention can occur with excess levels of this vitamin

6. Therapeutic treatment for clinical deficiency symptoms is a dosage of 10 mg/day PO

G. Vitamin B_6–pyridoxine

1. Roles and function in the body

a. Coenzyme in amino acid, lipid, and protein metabolism (gluconeogenesis); erythrocyte function; modulation of hormones; nervous system function; and direct conversion of tryptophan to niacin or to serotonin

b. There are three naturally occurring compounds comprising pyridines (pyridoxine, pyridoxal, and pyridoxamine)

c. It is also made by intestinal bacteria in the body

2. Dietary sources

a. Found in pork, organ meat, whole grains, wheat germ, and fortified cereals

b. Handling and preparation losses are seen with heat and storage (has a low bioavailability)

3. Recommendations in the diet

a. RDA for male and female clients up to age 50 is 1.3 mg/day

b. RDA for male clients above age 50 is 1.7 mg/day

c. RDA for female clients above age 50 is 1.5 mg/day

d. Increased intake is needed during growth states (pregnancy and lactation)

! 4. Deficiency states

a. Increased losses are seen in clients taking oral contraceptives (could possibly be due to increased estrogen levels), vitamin antagonists, and in clients with alcoholism

b. Drug interactions are seen with isoniazid (INH), hydralazine (Apresoline), dopamine (Intropin), and penicillamine (Depen) because they act as vitamin antagonists and form inactive compounds in the body

c. Can impair immune function in the elderly client due to its effect on protein metabolism (lymphocyte proliferation and interleukin production), which leads to decreased antibody formation

d. Peripheral neuropathy can be seen due to vitamin B_6 effect in neurotransmitter synthesis

e. Low vitamin B_6 levels are associated with an increase in serum homocysteine level that is associated with vascular atherosclerotic disease

f. Clinical deficiency symptoms manifest as neurological deficits (depression, confusion, headache, fatigue, and nerve damage to possible convulsions and abnormal brain activity), dermatologic lesions (scaly dermatitis), and microcytic anemia

g. Clinical deficiency states usually exist in the presence of deficiency of other B vitamins (Vitamin B_{12} and folic acid)

5. Excess states

a. Imposed peripheral neuropathy in high doses (2–6 grams/day)

b. UL (upper limit) of 100 mg per day to prevent nerve impairment symptoms

! **6.** Therapeutic treatment

a. Prophylactic use with isoniazid (INH) to prevent peripheral neuropathy due to vitamin antagonist effect of medication

b. Can be used in the treatment of depression and diabetic neuropathy

c. Vitamin B_6 supplements suggested usage includes beneficial effects on cardiac disease, carpal tunnel syndrome, premenstrual syndrome (PMS), proper immune function, and morning sickness

H. Folic acid or folate

1. Roles and function in the body

a. Folic acid is used in the synthesis of DNA (2/3 of plasma folate is protein bound) and it also helps to convert vitamin B_{12} to a coenzyme form in the body

b. Needed for growth and development of RBCs

c. Generic term for compounds is PGA (pteroylglutamic acid)

d. Folic acid helps to lower homocysteine levels in the body by breaking down amino acids

! **e.** Increased need is seen during the pre-pregnancy and antenatal periods for its effect on preventing neural tube defects by allowing normal spinal cord development

f. Folic acid in the body goes through the enterohepatic circulation (liver secretion to bile then reabsorbed in the intestine) to be regulated

g. Vitamin C (ascorbic acid) enhances folic acid conversion in the body

2. Dietary sources

a. Found in orange juice, liver, green leafy vegetables, and fruit

b. Enriched breads and cereals with fortification lead to improved bioavailability

c. Handling and preparation losses are seen with exposure to heat and light and can account for a loss of up to 50% of this vitamin

d. There are natural and synthetic forms of folic acid in food products and supplements that reflect the variation in bioavailability; these are used in calculating RDA requirements

3. Recommendations in the diet

a. RDA for male and female clients is 400 mcg/day that is measured in DFEs—dietary folate equivalents

b. Synthetic forms of this vitamin are absorbed at a higher rate than the natural form (1.7 times) due to a higher bioavailability

c. An equation that can be used to calculate conversion of DFE is mcg of food folate + (1.7 × mcg synthetic folate), which will provide an accurate folate level measurement

! **d.** Increased folic acid is needed (up to 400 mcg/day) during pregnancy and lactation

! **4.** Deficiency states

a. Neural tube defects are associated with folic acid deficiency in pregnant women and result in spinal deformities of the fetus

b. **Nutritional anemia: megaloblastic anemia** (large immature cells with a decreased oxygen-carrying capacity) can occur as a result of impaired DNA synthesis

Box 3-2

Listing of Drug Interactions with Folic Acid

- Aminosalicylic acid (ASA), phenytoin (Dilantin), sulfonamides, triamterene (Dyrenium), and trimethoprim (Bactrim) lead to decreased absorption of folic acid.
- Corticosteroids lead to increased folic acid requirements that can result in clinical deficiency if not corrected.
- Certain medications act as folic acid antagonists in the body (methotrexate [Rheumatrex], pyrimethamine, triamterene [Dyrenium], and trimethoprim [Bactrim]) leading to decreased absorption and clinical deficiency if not corrected.
- Folic acid can increase the risk of seizures in clients taking phenytoin (Dilantin).

c. There are numerous drug interactions seen with folic acid that lead to clinical deficiency because many drugs act as folate antagonists in the body in the treatment of cancers (see Box 3-2 for a listing of drug interactions)

d. Malabsorptive states seen in celiac disease (nontropical sprue), Crohn's disease, ulcerative colitis, and in clients with alcoholism lead to a deficiency state (remember that normal functioning of the GI tract is essential for absorption of folic acid in the body)

e. Low folate levels are associated with increased risk of cancer because this affects the development of epithelial cells of the body; grain products fortified with folate may decrease risk of heart disease

f. **Alpha-fetoprotein (AFP)** is used as a biochemical marker for both the correlation of the presence of neural tube defects and certain cancers in the body

g. Clinical deficiency states usually exist in the presence of other B vitamin deficiencies (vitamin B_6 and vitamin B_{12})

5. Excess states

a. Drug interactions with phenytoin (Dilantin) because of competition for binding sites can result in convulsions

b. UL (upper limit) is 1,000 mcg/day

c. Excess folate can mask vitamin B_{12} deficiency

6. Therapeutic treatment

a. Clients with malabsorption problems may have to take folic acid via IM, SubQ, or IV route (dosage 0.1 mg/day)

b. Correction with folic acid may only improve hematologic signs but not the underlying neurological manifestations associated with concurrent vitamin B_{12} deficiency

c. Folic acid can cause urine to turn a deep yellow color

d. Normally included in prenatal vitamins as mandated by the FDA (400 mcg/day)

I. Vitamin B_{12}–cobalamin or cyanocobalamin

1. Roles and function in the body

a. Coenzyme in the synthesis of hemoglobin, RBCs, and DNA

! **b.** Intrinsic factor and extrinsic factor

1) Intrinsic factor is secreted by the parietal cells in the stomach that allows the vitamin to be absorbed into the intestine

2) Extrinsic factor is vitamin B_{12} itself

2. Dietary sources
    a. Found in animal sources such as eggs, milk, meat, cheese, and in fortified cereals
    b. Vegetarians need fortified sources
    c. Handling and preparation losses are seen with heat, light, and air; microwave heating has been shown to inactivate this vitamin
3. Recommendations in the diet
    a. RDA for male and female clients is 2.4 mcg/day
    b. Increased needs are seen in growth states (pregnancy and lactation), renal and liver disease, hemorrhage, malignancy, and hyperthyroidism

!

4. Deficiency states
    a. Nutritional anemia: **pernicious anemia** (megaloblastic macrocytic normochromic) due to deficiency of intrinsic factor; can also be seen in response to the development of atrophic gastritis in the older adult client that leads to cell damage in the stomach (loss of intrinsic factor and HCl secretion)
    b. Disease states such as human immunodeficiency virus (HIV) and multiple myeloma are associated with low levels of vitamin B_{12}
    c. Strict vegetarian diets (without supplements/fortification) are associated with increased risk of clinical deficiency
    d. Gastric surgery (whereby parts of the stomach have been removed) is associated with clinical deficiency and may require lifelong parenteral vitamin B_{12} replacement therapy
    e. Symptoms associated with clinical deficiency include smooth beefy red tongue, fatigue, weakness, numbness, tingling, neurological abnormalities resulting in neuropathy, and dementia
    f. Elevated levels of homocysteine are seen with low levels of vitamin B_{12}
    g. Concurrent clinical deficiencies of other B vitamins can also be seen (vitamin B_6 and folic acid)
    h. Proximal ileostomies or lack of ileum can cause deficiency because vitamin B_{12} is absorbed in the ileum
5. Excess states
    a. High levels can be associated with acute liver disease
    b. High levels can be seen with leukocytosis because the serum-binding capacity of the vitamin is increased
6. Therapeutic treatment

!

    a. Injection therapy ranging from once a day to once a month (lifelong) depending on clinical indication (pernicious anemia–gastric surgery); refer to drug text for specific indications and dosages
    b. Oral form supplements can be used to support those with vegetarian diet preferences
    c. Side effects of injection therapy are pain and burning at the injection site; parenteral injections must be given deep IM and site rotation must be done to avoid skin sensitivities; a nasal form is now available
    d. Other B vitamin deficiencies may occur concurrently and may require drug therapy
    e. Numerous drugs can affect clients taking vitamin B_{12} therapy, leading to decreased absorption levels (chloramphenicol, cholestyramine [Questran], cimeti-

Table 3-3

	Vitamin	Role/function	Food Sources	Deficiency	Excess
Vitamin C	Ascorbic acid	Antioxidant Wound healing Hormone synthesis	Citrus fruits Green vegetables Potatoes	Scurvy Bleeding gums Perifollicular hemorrhage	GI distress Hot flashes Rashes Headache

Vitamin C assists in the conversion of folic acid and the absorption of iron in the body. Vitamin C helps with adrenal gland function and is involved with collagen synthesis.

dine [Tagamet], colchicine, neomycin, and potassium-released products); clients should be evaluated for potential drug interactions that could affect therapy and limit absorption

f. Schilling test (24-hour urine with radioisotope injection) can be used to check absorption and vitamin B_{12} levels in the body

J. Vitamin C–ascorbic acid

1. Roles and function in the body (see Table 3-3)
   - **a.** Performs an **antioxidant** function (compound that prevents damage caused by oxidation) in the body
   - **b.** Important in the synthesis of neurotransmitters (conversion of tryptophan to serotonin and norepinehrine), hormones (thyroxine), and bile acids; metabolism of amino acids; and the breakdown of fatty acids (carnitine)
   - **c.** Folic acid conversion and iron absorption are enhanced by the presence of vitamin C in the body
   - **d.** Vitamin C is a structural component involved in collagen formation in the body
2. Dietary sources
   - **a.** Found in citrus fruits and green vegetables
   - **b.** Orange juice is an excellent source of vitamin C
   - **c.** Handling and preparation losses are seen with heating and in the presence of air and alkaline solutions
3. Recommendations in the diet
   - **a.** RDA for males is 90 mg/day
   - **b.** RDA for females is 75 mg/day
   - **c.** Increased needs are seen in growth states (pregnancy and lactation), smokers (who need an additional 35 mg/day above the RDA guidelines), and in metabolic conditions in response to oxidative stress

! 4. Deficiency states
   - **a.** Scurvy is the clinical deficiency state that presents with bleeding gums, pinpoint hemorrhages, gingivitis, loosening of teeth, weakness, irritability, and joint pain
   - **b.** Clients with chronic inflammatory diseases and cancers (malignancies) may be prone to vitamin C deficiencies
   - **c.** Mouth presentations (bleeding gums) are one of the earliest symptoms seen with deficiency states
   - **d.** Drug interactions leading to decreased vitamin C levels are seen with the use of over-the-counter (OTC) medications including aspirin (ASA)
   - **e.** Numerous multisystem clinical symptoms can be seen throughout the body, including hematologic (microcytic anemia and pinpoint hemorrhages), oral

(bleeding gums and loose teeth), and altered healing and immune system function

! 5. Excess states

a. Clients with a history of kidney stone formation should not take increased vitamin C because it may precipitate stone formation

b. Clients with iron overload syndromes should not take increased vitamin C because this vitamin enhances iron absorption and can cause further overload

c. Dental erosion or damage to tooth enamel can be a result of excess vitamin C levels found in hidden sources such as food products (syrups and chewable gums)

d. Clients who have a history of clinical gout should not take increased vitamin C because this may predispose to a gouty flare-up

e. Clients who have sickle cell anemia should not take increased vitamin C because this can lead to an exacerbation of sickle cell crisis

f. High levels of vitamin C can result in inaccurate diagnostic test results

1) False positive test results can be seen in urine glucose tests with high levels of vitamin C

2) False negative test results can be seen in stool guaiac tests with high levels of vitamin C

g. Toxicity symptoms seen with high levels of vitamin C include diarrhea, nausea, abdominal cramps, hot flashes, rashes, headache, fatigue, and insomnia

Practice to Pass

What nutritional vitamin deficiencies would you expect to find in a client with alcoholism?

6. Therapeutic treatment

a. Minimum dosage of at least 10 mg/day is needed to prevent clinical symptoms of scurvy

b. Research has been done regarding the effect of vitamin C on the common cold, but no clear recommendations have been supported by the medical community; however, many people use vitamin C supplements as a form of alternative therapy to prevent, treat, and cure the common cold symptoms

III. FAT-SOLUBLE VITAMINS

A. See Table 3-4 for a summary of the role, food sources, and deficiency or excess states of fat-soluble vitamins

B. Vitamin A (and beta carotene)

1. Roles and functions in the body

a. Retinoids (preformed vitamin A compounds) include retinol, retinal, and retonic acid; these are found in animal sources

b. Retinol units/retinol equivalents are a measurement of vitamin A activity

c. Carotenoids (high provitamin A activity) include beta-carotene; they are found in plant sources and function as antioxidants

d. Transport of retinoids and carotenoids is done by chylomicrons in the body; retinoids bind to RBP (retinol binding protein) for specific transport, whereas carotenoids travel by lipoproteins

e. Visual adaptation to light and dark is a function of vitamin A activity

f. Healthy skin (epithelial tissue) and mucous membranes depend, in part, on adequate amounts of vitamin A in the body

Table 3-4

Fat-Soluble Vitamins

Vitamin	Role/function	Food Sources	Deficiency	Excess
A	Vision, bone and tissue growth, immune and reproductive function	Retinol: liver, milk, butter, cream, egg yolk, fortified foods Beta-carotene: green leafy vegetables, broccoli, carrots, peppers, sweet potatoes, peaches, watermelon, apricots	Night blindness, xerophthalmia Skin and mucous membrane problems Increased susceptibility to infection	Toxicity can result; birth defects in pregnancy; liver damage
D	Calcium and phosphorus metabolism, bone growth, along with other vitamins and minerals	Dairy products and fortified food sources, liver, fatty fish	Rickets Osteomalacia	Toxicity can result Kidney stones Calcification of soft tissues Death
E	Antioxidant and immune system function	Vegetable oil, nuts, fortified cereals, and margarine	Hemolysis of RBCs	May interfere with vitamin K activity
K	Blood clotting	Green leafy vegetables, cabbage (also synthesized in intestines)	Hemorrhagic disease of the newborn Hemorrhage	No toxic symptoms have been observed

Fat-soluble vitamins can cause significant damage to body systems in high concentrations (with the exception of vitamin E and vitamin K), therefore intake should be monitored closely to prevent cellular damage and possible teratogenic effects due to exposure.

   g. Vitamin A helps to regulate cell differentiation associated with reproduction (sperm in the male and fetal development in the female) and the immune response

2. Dietary sources
   a. Animal sources provide a rich source of preformed vitamin A–retinol (fish, liver oils, butter, eggs, and milk products that are fortified)
   b. Fruits and vegetables (dark green and deep orange) are good sources of vitamin A–beta-carotene
   c. Handling and preparation losses are seen with heating
3. Recommendations in the diet
   a. RDA for male client is 900 mcg RAE/day
   b. RDA for female client is 700 mcg RAE/day
   c. Vitamin A activity is now measured in retinol activity equivalents or RAE (1 mcg of retinol = 1 RAE and 12 mcg of beta-carotene = 1 RAE)
   d. Nutritional supplements also list vitamin A measurement in terms of international units (IU)

!

4. Deficiency states
   a. Night blindness is a clinical deficiency state due to lack of vitamin A at the back of the eye in the retina; this is the major cause of childhood blindness in the world

b. Xerophthalmia is a clinical deficiency state due to lack of vitamin A at the front of the eye that affects the cornea and can lead to total blindness
c. Keratomalacia is a clinical deficiency state in which softening of the cornea occurs, leading to blindness that is irreversible
d. Keratinization refers to changes in cell structures throughout the body that result in hard, inflexible skin due to secretion of the protein keratin

5. Excess states
a. Excess levels of carotenoids can result in yellowing of skin due to deposition in adipose tissue, which is reversible
! b. Teratogenic effects can occur with ingestion of vitamin A that can lead to fetal organ damage, birth defects, and even miscarriage
c. Increased levels leading to toxicity can be seen if binding proteins are saturated with ingestion of excess vitamin A products
d. Symptoms related to vitamin A toxicity range from headache, vomiting, and weight loss to birth defects, bone abnormalities (increased activation of osteoclasts), and liver damage

6. Therapeutic treatment
a. Beta-carotene is available in supplemental forms to avoid the toxic effects of preformed vitamin A
! b. Accutane and Retin-A are vitamin A derivatives that are used in the treatment of acne and skin aging effects; these medications should be managed under the direction of a dermatologist

C. Vitamin D–calciferol

1. Roles and function in the body
a. Vitamin D metabolites exist in the body and are used to synthesize this vitamin, unlike other vitamins
b. Vitamin D is also involved in the regulation of calcium and phosphorus balance in the body
c. Regulation by the kidney and parathyroid glands helps to maintain vitamin D balance (parathyroid hormone or PTH secretion is seen in response to low serum calcium levels so that the kidneys convert metabolites to active form)
! d. Sunlight activation enables vitamin D synthesis in the skin
e. Vitamin D also works with other vitamins (A, C, and K), hormones, and minerals (calcium, phosphorus, and magnesium) to affect bone growth

2. Dietary sources
a. Found naturally in fish, liver, and oils
b. Fortification (nutrients added to a food) of dairy products such as milk and margarine are seen in the Western diet
c. Handling and preparation losses are seen with heating

3. Recommendations in the diet
a. Depending on client's age, there is range of AI (allowable intake) with 5 mcg/day for male and female adult clients from 19–50 years of age
b. Depending on sun exposure, clients who follow a strict vegetarian diet may require supplementation and fortification to meet vitamin D levels
c. Measurement of vitamin D activity is now calculated in micrograms of cholecalciferol (vitamin D_3) as opposed to the older method that used international units (conversion factor 1 IU = 0.025 mcg cholecalciferol)

! **4.** Deficiency states

a. Rickets is the clinical deficiency state affecting children that results in structural deformities (bowed legs and pigeon breast) due to poor bone mineralization (as a result of decreased calcium) and growth retardation

b. Osteomalacia is the clinical deficiency state affecting adults that results in bone weakness, fragility, and increased bone fractures

c. Vitamin D deficiencies can be seen with clients who have intestinal, liver (cirrhosis), or parathyroid hormone disorders, chronic pancreatitis, renal disorders; also seen in breastfed infants

d. Associated deficiencies states seen with vitamin D include:

1) Tetany and muscle weakness due to hypocalcemia

2) Additionally, decreased levels of magnesium can be seen in clients with alcoholism along with vitamin D deficiency

e. Deficiency of vitamin D can lead to the development of osteoporosis in conjunction with calcium losses

f. Elderly clients are prone to develop Vitamin D deficiency due to limited intake of milk, aging of skin, limitation of outdoor activities, and less effective conversion in the skin

5. Excess states

a. Increased levels of vitamin D are associated with increased levels of calcium that can upset hormone balance and result in endocrine dysfunction

b. Hypervitaminosis D is the clinical excess state that is associated with calcium deposits, growth retardation, and kidney damage; clinical symptoms manifested are loss of appetite, nausea, vomiting, constipation, and death

6. Therapeutic treatment

a. Therapy maybe required for clients with fat malabsorption or chronic steroid use and for postmenopausal females who are at risk for osteoporosis

b. Vitamin D_2 and vitamin D_3 are available for use as dietary supplements and are usually part of multivitamin preparations (dosage ranging from 5 to 10 mcg/day)

c. Vitamin D treatment for clinical deficiency consists of vitamin D_2 (1,250 mcg once a week for 8 weeks)

d. This vitamin is contraindicated in clients who are hypercalcemic

! **e.** Precautions should be taken for clients who are taking cardiac glycosides (Digoxin) and supplemental vitamin D because development of associated hypercalcemia can predispose the client to cardiac arrhythmias (UL for adults is 50 mcg /day)

! **f.** Concurrent use of vitamin D (in therapeutic doses) along with thiazide diuretics can lead to development of hypercalcemia

g. Drug interactions can occur that may limit the absorption of vitamin D; these include cholestyramine (Questran), colestipol (Colestid), ketoconazole (Nizoral), mineral oil, orlistat (Xenical), phenobarbitol, and phenytoin (Dilantin)

D. Vitamin E–tocopherol

1. Roles and function in the body

a. Tocopherol compounds (D and L alpha-tocopherol) have the highest vitamin E activity in the body

b. Vitamin E has antioxidant properties that prevent oxidation of polyunsaturated fats or PUFAs and protect all cell membranes
c. Vitamin E has an immune system function as it protects all cell membranes
d. Vitamin E has an effect on oxygen and blood exchange in the lungs
e. Vitamin E is thought also to have an effect on neurotransmission, but the exact mechanism is not completely understood

2. Dietary sources
a. Found in vegetable oils, salad dressings, wheat germ, oil, and nuts
b. Use of polyunsaturated fats or PUFAs (such as margarine) in the diet can increase need for vitamin E

3. Recommendations in the diet
a. RDA for adult males and females is 15 mg/day
b. Measurement used expresses milligrams of tocopherol equivalents, which is related to vitamin E activity (mg TE)
c. Handling and preparation losses are seen in cooking and oxygenation

! 4. Deficiency states
a. Clinical deficiency results in erythrocyte hemolysis (seen in premature infants because maternal vitamin E is transferred to the fetus during the last weeks of pregnancy), which can lead to the development of hemolytic anemia if not corrected by vitamin E treatment
b. Clinical deficiency can be seen in clients who are immunosuppressed or who have fat malabsorption states such as cystic fibrosis
c. Research findings have raised the possibility of fertility and sterility issues with vitamin E deficiency; however, this has not been proven in humans and may relate only to current animal research studies
d. Prolonged clinical deficiency can result in neurological/muscular symptom development (loss of coordination, reflexes, fatigue, and impaired vision and speech)

5. Excess states
a. High doses of vitamin E may impair absorption of other fat-soluble vitamins
! b. High doses of vitamin E may potentiate anticoagulant effects of sodium warfarin (Coumadin)

6. Therapeutic treatment
a. Correction of hemolytic anemia seen in infants
b. Has been used in the treatment of fibrocystic breast disease (fibrous nonmalignant lumps)
c. Has been used in the treatment of intermittent claudication (calf pain at intervals caused by poor blood supply)
d. Drug interactions can occur that may limit absorption of vitamin E (anticonvulsants, cholestyramine [Questran], colestipol [Colestid], isoniazid [INH], mineral oil, neomycin, orlistat [Xenical], and sulcrafate [Carafate]), potentiate drug–drug effects (antiplatelets and warfarin), or decrease side effects (vitamin E taken with zidovudine decreases myelosuppressive action)

E. Vitamin K

1. Roles and function in the body

a. Vitamin K belongs to a family of compounds called quinones (phylloquinones in plants and menaquinones in animal sources)

b. Vitamin K is involved in the clotting cascade as it is needed for production of prothrombin that is converted to thrombin and for the conversion of fibrinogen to fibrin (active form)

c. Vitamin K affects clotting factors (II, VII, IX, and X) in the liver and is measured by the PT (prothrombin time) in the clinical setting

d. Bacteria in the intestines (menaquinone) synthesize vitamin K; it requires bile acids to effectively function in the body

! e. Newborns require vitamin K injection at birth to stimulate intestinal synthesis to prevent hemorrhagic disease of the newborn (due to the newborn's sterile gut)

! f. Vitamin K acts as an antagonist to the action of sodium warfarin (Coumadin)

2. Dietary sources
   a. Found in green leafy vegetables, cabbage, and milk
   b. Bacterial synthesis in the intestine provides about one-half of the body's needs
3. Recommendations in the diet
   a. AI (allowable intake) levels are 120 mcg/day for adult males
   b. AI levels are 90 mcg/day for adult females

! 4. Deficiency states
   a. Hemorrhagic disease of the newborn reveals a clinical vitamin K deficiency state (failure to clot)
   b. Clients who have liver disease and fat malabsorption are prone to develop clinical deficiency due to decreased bile production that will in turn affect vitamin K absorption
   c. Clients who are on long-term broad-spectrum antibiotics are at risk for clinical deficiency because normal intestinal flora is destroyed, which leads to decreased bacterial synthesis of vitamin K
5. Excess states: no toxic symptoms have been observed

! 6. Therapeutic treatment
   a. Subcutaneous injection of phytonadione (Aqua-Mephyton) is required for all newborns
   b. Vitamin K can be given both pre- and postoperatively to regulate the blood coagulation pathway
   c. PT (prothrombin time) can measure vitamin K action in the clinical setting; these results can be trended along with international normalized ratio (INR) results to evaluate client outcomes when using anticoagulation therapy
   d. Vitamin K is used to reverse the action of warfarin sodium (Coumadin) in the clinical setting
   e. Heparin can be used to reverse the action of vitamin K in the clinical setting
   f. Drug interactions can be seen that decrease absorption (broad-spectrum antibiotics, cholestyramine, colestipol, mineral oil, orlistat, and sucralfate), increase requirements (quinidine and sulfonamides), and oppose action (oral anticoagulants)
   g. Vitamin K may be included in treatment regimens for clients undergoing total parenteral nutrition (TPN) therapy

Practice to Pass

What vitamin deficiency would you expect to see in a client who is receiving antibiotic therapy?

h. Additional probiotic food sources may be added to the diet (e.g., yogurt) to minimize alteration of intestinal synthesis of normal flora during the course of antibiotic therapy

IV. WATER

A. Roles and function in the body

1. Component of body weight
   a. 60% of body weight in adult
   b. Newborns have a larger percentage of water in the body weight and therefore are more likely to be affected by changes in diet and water balance
   c. 2/3 of body water is intracellular and 1/3 is extracellular
2. Transport and participant in chemical reactions
   a. Water will freely move (by osmosis) to equalize solute concentrations in the body to maintain balance
   b. Chemical reactions in the body exist in a fluid medium
3. Fluid and electrolyte regulation
   a. Exchange occurs via sodium–potassium pump as the body attempts to balance cations (+) with anions (−)
   b. Association with sodium (Na^+) leads to involvement of renal and hormonal regulation (blood volume/blood pressure, osmolality/extracellular volume, antidiuretic hormone/H_2O retention, angiotensin/renin, and aldosterone/Na^+ retention)
4. Acid-base balance
   a. Maintained by the ability to balance electrolytes by acting as a solvent
   b. Participates in buffer systems in the body

B. Dietary sources

1. Water is part of most food sources (naturally occurring) and is in itself considered a food product because it is bought and packaged separately
2. Water is added to most food products during the cooking process
3. Water is available in homes through public water systems and wells and in the commercial setting as packaged items
4. Water can be found in most solid foods ranging from 0% in oil to almost 100% in lettuce
5. Water is also provided to the body as an end product of metabolism of macronutrients

C. Recommendations in the diet

1. Accepted water (fluid) intake is 2 L/day (eight 8-ounce glasses a day)
2. Most clients do not meet their daily water (fluid) needs
3. Increased intake is required for increased losses (e.g., sweating during physical activity, high temperatures, nasogastric tube output, and diarrhea), high-protein diets, high-sodium intake, and caffeine intake
4. Fluid needs are increased during pregnancy/lactation and infancy
5. Fluids such as alcoholic beverages, tea, and coffee can act as diuretics and should constitute a part but not all of the daily fluid intake

! D. **Deficiency states**

1. Altered fluid and electrolyte balance can occur from fluid losses (both insensible and sensible), which will place the client in a state of dehydration
2. Altered acid/base balance can occur as fluid losses change the environment for chemical reactions
3. Dehydration
   a. Can occur due to fluid loss and can be isotonic, hypotonic, or hypertonic, depending on relative concentration of electrolytes
   b. Dehydration states manifest as presence of thirst, poor skin turgor, decreased activity tolerance, weakness, disorientation, and confusion
   c. Children (newborn, infants, toddlers, and school-age) and elderly clients are more at risk to develop clinical symptoms even with small fluid losses

! E. **Excess states**

1. Altered fluid and electrolyte balance due to fluid retention affects serum concentration of electrolytes and can result in hypervolemia, water intoxication, or hyponatremia
2. Altered acid-base balance can occur due to fluid retention that alters the chemical environment as a consequence of altered electrolyte status
3. Edema states manifest with skin changes (pitting or nonpitting) and mental status changes (disorientation to coma) that can be severe if cardiac and respiratory systems become involved, leading to heart failure

! F. **Therapeutic treatment**

1. Oral rehydration therapies are the first line of treatment used to replace fluid losses in a client who is conscious
2. If fluid losses are more severe or if the client is unconscious, the use of IV solutions is required to restore water balance
3. Careful correction of fluid therapy is necessary in order to prevent further fluid shifting and possible fluid, electrolyte, and acid/base disturbances
4. Water (fluid) restriction may be indicated for clients who are at risk for the development of edematous states that could lead to heart failure
5. Clients who have underlying health problems such as cardiac, liver, renal, or respiratory conditions may have to monitor their fluid intake in order to prevent fluid overload that would lead to further compromise

Practice to Pass

List factors that would increase the amount of water needed in the diet.

V. MAJOR MINERALS

A. **Sodium**

1. Roles and function in the body
   a. Sodium is involved in fluid balance (maintaining osmolality) via antidiuretic hormone (ADH) and aldosterone secretion
   b. Sodium is involved in nerve transmission and neurological function (think brain!)
   c. There is a cerebral cellular response to sodium that responds by shrinkage or edema formation to corresponding sodium levels (high serum Na^+ levels—cells shrink; low serum Na^+ levels—cells swell)
   d. Sodium helps to maintain acid-base balance in conjunction with chloride

2. Dietary sources
   a. Found in high concentrations in processed or prepared foods
   b. Can be used as a preservative or flavoring agent in food products
   c. Hidden sources in the diet can be found in medications, since sodium can be a constituent part of certain drugs
3. Recommendations in the diet
   a. The RDA for sodium for clients 19–50 years of age is 1.5 grams/day
   b. Most Western diets contain too much sodium
   c. It is recommended that clients be instructed not to routinely add salt to foods during the cooking process or to routinely salt their food prior to tasting in order to decrease sodium intake in the diet
   d. The upper limit for sodium is 5.8 grams/day
4. Deficiency states
   a. Altered fluid and electrolyte balance can lead to hyponatremia and may be seen with syndrome of inappropriate antidiuretic hormone (SIADH) in the clinical setting
   b. Altered acid-base balance is usually associated with volume depletion states
   c. Symptoms manifested by low sodium (deficiency) are nausea, vomiting, diarrhea, muscle cramps, and mental status changes (confusion and disorientation)
5. Excess states
   a. Altered fluid and electrolyte balance leads to hypernatremia and possible association with diabetes insipidus (DI) in the clinical setting
   b. Increased sodium levels contribute to the development of edema and hypertension and lead to neurological signs (confusion, seizures)
6. Therapeutic treatment
   a. To replace deficiency, use added salt in the diet, salt tablets, and broth to restore sodium levels
   b. If sodium deficit is severe, then use of IV solutions (hypertonic) may be indicated to restore balance
   c. To correct excess, salt restriction, use of diuretics and appropriate IV fluids (hypotonic and isotonic) may be indicated to restore balance
   d. Sodium-restricted diets may be utilized in clients whose medical condition predisposes them to fluid volume excess (such as heart failure, renal failure)

B. Chloride

1. Roles and function in the body
   a. Chloride is involved in fluid balance because it works with sodium
   b. Chloride is involved in acid-base balance and moves across the cell to membrane to interact with potassium
   c. Chloride works in the stomach to help maintain gastric acidity as it is a constituent part of hydrochloric acid (HCl)
2. Recommendations in the diet
   a. As for sodium, there is only a minimum recommended level of chloride in the diet—750 mg/day
   b. Since chloride is often linked with sodium in foods, most Western diets contain adequate amounts of chloride

3. Deficiency state
   a. Chloride deficiency is seen in infants who have the clinical condition of failure to thrive (FTT)
   b. Losses occur through the gastrointestinal tract (emesis, NGT output, etc.) and can result in acid-base imbalance
4. Excess state
   a. Increased chloride levels are associated with dehydration
   b. Excess levels are not usually seen unless there are underlying disease states
5. Therapeutic treatment
   a. To correct deficiency, include foods that are high in sodium content as sodium and chloride are often used together in food processing
   b. To correct excess, increase fluid level to restore balance

C. Potassium

1. Roles and function in the body
   a. Potassium is important in nerve transmission and muscle contraction
   b. Potassium helps to maintain acid-base balance by transcellular shifting in response to acid-base changes in the body
   ! c. Potassium significantly affects cardiac muscle (think heart!), and potential serious health consequences can occur, ranging from arrhythmias to heart block and possibly death if levels become abnormal
2. Dietary sources
   a. Potassium is found in large quantities in cooked dried beans, milk, fruits, and vegetables
   b. Potassium is found in large quantities in most fresh foods and in low quantities in most processed foods
   c. Large amounts of licorice in the diet can lead to hypokalemia (deficiency of potassium) and sodium-water retention
3. Recommendations in the diet: the RDA is 4.7 grams/day, and there is no upper limit
4. Deficiency states
   ! a. Clinical deficiency is often seen coexisting with deficiencies of other electrolytes such as magnesium and calcium
   b. Deficiency states do not usually arise from dietary factors (unless excess natural licorice is ingested) but rather from use of certain medications that promote K^+ excretion (diuretics, laxatives, and steroids)
   c. Low levels of potassium can also serve to potentiate drug actions as in the case of digitalis toxicity
   d. Deficiency is also associated with refeeding syndrome, which occurs when malnourished clients receive increased calories
5. Excess states
   ! a. Excess states do not usually arise from dietary ingestion unless clients use salt substitutes or potassium supplements
   b. Certain medications can lead to retained levels of potassium in the body, such as ACE inhibitors, steroids, and potassium-sparing diuretics

6. Therapeutic treatment

! a. Oral replacement of potassium (liquid or pills) can be used to restore potassium serum levels; it is important to take this medication with food so as to minimize gastrointestinal side effects

! b. IV replacement can be given as an additive in solution (*Never* give as IVP as this can cause the client to have cardiac arrest!)

c. Kayexalate exchange resin and diuretic therapy can be used to promote K^+ loss

d. Dialysis maybe indicated for significantly high serum levels (intractable hyperkalemia) due to renal failure

D. Calcium

1. Roles and function in the body

a. Calcium is a constituent part of bones and teeth in the body

b. Calcium is necessary for nerve conduction (neurotransmitters) and muscle contraction (actin/myosin)

c. Calcium is involved in the coagulation pathway

d. Active and inactive forms exist in the body (ionized and nonionized) and are affected by protein binding

e. A complex regulation system that includes vitamin D, phosphorus (inverse relationship), PTH (increases serum Ca^{++}), and calcitonin (decreases serum Ca^{++}) helps to maintain calcium balance

2. Dietary sources

a. Found in sardines, milk and other dairy products (cheese and yogurt), and fortified foods and beverages

! b. **Phytates** (phytic acid—nuts, seeds and grain) in foods decrease calcium absorption

! c. **Oxalates** (oxalic acid—spinach, beets, rhubarb, and chocolate) in foods decrease calcium absorption

d. High-fiber diets decrease calcium absorption

e. The inclusion of lactose, acidic foods, and fat in the diet leads to increased absorption

3. Recommendations in the diet

a. AI (adequate intake) is set at 1,000 mg/day for adults 19–50 years of age

b. AI is set at 1,200 mg/day for adults 51 years of age and over

c. Additional increases in calcium requirements in the diet may be seen—there is significant research directed at the benefits of calcium in preventing the development of osteoporosis and osteopenia (in premenopausal and postmenopausal age groups)

! 4. Deficiency state

a. Clinical signs associated with calcium deficiency can result in development of Chvostek (facial nerve grimace) and Trousseau (carpopedal spasm) signs

b. Associated electrolyte deficiencies can be seen with potassium and magnesium in the clinical setting

c. Development of tetany symptoms can occur

d. Osteoporosis can develop due to decreased levels of calcium throughout one's lifetime

e. Deficiency state leads to bone demineralization and relaxed nerve and muscle coordination

5. Excess states
   a. Increased calcium levels can be seen in the clinical setting as part of a metastatic process or kidney stone formation
   b. Increased intake is associated with constipation
   c. Excess levels may interfere with absorption of other electrolytes/minerals
   d. Milk-alkali syndrome (alkalotic condition due to increased amounts of milk or antacid products) can lead to development of excess levels of calcium
   ! e. Excess serum levels can lead to development of hypercalcemic crisis that is a medical emergency and must be treated promptly
6. Therapeutic treatment
   a. To correct deficiency, increase dietary sources and use calcium supplements as prescribed (calcium carbonate, citrate, malate, and phosphate preparations)
   b. Calcium supplements vary in their bioavailability; refer to drug text for specific absorption information
   c. The use of calcium-containing antacids (such as Tums™) maybe recommended as a form of calcium supplement; however, it is important to assess the client for excessive intake patterns of antacids that contain aluminum or magnesium because this can lead to further imbalance and GI symptoms
   ! d. To correct excess levels (hypercalcemic crisis) use hydration, loop diuretics, and possibly antineoplastic agents

E. Phosphorus

1. Roles and function in the body
   a. Phosphorus is a structural component of bones, teeth, and phospholipids throughout the body
   b. Phosphorus is involved in the synthesis of DNA and RNA, and it functions as a coenzyme in many chemical reactions in the body
   c. Phosphorus participates in the buffer system as a phosphate
   d. Phosphorus has an inverse relationship with calcium in the body
2. Dietary sources
   a. Phosphorus is found in high amounts in dairy and meat products
   b. It is also found in processed foods because it is often used as an additive
3. Recommendations in the diet
   a. RDA for adults (male and female) is 700 mg/day
   b. Upper level is listed as 4,000 mg/day for adults 19–70 years of age
4. Deficiency states
   a. Deficiency states are associated with bone loss and muscle weakness
   b. Due to inverse relationship with calcium, high levels of calcium accompany low levels of phosphorus
   c. Clients at risk for clinical deficiency of phosphorus are those who have underlying wasting disease, hyperparathyroidism, or refeeding syndrome, which can occurs when malnourished clients are started on enteral or TPN feedings (low phosphate and magnesium levels occur because of cellular movement if feedings are started too quickly, and minerals are not replaced in solution to balance deficits)

5. Excess states
    a. Excess levels are associated with low serum calcium levels and the client may exhibit tetany symptoms
    b. Clients with compromised renal status (renal failure) will have elevated phosphorus levels that will require therapeutic treatment
    c. Clients who chronically use sodium phosphate laxatives will be at risk for elevated levels
6. Therapeutic treatment
    a. Maintain dietary intake of adequate sources to correct deficiency states
    b. Correct underlying clinical conditions that predispose client to phosphorus imbalances and restrict use of medication therapy that interferes with phosphorus balance

F. Magnesium

1. Roles and function in the body
    a. Magnesium is found mainly in the bones in the body
    b. Magnesium is reported to be nature's calcium channel blocker—it acts to decrease blood pressure and smooth muscle contraction
    c. Magnesium functions as a coenzyme in energy metabolism (needed for ATP production) and a neurotransmitter in the central nervous system (decreases sensitivity to acetylcholine and excitability at motor junction)
    d. Magnesium and calcium (in conjunction) act to regulate blood pressure and blood clotting by balancing these effects (magnesium decreases and calcium increases)
    e. Magnesium is being evaluated for possible clinical use in the treatment of myocardial infarction (MI) due to its relaxing effect on smooth muscle tissues
2. Dietary sources
    a. Magnesium is found in sunflower seeds, legumes, and dark green leafy vegetables
    b. Magnesium is also found in chocolate, cocoa, nuts, seafood, and whole grain breads and cereals
    c. Magnesium absorption is increased with active forms of vitamin D
    d. Increased magnesium in the diet does not necessarily lead to increased absorption; and it is also possible for magnesium levels to become toxic in the presence of renal dysfunction
3. Recommendations in the diet
    a. RDA for adult males is 400–420 mg/day
    b. RDA for adult females is 310–320 mg/day
4. Deficiency states
    a. Decreased absorption of magnesium can occur when there is a high intake of fat, phosphorus, calcium, and protein in the diet
    b. Decreased magnesium levels are seen in clients who have malabsorption problems or chronic alcohol abuse
    c. Deficiency states of magnesium can occur in response to either increased magnesium excretion (chronic use of laxative products) or through decreased magnesium absorption
    d. It is important to check the serum potassium and phosphorus levels of clients who take diuretic therapy or who have protein malnutrition; often when mag-

nesium deficits occur, it is in conjunction with phosphorus and potassium deficits (if you do not correct all three deficits together, then normal balance will not be restored)

e. Clinical manifestations associated with magnesium deficiency include muscle weakness, mental status changes (confusion leading to convulsions), and, in severe cases, tetany-like symptoms (which are usually due to co-existing low calcium levels)

f. Rapid refeeding to treat malnutrition leads to low magnesium levels (with concurrent low phosphate and potassium levels)

5. Excess states

Practice to Pass

Why is magnesium considered to be "nature's calcium channel blocker"?

a. Dietary factors usually do not play a significant part in the development of excess states; excess is more often related to underlying clinical conditions such as renal failure, dehydration states, diarrhea, and alkalotic imbalances

b. Excess levels can be seen with use of medications that contain magnesium, such as laxatives and antacids, or more likely with the administration of magnesium sulfate ($MgSO_4^-$), which is used as an anticonvulsant for the treatment of toxemia of pregnancy and to stop preterm labor

c. Excess levels of serum magnesium in the body can lead to respiratory depression, loss of reflexes, and ultimately coma and death; it is crucial that magnesium levels are trended and clients assessed for potential excess magnesium levels, either as a part of their underlying condition or as a part of their therapeutic treatment

6. Therapeutic treatment

a. To correct deficiency, increase content of magnesium-rich foods in the diet

b. Since low calcium levels usually accompany magnesium deficiency and oftentimes low potassium levels, it is important to correct all electrolyte imbalances in order to restore effective serum levels

c. If deficiency is more severe, then oral administration of magnesium oxide can be used, but be alert to potential side effects such as diarrhea and nausea

d. If deficiency is extremely severe or if magnesium is being used as a medication, then IV titration of $MgSO_4$ is indicated; this will require monitoring of serum levels, respiratory status, blood pressure, and reflexes during the course of clinical treatment; refer to specific drug texts for protocols for administering $MgSO_4$ in the clinical setting

e. If excess levels are seen, then correction of underlying clinical condition must be attempted or, in the case of renal failure, the client may have to undergo dialysis

f. It is important to remove all sources of excess magnesium from the diet and/or treatment regimen

VI. TRACE ELEMENTS

A. Iron

1. Roles and function in the body

a. Iron is involved as a component of RBCs in hemoglobin formation and as a component of muscles in the form of myoglobin

b. Iron is stored and transported in the body through a series of blood-carrying proteins (ferritin reflects body iron stores and transferrin and pretransferrin are carriers)

c. **Heme** is the iron-holding part of the hemoglobin molecule and is usually found in animal sources

d. **Nonheme** sources of iron are found in plants and animals; these are not considered to be as good an iron source as heme sources due to differences in absorption

e. Bioavailability and intestinal absorption of iron are regulated by a number of factors in the body and reflect the body's ability to respond to the two iron states—ferrous iron ++ (reduced) and ferric iron +++ (oxidized)—that occur in the body

! 2. Dietary sources

a. Heme sources of iron include meat, poultry, and fish that can be absorbed in the body; in addition, these sources contain a factor known as MFP (meat, fish, and poultry) factor that helps to enhance iron absorption of nonheme sources as well in the diet

! b. Eating vitamin C at the same time with iron sources in the diet also helps to promote iron absorption

c. Nonheme sources of iron are found in plant and animal foods and are not absorbed as well in the body

d. Certain sugars and wine (containing sugars) also help to enhance absorption of nonheme iron sources

e. A decrease in stomach acid, phytates, oxalates, tannins, and other mineral excesses (calcium, copper, zinc, or manganese) can lead to decreased absorption

3. Recommendations in the diet

a. RDA for the adult male is 8 mg/day

b. RDA for the adult female is 18 mg/day for ages 19–50 years and 8 mg/day for ages 51 and over

c. Growth states (pregnancy, lactation, and childhood) require increased iron levels, but this is usually achieved with use of multivitamin preparations and/or prenatal vitamins

! 4. Deficiency state

a. Nutritional anemia—iron deficiency anemia (IDA—microcytic hypochromic anemia) presents with fatigue, weakness, headache, pallor, temperature intolerance, and behavioral changes; it is the most common type of nutritional anemia seen

b. **Pica** represents the ingestion of nonfood substances that is associated with a clinical iron deficiency and may actually be the first sign of a problem; client will eat a wide range of nonfood items including ice, clay, dirt, and paste; iron deficiency may be a cause or effect of pica

c. At-risk populations for iron deficiency include females due to menses (blood loss due to menstrual flow), pregnant females due to dilutional anemia of pregnancy (as a result of increased blood volume), and strict vegetarians

d. In addition, athletes may be at risk to develop sports anemia that can lead to iron deficiency states

e. Factors that decrease iron absorption—such as phytate fibers (grains and vegetables), tannic acid (found in tea and coffee), oxalic acid (spinach), calcium and phosphorus (milk), and EDTA (food additive)—can contribute to iron deficiency

! **5.** Excess states

a. Iron overload symptoms include tissue damage, infections, and liver damage due to deposition of iron in the body

b. Hemochromatosis is an autosomal recessive genetic syndrome whereby iron absorption is increased, leading to significant joint pain and impairment of liver function and blood glucose level

c. Hemosiderosis reflects the deposition of excess iron in the liver and body tissues, which causes significant impairment

d. Clients with alcoholism are at risk for developing increased iron levels due to ingestion of beverages containing extra iron (wine)

e. Pediatric clients are at risk for iron toxicity due to accidental ingestion (iron poisoning) of iron-containing products; clinical manifestations of iron poisoning include nausea, vomiting, and diarrhea with cardiac effects (tachycardia and weak pulse) that can lead to shock and death

f. Use of iron-containing cookware products can lead to increased iron levels in the body from nonfood sources

6. Therapeutic treatment

a. For microcytic anemia deficiency state, increase heme sources of iron in the diet and be alert for dietary factors that will increase iron absorption in the body

b. Oral replacement in the form of iron sulfate pills may be indicated in clients who have deficiency symptoms (anemia), but be aware of gastrointestinal side effects and change in stool color (darkened) as a consequence of therapy

! **c.** Intramuscular or IV replacement may be needed with iron dextran (Dexferrum) if the clinical situation is more severe; use Z-track technique for IM injection to prevent skin staining at injection site

d. Check reticulocyte count for response to therapeutic treatment; folate and/or vitamin B_{12} deficiency can cause macrocytic anemia

e. Clients who have iron excess should limit their intake of iron-enriched foods and avoid using iron-containing cookware that may further aggravate the problem

B. Iodine

1. Roles and function in the body

a. Iodine is an important component of the thyroid hormones (T_3, T_4, and TSH)

b. Iodine is needed for growth and development, reproduction, and balance of metabolic rate and temperature in the body

2. Dietary sources

a. Iodine is found in saltwater fish and shellfish

b. Iodine is also found in iodized salt (fortified) in many other fortified food products (bread, milk, and red dye #3)

! **c.** Foods such as broccoli, brussel sprouts, cabbage, and cauliflower act as goitrogens or thyroid antagonists in the body; overconsumption of these can lead to the development of a toxic goiter because they interfere with the body's absorption or utilization of iodine

3. Recommendations in the diet

a. RDA is 150 mcg for adult males and females; the average adult consumes more than the RDA for iodine

b. Monitor dietary intake for excess use of foods in the cabbage family that are goitrogens as described above

! 4. Deficiency states

a. Clinical deficiency results in goiter formation (enlarged thyroid gland)

b. Hypothyroid clinical states exist due to insufficient hormones; this can lead to cretinism (congenital condition seen in newborn infants due to maternal deficiency) and may present as myxedema (deficiency seen in children and adults due to decreased thyroid activity)

c. Clinical manifestations include slowing down of body metabolism, weight gain, temperature intolerance (cold), hypotension, bradycardia, and constipation

! 5. Excess states

a. Excess states can also lead to goiter development

b. Hyperthyroidism leads to increased hormone levels that increase metabolic rate, promote weight loss, and lead to intolerance to heat and tachycardia

c. Accidental exposures to excess iodine levels during pregnancy can lead to teratogenic effects that compromise fetal development

d. Excess iodine therapy can lead to adverse clinical effects; clients who are being treated for hypothyroidism are at risk to develop excess states if their medication therapy is not adequately titrated

e. Fortified iodine sources in the diet and extensive use of iodized salt may lead to excess levels; clients should be aware of the hidden iodized salt content of foods selected in the diet

6. Therapeutic treatment

a. To correct iodine deficiency in the diet, use iodine-fortified food sources such as iodized salt

b. If a client is found to have endocrine dysfunction (thyroid problems), then correction of underlying clinical condition is necessary to maintain iodine balance in the body

c. To prevent iodine excess, limit the amount of iodized salt in the diet (1/2 tsp daily in diet provides more than the RDA)

C. Copper

1. Roles and function in the body

a. Copper acts as a co-factor in hemoglobin, blood clotting, and collagen formation in the body

b. Copper participates in iron metabolism (oxidates the ferrous form to ferric form) and participates as an antioxidant with zinc to help support immune system function

2. Dietary sources

a. Copper is found in organ meats and seafood

b. Copper is also found in nuts, seeds, legumes, and whole grain products

3. Recommendations in the diet: the RDA is 900 mcg/day

4. Deficiency state

a. Rare; is associated with increased intake of zinc, iron, calcium, manganese, phytates, antacids, vitamin C, diets high in fructose, and TPN solutions that are deficient in copper

b. Deficiency results in anemia (hypochromic microcytic) and possible development of neutropenia

c. Deficiency leads to skeletal demineralization (osteoporosis), skin changes (due to decreased pigments), and hair changes (kinky hair)

d. Menkes disease is a genetic X-linked recessive disorder that affects cerebral function and is due to a defect in the absorption of copper (can be fatal)

5. Excess states

! a. Wilson's disease is an autosomal recessive (congenital) disease that affects copper excretion, leading to accumulation of copper deposits in organs of the body (can be fatal)

b. Excess states can manifest with nausea, vomiting, diarrhea, and abdominal cramps

6. Therapeutic treatment

a. Replacement of deficiencies can be done with copper supplements (cupric oxide, copper gluconate, copper sulfate, and copper amino acid chelates) with daily dosages ranging from 1.5 to 3.0 mg

b. Copper is seen in multivitamin products in sufficient quantity, so supplemental use may not be indicated unless there is some underlying clinical indication

c. To decrease excess levels of copper, reduce dietary intake and use chelating agents such as penicillamine (used in the treatment of Wilson's disease) and phlebotomy

D. Zinc

1. Roles and function in the body

a. Zinc works to accomplish growth and repair in the body by participating in DNA and RNA synthesis and heme formation for the protein hemoglobin

b. Zinc also participates in carbohydrate metabolism (insulin) and release of energy and in essential fatty acid metabolism

c. Zinc participates in the activation of vitamin A in the body and attaches albumin and transferrin for transport in the body

d. Zinc participates in the immune response by stabilizing cell membranes and preventing the damage of free radicals

e. Zinc works throughout the body as an important coenzyme

f. Current research indicates that adequate zinc levels are now being associated with an easier labor and delivery experience due to its overall metabolic effects

g. Zinc can be stored in the body's liver cells as metallothionein (storage binding protein) until it is needed for metabolic processes

h. Zinc also participates in hormone action (insulin and thyroid) and helps to maintain metabolic rate function

2. Dietary sources

a. Found in shellfish (oysters and crabmeat), red meat (beef sirloin), and poultry

b. Found in wheat germ, green peas, yogurt, and whole grain products

c. Caffeine, oxalic acid, fiber, phytic acid, tea, and increased iron lead to a decrease in zinc absorption

3. Recommendations in the diet

a. RDA for the adult male is 11 mg/day

b. RDA for the adult female is 8 mg/day

4. Deficiency states
    a. Various food products (as noted above) affect the bioavailability and lead to reduced absorption of zinc
    b. Calcium acts as a chelating agent that leads to decreased levels of zinc
    c. ! Deficiency can manifest as decreased growth, decreased immune function, poor wound healing, altered taste perception, and altered metabolic rate
    d. Clients present with a multitude of symptoms related to clinical deficiency ranging from weakness and irritability to growth retardation; since zinc participates as a coenzyme in many of the body's metabolic processes, there will be alterations in all of these reactions leading to altered hormone activity and overall decreased immune response
    e. Clients at risk for zinc deficiency include pregnant adolescents, vegetarians, the elderly, low-income clients prone to malnutrition, clients with high output ileostomies, and those in stress states due to clinical conditions such as myocardial infarction, severe burns, Crohn's disease, and lymphoma
5. Excess states
    a. Increased levels of zinc lead to a clinical deficiency of copper and anemia
    b. Clinical manifestations include vomiting, diarrhea, fever, and possible renal failure with toxic levels
    c. Increased levels also promote the process of atherosclerosis
6. Therapeutic treatment
    a. Zinc is found as an ingredient in certain lozenges that are used to treat cold symptoms and may cause altered taste perception
    b. Zinc is available in several forms (glutonate, oxide, aspartate, piccolinate, citrate, monomethionine, and histidine) and is available as a separate preparation or in combination products
    c. To treat clinical deficiency, include adequate sources in the diet and be aware of limiting foods and other trace elements (calcium and copper) that affect bioavailability and absorption
    d. To treat clinical excess, decrease intake of supplemental zinc in the diet and be aware of medications and other products that contain zinc as a hidden source

E. Selenium

1. Roles and function in the body
    a. Selenium functions as an antioxidant (part of enzyme glutathione peroxidase) in the body and with vitamin E provides a synergistic effect to increase immune activity
    b. Selenium is involved in iodine metabolism and functions as a protein component in amino acids
    c. Current research suggests that selenium may be effective against prostate cancer
2. Dietary sources
    a. Found in Brazil nuts, seafood, liver, meats, green vegetables, and dairy products
    b. Amount of selenium found in foods may vary, as it is dependent on selenium content of soil and water in which foods are grown
3. Recommendations in the diet
    a. RDA for adults is 55 mcg/day

b. UL (upper limit) is 400 mcg/day

c. Increased needs occur in adolescent, pregnant, and lactating clients

d. Increased vitamin E in the body leads to decreased selenium requirements

4. Deficiency states

a. Clinical deficiency disease is called Keshan disease (found in China), which causes the development of cardiomyopathy leading to heart failure; this clinical condition resulted from soil that was lacking in selenium

b. Prolonged use of TPN solutions that do not include selenium can cause deficiency in the clinical setting

5. Excess states

a. Clinical manifestations related to excess levels include fatigue, nausea, vomiting, diarrhea, loss of hair, garlic or sour-milk breath odor, and nail and skin lesions

b. High doses (even in small amounts) can prove to be toxic and can cause clinical symptoms that affect the CNS

6. Therapeutic treatment

a. Inclusion of selenium in TPN solutions is advised to prevent deficiencies in the clinical setting

b. Dietary deficiency is usually not seen in the United States

c. Supplemental use of selenium must be monitored so as to avoid toxic effects of overdosage

F. Manganese

1. Roles and function in the body

a. Functions as a cofactor in energy metabolism and bone formation

b. The liver and the pancreas have the highest content in the body

2. Dietary sources

a. Found in wheat bran, legumes, cereal grains, and green leafy vegetables

b. Found in coffee and tea

c. Adequate amounts are found in plant sources in the diet

3. Recommendations in the diet

a. Adequate intake (AI) for adult males is 2–3 mg/day

b. AI for adult females is 1.8 mg/day

4. Deficiency state

a. Clinical deficiency is seen in clients who have diabetes, protein-energy malnutrition (PEM), and epilepsy

b. Clinical manifestations of deficiency include weight loss, nausea, vomiting, diarrhea, changes in hair color, and increased cholesterol levels

c. Phytic and oxalic acids lead to decreased absorption of manganese in the diet

d. High intakes of calcium, magnesium, and iron can lead to decreased absorption of manganese

e. Use of antacids and tetracyclines can lead to decreased absorption

5. Excess state

a. High levels have been seen with mine workers due to dust inhalation; this can lead to toxic levels (manganese dust); and in clients receiving long-term TPN

!

b. Increased levels are associated with liver and CNS damage, leading to cerebral abnormalities

6. Therapeutic treatment
   a. Manganese is available in several forms (gluconate, sulfate, ascorbate, and amino acid chelates) and can be given separately or in a combination product
   b. Some supplements contain hidden manganese and should be not be given to clients who have liver disease because altered liver function can lead to retention and high manganese levels

G. Fluoride

1. Roles and function in the body
   a. Functions as part of dental structure in the formation of tooth enamel, teeth, and bones
   b. Fluorapatite (calcium, phosphorus, and fluoride) is a substance that makes bone and teeth stronger in the body
   c. Fluoride helps to strengthen resistance to bacterial acid in the body
2. Dietary sources
   a. Found in fluoridated water and supplements in the United States
   b. Concentration is 1 PPM (one part per million = 1 mg per liter of water)
3. Recommendations in the diet
   a. AI for adult male is 4.0 mg/day
   b. AI for adult female is 3.0 mg/day
4. Deficiency state
   a. Due to fluoridation of water supply and inclusion of fluoride in toothpaste and other health products, clinical deficiency states do not usually occur in the United States
   b. In developing countries without adequate fluoridation, deficiency can occur that results in tooth decay and increased dental caries
5. Excess states
   a. Fluorosis is a clinical condition caused by prolonged fluoride ingestion leading to mottled teeth, headache, and gastric distress
   b. Continued ingestion of increased fluoride can lead to the development of systemic fluorosis that can cause the development of osteosclerosis and spinal deformities
6. Therapeutic treatment
   a. Clinical deficiency is rare in the United States due to fluoridated water supply and health products
   b. To decrease excess levels, check water source for fluoride content and limit or avoid use of products containing fluoride

H. Chromium

1. Roles and function in the body
   a. Functions in CHO metabolism (enhances the action of insulin) and lipid metabolism
   b. Participates in RNA and DNA and as a cofactor in fat and cholesterol metabolism
2. Dietary sources
   a. Found in spices (thyme and black pepper), brewers yeast, and broccoli
   b. Found in unrefined foods and meat, liver, fats, and vegetable oils

3. Recommendations in the diet
   a. AI for adult male is 35 mcg/day
   b. AI for adult female is 25 mcg/day
   c. Increased needs are seen in response to exercise, infection, and trauma
4. Deficiency state
   a. Antacids and phytates decrease absorption
   b. Clinical deficiency manifests as a "diabetes-type condition" with abnormal response to glucose that can become symptomatic (hypoglycemic)
5. Excess state
   a. Vitamin C can lead to increased absorption of chromium in the diet
   b. Excess levels can result in a metallic taste in the mouth
6. Therapeutic treatment
   a. Chromium is available in many supplemental forms (picolinate, chloride, and yeast) and can be given alone or in a combination product
   b. Chromium picolinate supplements are being marketed for promotion of fat loss and building up of protein in the body but clinical evidence has not supported this claim

I. Molybdenum

1. Roles and function in the body
   a. Involved as a cofactor in protein synthesis
   b. Involved in the working part of many metal-containing enzymes in the body
   c. Found in the liver, kidneys, bone, and adrenal glands
2. Dietary sources
   a. Found in organ meats
   b. Found in legumes, grains, and milk
3. Recommendations in the diet
   a. RDA for adults is 45 mcg/day
   b. Daily intake often averages 200 to 500 mcg/day
4. Deficiency state
   a. Dietary deficiencies are rarely seen in the typical Western diet since such a small amount is needed to meet daily needs
   b. Clients receiving TPN feedings without supplementation can be at risk to develop clinical deficiency
   c. Clients with an inability to process sulfa-containing amino acids can be at risk to develop clinical deficiency
   d. Deficiency symptoms can manifest as increased pulse and respirations, visual defects, and coma
5. Excess states
   a. Increased levels may be associated with hyperuricemia and gout-like symptoms
   b. In animal studies, excess levels have caused renal damage and affect reproduction
   c. High levels of molybdenum can cause several drug interactions such as reduced effect of acetaminophen and decreased absorption of copper

Practice to Pass

Explain the importance of trace elements in the body despite the fact that only small amounts are needed to affect metabolic activity.

6. Therapeutic treatment
   a. Molybdenum is available in sodium and ammonium forms and is usually found in combination products
   b. Ongoing research is looking into the health benefits of molybdenum in treating other clinical conditions such as Wilson disease or cancer

Case Study

A 20-year-old client wants to know the best way to get an adequate supply of vitamins and minerals through dietary intake. The client has no significant medical history and no reported allergies or food sensitivities. Currently, the client is a college student and shares an apartment with two other female roommates.

1. What background information would you obtain from the client in order to assist you with dietary recommendations?
2. What methods of food preparation would you suggest to enhance dietary absorption of nutrients?
3. What referral would you make for this client?
4. Would you encourage the client to use supplements to meet dietary goals?
5. How would you advise this client when she asks you about the use of megavitamin therapy?

For suggested responses, see pages 317–318.

POSTTEST

POSTTEST

1 A client informs the nurse he takes 3 grams of vitamin C a day to prevent "catching a cold." Which of the following client conditions would be of concern to the nurse?

1. An iron deficiency anemia
2. A history of kidney stones
3. Occasional anginal episodes
4. A history of cholecystitis

2 The nurse would encourage which of the following foods to the client with a deficiency in thiamine? Select all that apply.

1. Sunflower and sesame seeds
2. Citrus fruits
3. Lean pork, beef, and liver
4. Strawberries
5. Peanuts

3 A client who abuses alcohol presents with significant mental status changes and loss of balance. Which vitamin deficiency does the nurse suspect as the possible cause of this presentation?

1. Vitamin C
2. Thiamin
3. Riboflavin
4. Niacin

4 The nurse determines that dietary teaching has been effective when a client states that which of the following food items has the highest sodium content?

1. Milk
2. Fresh fruit
3. Meats
4. Chocolate pudding

5 The nurse is teaching a client with type 2 diabetes mellitus about blood glucose control. The nurse would include in the discussion that it is important to take adequate amounts of which of the following in the diet or in supplements?

1. Chromium
2. Biotin
3. Niacin
4. Sodium

6 The clinic nurse is completing a history and physical examination on a client who has a history of thyroid problems. The nurse assesses this client for signs of which potential mineral imbalance?

1. Magnesium
2. Iodine
3. Zinc
4. Selenium

7 During a routine history and physical examination, the client reports the desire to eat large amounts of ice (two 8-ounce cups) during the day. This nurse assesses the client for other manifestations of which of the following possible underlying clinical conditions?

1. Water deficiency due to dehydration
2. Iron deficiency associated with pica
3. Malnutrition due to protein deficiency
4. Sodium deficiency due to ingestion of ice

8 The nurse who is teaching a prenatal class about the need for vitamin supplements includes that deficiency of folic acid can lead to which of the following?

1. Masking of vitamin B_{12} deficiency
2. Decreased homocysteine levels
3. Microcytic anemia
4. Neural tube defects

9 When conducting discharge teaching for a client who is at risk for pernicious anemia because of gastrectomy, the nurse reinforces that the client will require which of the following for preventive treatment?

1. Niacin supplementation for lifetime
2. Vitamin B_{12} injections for lifetime
3. A single dose injection of ferrous sulfate to correct the condition
4. Riboflavin injections monthly for at least a year

10 A client taking folate supplements reports to the nurse that her urine is very dark yellow and she is quite concerned. Which response by the nurse is appropriate?

1. "You probably need to drink more water."
2. "You probably need to reduce the amount of folate you are taking."
3. "Folate can cause your urine to be a deep yellow color."
4. "You should report this finding to your physician."

ANSWERS & RATIONALES

Pretest

1 **Answer: 2** Vitamin B_{12} deficiency can result in the development of a macrocytic nutritional anemia because it is necessary for red blood cell production in the body. Option 1 is incorrect because a deficiency of calcium leads to bone demineralization. Option 3 is incorrect because iron deficiency results in a nutritional anemia that is microcytic. Option 4 is incorrect—vitamin B_1 (thiamin) clinical deficiency results in beriberi.
Cognitive Level: Application **Client Need:** Health Promotion and Maintenance **Integrated Process:** Nursing Process: Implementation **Content Area:** Foundational Sciences: Nutrition **Strategy:** Recall knowledge of macrocytic anemia to answer to direct you to option 2. **Reference:** Adams, M., Josephson, D., & Holland, L. (2005). *Pharmacology for nurses: A pathophysiologic approach.* Upper Saddle River, NJ: Pearson/Prentice Hall, pp. 553–554.

2 **Answer: 1** Infants receive an injection of vitamin K to protect them against the development of hemorrhagic disease of the newborn. Infants are born with a sterile gut and are therefore unable to synthesize vitamin K in the small intestines. A single injection of vitamin K helps to introduce enough of the vitamin so that the infant is afforded protection. All of the other options are incorrect—this drug has no clinical impact on these clinical conditions.
Cognitive Level: Application **Client Need:** Health Promotion and Maintenance **Integrated Process:** Teaching and Learning **Content Area:** Foundational Sciences: Nutrition **Strategy:** Recognize Aqua-Mephyton is vitamin K, which plays a role in the clotting process to direct you to option 1. **Reference:** Nix, S. (2005). *Williams' basic nutrition & diet therapy* (12th ed.). St. Louis, MO: Elsevier Mosby, p. 97.

3 **Answer: 3** Clients who take more than 1 gram of vitamin C daily may have a false negative result on stool guaiac testing. It is important for the nurse to understand that the test results will be inconclusive and should be repeated in a few days once the client has stopped taking the additional vitamin C. Option 1 is incorrect because there is a relationship between the testing chemical reaction. Option 4 is incorrect—the results

are not valid and not open to interpretation due to drug interactions.

Cognitive Level: Application **Client Need:** Health Promotion and Maintenance **Integrated Process:** Nursing Process: Analysis **Content Area:** Foundational Sciences: Nutrition **Strategy:** The question asks what effect the vitamin C will have, implying an effect will occur, so eliminate option 1. Eliminate option 4 as being too vague. Recall knowledge of vitamin C to choose option 2. **Reference:** Adams, M., Josephson, D., & Holland, L. (2005). *Pharmacology for nurses: A pathophysiologic approach.* Upper Saddle River, NJ: Pearson/Prentice Hall, pp. 557–559.

4 **Answer: 2** A clinical deficiency of vitamin D during childhood can result in structural deformities that result in a clinical diagnosis of rickets. The other options will not cause this type of structural deformity.

Cognitive Level: Analysis **Client Need:** Health Promotion and Maintenance **Integrated Process:** Nursing Process: Assessment **Content Area:** Foundational Sciences: Nutrition **Strategy:** Critical words are *bowed legs* and *pigeon chest,* indicating a bone malformation. Recall knowledge of bone development to choose option 2. **Reference:** Nix, S. (2005). *Williams' basic nutrition & diet therapy* (12th ed.). St. Louis, MO: Elsevier Mosby, p. 92.

5 **Answer: 1** Baked potato and broccoli are high in potassium. All of the other options reflect food sources that are lower in potassium.

Cognitive Level: Analysis **Client Need:** Health Promotion and Maintenance **Integrated Process:** Nursing Process: Evaluation **Content Area:** Foundational Sciences: Nutrition **Strategy:** Option 1 includes two sources of potassium and therefore a more comprehensive answer. **Reference:** Nix, S. (2005). *Williams' basic nutrition & diet therapy* (12th ed.). St. Louis, MO: Elsevier Mosby, p. 137.

6 **Answer: 1** Whole grain products can contain large amounts of phytic acid (phytates), which can limit the absorption of several nutrients: calcium, zinc, iron, and magnesium. Options 2 and 3 are incorrect because phytic acid is composed of inorganic phosphate compounds. Option 4 is incorrect because phytic acid does not affect either sodium or chloride levels.

Cognitive Level: Application **Client Need:** Health Promotion and Maintenance **Integrated Process:** Nursing Process: Assessment **Content Area:** Foundational Sciences: Nutrition **Strategy:** Critical words are *nutrient deficiencies* and *grain products.* Recall specific information on phytates to choose option 1. **Reference:** Nix, S. (2005). *Williams' basic nutrition & diet therapy* (12th ed.). St. Louis, MO: Elsevier Mosby, p. 21.

7 **Answer: 3** Anemic clients who do not respond to iron replacement therapy and present with symptoms associated with neuropathy are likely to be suffering from an underlying vitamin B_{12} deficiency. Option 1 is incorrect because, even if the client were not being compliant, these types of symptoms would be due to an associated clinical deficiency. Option 2 is unrelated to any information presented in the question. Option 4 is incorrect because the use of vitamin C supplements would cause symptoms of iron overload since it enhances the absorption of iron.

Cognitive Level: Application **Client Need:** Health Promotion and Maintenance **Integrated Process:** Nursing Process: Assessment **Content Area:** Foundational Sciences: Nutrition **Strategy:** Recognize the symptoms are indicative of peripheral neuropathy to direct you option 3. **Reference:** Adams, M., Josephson, D., & Holland, L. (2005). *Pharmacology for nurses: A pathophysiologic approach.* Upper Saddle River, NJ: Pearson/Prentice Hall, pp. 364–366.

8 **Answer: 2** Peptic ulcer disease can be aggravated by niacin, and the clients' complaints of heartburn are indicative of GI irritation. Flushing is a side effect and although uncomfortable, it would not be as serious as gastric irritation. Dryness of the mouth is not life threatening. Diarrhea would be a symptom of niacin deficiency.

Cognitive Level: Analysis **Client Need:** Health Promotion and Maintenance **Integrated Process:** Nursing Process: Implementation **Content Area:** Foundational Sciences: Nutrition **Strategy:** The critical words in the stem of the question are *of most concern.* This tells you that more than one option may be correct and that you must choose the most important option. Recall niacin causes GI irritation to direct you to option 2. **Reference:** Adams, M., Josephson, D., & Holland, L. (2005). *Pharmacology for nurses: A pathophysiologic approach.* Upper Saddle River, NJ: Pearson/Prentice Hall, pp. 364–366.

9 **Answer: 1** Avidin is a protein found in raw eggs that binds with biotin and decreases absorption of this vitamin. Options 2 and 3 represent foods that are high in biotin; option 4 is high in vitamin C.

Cognitive Level: Application **Client Need:** Health Promotion and Maintenance **Integrated Process:** Nursing Process: Analysis **Content Area:** Foundational Sciences: Nutrition **Strategy:** Critical words are *frequent intake* and *biotin deficiency.* If specific recall of biotin is poor, recognize raw eggs are not advised to choose option 1. **Reference:** Stanfield, P., & Hui, Y. (2003). *Nutrition and diet therapy self-instructional modules* (4th ed.). Sudbury, MA: Jones & Bartlett, p. 75.

10 **Answer: 2** Heme iron is considered to be the most absorbable form of iron in the body. In order to maximize absorption of iron, meat, fish, poultry, and ascorbic acid (vitamin C) can be used. Milk would interfere with absorption of the iron, some green leafy vegetables con-

tain oxalate, which also interferes with absorption. Water would not increase absorption.
Cognitive Level: Application **Client Need:** Health Promotion and Maintenance **Integrated Process:** Nursing Process: Implementation **Content Area:** Foundational Sciences: Nutrition **Strategy:** Critical words in the question are *increased absorption.* Recall iron absorption is increased by ascorbic acid to choose option 2. **Reference:** Adams, M., Josephson, D., & Holland, L. (2005). *Pharmacology for nurses: A pathophysiologic approach.* Upper Saddle River, NJ: Pearson/Prentice Hall, pp. 379–382.

Posttest

1 **Answer: 2** Increased intake of vitamin C can increase risk for stone formation. The daily recommended dose is 90 mg per day. The increased vitamin C intake would not impact the other options.
Cognitive Level: Analysis **Client Need:** Health Promotion and Maintenance **Integrated Process:** Nursing Process: Analysis **Content Area:** Foundational Sciences: Nutrition **Strategy:** Knowledge of normal requirements is necessary. Recognize 3 grams is excessive and, being water soluble, the vitamin will be excreted via the kidneys to direct you to option 2. **Reference:** Adams, M., Josephson, D., & Holland, L. (2005). *Pharmacology for nurses: A pathophysiologic approach.* Upper Saddle River, NJ: Pearson/Prentice Hall, p. 554.

2 **Answers: 1, 3, 5** Good food sources of thiamine include wheat germ, lean pork, beef, liver, whole and enriched grains, seeds, nuts, and a few vegetables.
Cognitive Level: Application **Client Need:** Health Promotion and Maintenance **Integrated Process:** Nursing Process: Implementation **Content Area:** Foundational Sciences: Nutrition **Strategy:** Refer to the similar options of 4 and 2, including fruits. In this case the similar options are incorrect and should be eliminated. **Reference:** Roth R., & Townsend, C. (2003). *Nutrition and diet therapy* (8th ed.). Albany, NY: Thomson Delmar Learning, p. 126.

3 **Answer: 2** Clients who abuse alcohol are prone to develop thiamin deficiency because ethanol affects the intestinal absorption of thiamin. Wernicke-Korsakoff syndrome is associated with a state of encephalopathy that is seen in clients with alcoholism and presents with mental status changes, psychosis, and coma. Option 1 is incorrect—vitamin C deficiency is associated with scurvy. Option 3 is incorrect—riboflavin deficiency is associated with ariboflavinosis. Option 4 is incorrect—niacin deficiency is associated with pellagra.
Cognitive Level: Application **Client Need:** Health Promotion and Maintenance **Integrated Process:** Nursing Process: Assessment **Content Area:** Foundational Sciences: Nutrition **Strategy:** Critical items in the question are *alcohol* and neuronal symptoms. Recall knowledge of vitamin absorption and alcohol intake to choose option 2. **Reference:** Adams, M., Josephson, D., & Holland, L. (2005). *Pharmacology for nurses: A pathophysiologic approach.* Upper Saddle River, NJ: Pearson/Prentice Hall, p. 548.

4 **Answer: 4** Processed foods have the highest sodium content. Chocolate pudding is the only option that reflects a processed food item. Meat and milk are animal products and as such have physiological saline. Fresh fruit is lowest in sodium.
Cognitive Level: Analysis **Client Need:** Health Promotion and Maintenance **Integrated Process:** Teaching and Learning **Content Area:** Foundational Sciences: Nutrition **Strategy:** Recall sodium is found in processed foods and many snack foods to direct you to option 4. **Reference:** Nix, S. (2005). *Williams' basic nutrition & diet therapy* (12th ed.). St. Louis, MO: Elsevier Mosby, p. 356.

5 **Answer: 1** Chromium is helpful in maintaining glucose homeostasis by enhancing the activity of the hormone insulin. The other options are sources of vitamins and not minerals.
Cognitive Level: Application **Client Need:** Health Promotion and Maintenance **Integrated Process:** Teaching and Learning **Content Area:** Foundational Sciences: Nutrition **Strategy:** Identify the unique option 1 and associate it with the core issue (mineral) in the stem of question. **Reference:** Rolfes, S., Pinna, K., & Whitney, E. (2006). *Understanding normal and clinical nutrition* (7th ed.). Belmont, CA: Wadsworth & Thomson Learning, p. 456.

6 **Answer: 2** Iodine is predominately found in the thyroid gland, which secretes thyroid hormones that affect the body's metabolic rate. The other options are not associated with thyroid problems. Other minerals that might be affected include sodium, potassium, iron, and calcium, depending on the underlying presentation.
Cognitive Level: Application **Client Need:** Health Promotion and Maintenance **Integrated Process:** Nursing Process: Assessment **Content Area:** Foundational Sciences: Nutrition **Strategy:** Recall normal thyroid function requires iodine to produce the hormone thyroxine to choose option 2. **Reference:** Nix, S. (2005). *Williams' basic nutrition & diet therapy* (12th ed.). St. Louis, MO: Elsevier Mosby, pp. 143–145.

7 **Answer: 2** Clients who exhibit behaviors of eating nonfood items such as ice, clay, and dirt are likely to have iron deficiency. This odd symptom presentation is often the first indicator that there may be a potential problem. Option 1 is incorrect—a client who is dehydrated would be more apt to drink fluids than ice chips. Option 3 is incorrect because there is nothing to indicate that the client is suffering from a protein deficiency. Option

4 is incorrect because the client is not ingesting sufficient fluid to dilute the serum sodium level.
Cognitive Level: Analysis **Client Need:** Health Promotion and Maintenance **Integrated Process:** Nursing Process: Assessment **Content Area:** Foundational Sciences: Nutrition
Strategy: Critical phrases *desire to eat,* indicating a craving and also *possible,* indicating there is not an absolute cause and effect. Eliminate option 4 since the sodium deficiency would be caused by the excessive water intake and not produce a craving for it. Eliminate option 3 as ice is not a source of protein. Recall pica is food craving for nonfood items to choose option 2. **Reference:** Rolfes, S., Pinna, K. & Whitney, E. (2006). *Understanding normal and clinical nutrition* (7th ed.). Belmont, CA: Wadsworth & Thomson Learning, p. 443.

8 **Answer: 4** Folic acid deficiencies have been proven to cause neural tube defects in the developing fetus. Option 1 is incorrect because high levels of folic acid can prevent identification of vitamin B_{12} deficiency. Option 2 is incorrect because high homocysteine levels are associated with folic acid and other B vitamin deficiencies. Option 3 is incorrect because folic acid deficiency results in a macrocytic anemia.
Cognitive Level: Application **Client Need:** Health Promotion and Maintenance **Integrated Process:** Teaching and Learning **Content Area:** Foundational Sciences: Nutrition
Strategy: Recall functions of folic acid in the body to choose option 4. **Reference:** Rolfes, S., Pinna, K. & Whitney, E. (2006). *Understanding normal and clinical nutrition* (7th ed.). Belmont, CA: Wadsworth & Thomson Learning, p. 336.

9 **Answer: 2** Pernicious anemia is due to a clinical deficiency of intrinsic factor that prevents the absorption of vitamin B_{12} in the body. This commonly occurs following gastrectomy. Thus, for treatment to be effective, vitamin B_{12} must be administered via injection for the rest of the client's life. Options 1 and 3 are incorrect because niacin is unrelated to pernicious anemia, and iron will not correct pernicious anemia. Option 4 is incorrect because riboflavin is not related to the issue of pernicious anemia and riboflavin is administered orally.
Cognitive Level: Application **Client Need:** Health Promotion and Maintenance **Integrated Process:** Teaching and Learning **Content Area:** Foundational Sciences: Nutrition
Strategy: Refer to the core issue in the question of the client with pernicious anemia. Pernicious anemia is associated with the intrinsic factor as well as vitamin B_{12} itself. **Reference:** Rolfes, S., Pinna, K. & Whitney, E. (2006). *Understanding normal and clinical nutrition* (7th ed.). Belmont, CA: Wadsworth & Thomson Learning, p. 340.

10 **Answer: 3** This is a normal finding with folate. Increasing water intake might dilute the urine and make it less yellow, but this response does not provide reassurance this is a normal reaction. Reducing amount of folate may not reduce the color. It does not need to be reported.
Cognitive Level: Application **Client Need:** Health Promotion and Maintenance **Integrated Process:** Communication and Documentation **Content Area:** Foundational Sciences: Nutrition **Strategy:** Eliminate option 1 since the question relates to the intake of folate. Eliminate option 4 since it is not a serious threat. Knowledge of normal folate action directs you to option 3. **Reference:** Rolfes, S., Pinna, K. & Whitney, E. (2006). *Understanding normal and clinical nutrition* (7th ed.). Belmont, CA: Wadsworth & Thomson Learning, p. 52.

References

Cataldo, C., DeBruyne, L., & Whitney, E. (2006). *Nutrition and diet therapy* (7th ed.). Belmont, CA: Wadsworth & Thomson Learning, pp. 169–332.

Dudek, S. G. (2006). *Nutritional essentials for nursing practice* (5th ed.). Philadelphia: Lippincott, pp. 93–150.

Grodner, M., Anderson, A. L., & DeYoung, S. (2004). *Foundations and clinical applications of nutrition: A nursing approach* (3rd ed.). St. Louis: Mosby, pp. 166–237.

Institutes of Medicine. Dietary Reference Intakes. http://www.iom.edu, accessed 10/7/05.

Kozier, B., Erb, G., Berman, A. J., & Burke, K. (2004). *Fundamentals of nursing: Concepts, process, and practice* (7th ed.). Upper Saddle River, NJ: Prentice Hall, pp. 1118, 1312–1318.

LeMone, P., & Burke, K. (2004). *Medical-surgical nursing: Critical thinking in client care* (3rd ed.). Upper Saddle River, NJ: Prentice Hall, pp. 118–149, 422–430.

Lutz, C., & Przytulski, K. (2006). *Nutrition and diet therapy* (4th ed.). Philadelphia: F. A. Davis, pp. 97–156.

Nix, S. (2005). *Williams' basic nutrition & diet therapy* (12th ed.). St. Louis, MO: Elsevier Mosby, pp. 87–122.

Rolfes, S., Pinna, K. G. & Whitney, E. (2006). *Understanding normal and clinical nutrition* (7th ed.). Belmont, CA: Wadsworth, pp. 321–460.

Roth, R. A. & Townsend, C. E. (2000). *Nutrition and diet therapy* (7th ed.). Albany, NY: Delmar, pp. 108–165.

Stanfield, P., & Hui, Y. (2003). *Nutrition and diet therapy self-intruction modules* (4th ed.). Sudbury, MA: Jones & Bartlett, p. 75.

Thomson Micromedex. *Micromedex®* Healthcare Series. Vol. 126, accessed 10/9/05.

Nutritional Biochemistry

4

Chapter Outline

Objectives

- Review concepts of digestion, absorption, and transport of macronutrients.
- Identify specific enzymes that facilitate digestion, transport, and absorption of nutrients.
- Explain the complexities of digestion that can affect nutritional intake.
- Review concepts of metabolism for macronutrients.
- Describe the process of catabolism and anabolism.
- Identify the nutritional concerns for clients with altered metabolism.

NCLEX-RN® Test Prep

Use the CD-ROM enclosed with this book to access additional practice opportunities.

Review at a Glance

absorption the process whereby nutrients and chemical substances are taken in and utilized by the body

acetyl-coenzyme A (acetyl-coA) a two-carbon molecule that serves as the common intermediate pathway for entry into the TCA cycle

aerobic metabolism chemical processes that require oxygen to yield energy

anabolism building-up process in the body that is a result of combining substances leading to more complex entities and that requires energy

anaerobic metabolism chemical processes that do not require oxygen to yield energy

beta-oxidation a form of catabolism whereby fatty acids are used as an energy source in the body as a result of oxygenation

catabolism breaking-down process in the body that leads to breakdown of complex entities and that releases energy

digestion the combination of mechanical and chemical factors leading to breakdown of nutrients for absorption

digestive enzymes chemical substances that aid in the digestive process to break down nutrients into constituent parts

electron transport chain (ETC) a series of chemical enzyme reactions whereby electrons are transferred from one protein to another assisted by B vitamins that function as coenzymes to release water and energy in the form of ATP production

gluconeogenesis formation of glucose and glycogen from protein and lipid sources in the body (anabolic process)

glycogenesis formation of glycogen from glucose (anabolic process)

glycolysis enzymatic breakdown process (catabolism) whereby glucose is broken down to form lactic acid or pyruvic acid depending on whether oxygen is required to yield energy

ketone bodies a group of three naturally occurring chemical compounds in the body as a result of normal metabolism (acetoacetic acid, acetone, and β-hydroxybutyric acid) that share a similar structure

malabsorption impaired absorption of nutrients in the GI tract that can arise due to a variety of clinical conditions

metabolism the sum of chemical reactions in the body that are involved in building up (anabolism) and breaking down (catabolism) substances leading to energy formation

transport the movement of substances throughout the body, accomplished by active or passive transport

PRETEST

1 The client with Crohn's disease is not following dietary recommendations. The nurse would expect to assess which of the following clinical manifestations in this client? Select all that apply.

1. Diarrhea
2. Abdominal pain
3. Weight loss
4. Uremia
5. Constipation

2 The nurse would make which of the following statements in explaining how dietary fiber aids in the processes of digestion, transport, and absorption?

1. "Fiber helps to coat the gastric lining of the stomach in order to decrease the acidic environment."
2. "Soluble fiber adds weight to feces, and insoluble fiber acts as a bulking agent to assist in the elimination process."
3. "A large amount of fiber in the diet has no effect on the digestion of nutrients."
4. "Dietary fiber must be taken with mineral oil to be effective in facilitating nutrient digestion, transport, and absorption."

3 Which of the following clients is at greatest risk for developing a digestive problem related to the oral cavity?

1. A 48-year-old male client with a history of gastric reflux
2. An 18-year-old college student eating "fast" food for lunch
3. A 20-year-old client who has past medical history of wisdom teeth removal
4. A 50-year-old client with a history of temporomandibular joint (TMJ) disorder

4 The nurse is performing a gastrointestinal assessment on a client. Which of the following clinical findings would the nurse associate with malabsorption of fat?

1. Steatorrhea
2. Increased gastric emptying
3. Constipation
4. Pallor

5 What client statement would indicate that dietary teaching has been effective in a client with gastroesophageal reflux disease (GERD) regarding dietary practices to facilitate digestion?

1. "I will continue to use antacids on a daily basis."
2. "I will limit late night snacking to prevent GI symptoms."
3. "I will cut up my food into very small pieces to make it easier to chew."
4. "I will limit the amount of fluid and fiber in my diet."

6 The nurse anticipates that which of the following clients admitted to the nursing unit is in the most severe catabolic pattern of metabolism?

1. A 12-year-old adolescent with acute appendicitis
2. A 22-year-old pregnant client with slight painless vaginal bleeding
3. A client who is 5 days postoperative for femoropopliteal bypass
4. A client who was admitted 3 days ago with multiple trauma

7 The nurse expects that a client experiencing which metabolic process will develop lactic acidosis?

1. Glycolysis
2. Anaerobic metabolism
3. Gluconeogenesis
4. Oxidative phosphorylation

8 A client with a history of lactose intolerance confides to the nurse she consumed a large amount of ice cream at a social event. The nurse can expect the client to experience:

1. Bloating and diarrhea
2. Constipation for 2–3 days
3. Foul smelling, bulky stools
4. A headache

9 A client's urine tests positive for presence of ketone bodies. The nurse concludes that this test result indicates which of the following?

1. Excessive intake of simple sugars in diet
2. Decreased lipids in the diet
3. An alkaloid condition in the body
4. Inadequate carbohydrate intake in the diet

10 The nurse would explain to a client with celiac disease that which foods are best to avoid to reduce flares of the disease?

1. Wheat, corn, and rice
2. Barley, soybeans, and corn
3. Wheat, barley, and rye
4. Rice, oats, wheat

See pages 101–103 for Answers and Rationales.

I. CONCEPTS OF DIGESTION, ABSORPTION, AND TRANSPORT OF MACRONUTRIENTS

A. Refer to Box 4-1 for a listing of organs involved in digestion, absorption, and transport of macronutrients

B. Digestion

1. Is the process of breaking down food components as they progress down the gastrointestinal (GI) tract for absorption
2. Muscular actions of peristalsis, segmentation, and sphincter contractions propel food through the GI tract

Box 4-1

Organs Involved in the Digestion, Absorption, and Transport of Macronutrients

- Mouth
- Esophagus
- Stomach
- Small intestine
- Large intestine
- Rectum

3. Secretions in the form of **digestive enzymes** (substances that break down food into smaller compounds) facilitate the process of digestion and act in response to the pH environment of the body
4. The stomach is acidic in nature and the intestines are alkaline in nature
   a. pH of saliva is 7
   b. pH of gastric juice is 2
   c. pH of pancreatic juice is 8
5. Mechanical action in the form of chewing works in conjunction with chemical enzymes to facilitate digestion
6. Bile emulsification of fats occurs in the duodenum and facilitates enzymatic action

C. Absorption

1. Is the process whereby nutrients are absorbed into blood or lymph circulation
2. The increased surface of villi and microvilli on the brush border of the small intestine are the major sites of absorption in conjunction with enzymes
3. Mechanisms such as simple diffusion and facilitated and active transport move nutrients through the GI tract
4. Electrolytes and water are absorbed as the principal end products of digestion along with glucose, amino acids, fatty acids, monoglycerides, glycerol, nucleic acids, cholesterol, vitamins, and minerals
5. Differences in absorption can be influenced by dietary factors (phytates and oxalates) and chemical composition of vitamin structures (water-soluble and fat-soluble)

Practice to Pass

What factors are needed to assist the body in the digestion, absorption, and transport of nutrients?

D. Transport

1. Is the process of delivery of nutrients to all tissues of the body via vascular and lymphatic channels
2. The liver and hepatic circulation are of primary importance in the transport of nutrients
3. Specific transport carriers exist in the body to facilitate transport of needed nutrients
   a. The bloodstream helps to transport water-soluble vitamins and smaller fat molecules
   b. The lymphatics help to transport fat-soluble vitamins and larger fat molecules using chylomicrons and other lipoproteins as carriers

II. DIGESTIVE ENZYMES

A. Summarized in Table 4-1: Physiology of digestion

B. Carbohydrates and fiber

1. Mouth
   a. Salivary glands secrete salivary amylase to start the digestive process of carbohydrate (CHO), changing starch to maltose, and break down starch into smaller products
   b. Mechanical aspects of digestion moisten ingested foods
2. Stomach
   a. Hydrochloric acid (HCl) hydrolyzes CHO into maltose and sucrose
   b. Fiber remains unchanged
3. Small intestine
   a. Pancreatic enzymes (maltase, sucrase, and lactase) break down disaccharides (maltose, sucrose, and lactose) into monosaccharides (building blocks)
   b. Cholecystokinin (CCK) stimulates the hydrolysis of starch
   c. Fiber remains unchanged
4. Large intestine
   a. No further enzyme action of CHO occurs
   b. Bacterial enzyme action breaks fiber down into small chain fatty acids and gas

Table 4-1 Physiology of Digestion

Organ	Fiber	Carbohydrate	Lipid	Protein	Vitamins	Minerals/Water
Mouth	Mechanical action Moisten	Salivary glands Amylase starch	Lingual lipase	Chewing Moisten	No action	Salivary glands add water
Esophagus	Unchanged	Starch	Unchanged	No action	No action	No action
Stomach	Unchanged	HCl hydrolyzes maltose and sucrose	Triglycerides to diglycerides and fatty acids	Pepsin HCl Gastrin	Intrinsic factor vitamin B_{12}	HCl → makes Fe more absorbable Water secretion CHYME
Small intestine	Unchanged	Pancreatic amylase Intestinal secretions Monosaccharide absorption Portal circulation	Fat → bile Emulsified fat Pancreatic lipase → monoglycerides, glycerol, and fatty acids	Amino acid absorption (sodium dependent channels)	Bile emulsifies fat-soluble vitamins Water-soluble vitamins absorbed	Secretion of fluid helps with mineral absorption and vitamin D helps with calcium absorption
Large intestine	Bacterial enzymes Regulation of bowel activity	No action	Cholesterol and fat (bound to fiber) are eliminated through feces	No action	Intestinal synthesis of vitamin K	Water and remaining minerals are absorbed

c. Binding capacity of fiber in the elimination process leads to excretion of cholesterol and other minerals

C. Lipids

1. Mouth
   a. Lingual lipase begins digestion of fat
   b. Temperature in the mouth causes certain fats to melt in the oral cavity
2. Stomach
   a. Enzyme action of lingual lipase leads to breakdown of fats to glycerol and fatty acids
   b. Enzyme action of gastric lipase leads to breakdown of lactose
3. Small intestine
   a. Pancreatic enzymes (pancreatic lipase) break down emulsified fat to glycerol, monoglycerides, and fatty acids
   b. Lipolysis takes place, during which the digestive action of lipase aids decomposition of fats into fatty acids
   c. Bile (from the gallbladder and liver) aids in the emulsification of fat
   d. CCK is secreted in the small intestine in response to dietary proteins and fats and acts on the pancreas to release enzymes and on the gallbladder to release bile salts
   e. CCK aids in hydrolysis of fats and works synergistically with secretin to improve gastric functioning
4. Large intestine
   a. Fat and cholesterol bind to fiber and are eliminated in the feces
   b. Insoluble fiber acts to increase the weight of feces in the body
   c. Soluble fiber acts as a bulking agent because it holds onto water
   d. Adequate hydration helps to move fats for elimination from the body

D. Proteins

1. Mouth
   a. Mechanical digestion of protein occurs in the mouth as saliva helps to moisten food and chewing facilitates the movement of food through the GI tract
   b. No enzyme action of protein takes place in the mouth
2. Stomach
   a. HCl in the stomach converts pepsinogen to pepsin (active form) and further enzymatic action aids breakdown of protein into smaller polypeptide chains
   b. Denaturation occurs under the acidic conditions in the stomach
   c. Hydrolysis of proteins begins with HCl acid activation
   d. Casein (milk protein) and renin help with breakdown of substances
   e. The hormone gastrin is secreted by the gastric mucosa in response to food (sight, smell, and taste), causing activation of gastric juice that is acidic and is needed to activate pepsin
3. Small intestine
   a. Pancreatic enzyme secretion (proteolytic enzymes—trypsin, chymotrypsin, elastin, and carboxypeptidase) leads to breakdown of dipeptides to amino acids
   b. CCK stimulation leads to enzymatic breakdown of proteins

Practice to Pass

What is the clinical significance of digestive body organs having different pH levels?

c. Absorbed amino acids are then taken into the portal vein circulation and liver

4. Large intestine
   a. No enzymatic action takes place in the large intestine
   b. Water is absorbed

III. COMPLEXITIES OF DIGESTION

A. Mouth

1. Swallowing
   a. Structural deformities (cleft lip, cleft palate, temporomandibular joint disorder, poor oral dentition) place clients at risk for swallowing problems
   b. Disease states (cerebrovascular accident [CVA], xerostomia, or oral cavity disease—fungal, herpes simplex) place clients at risk for swallowing problems
2. Esophagus
   a. Structural deformities (achalasia, hiatal hernia) place clients at risk for having esophageal problems
   b. Disease states (gastroesophageal reflux disease [GERD], esophageal cancer, esophageal varices, and Barrett's esophagus) place clients at risk for having esophageal problems
   c. ! Decreased lower esophageal sphincter (LES) pressure correlates with exacerbation of reflux and is associated with dietary intake of alcohol, coffee, tea, chocolate, spearmint, and peppermint

B. Stomach

1. Peristalsis
   a. Is the action of food being pushed through the GI tract under involuntary muscle contraction
   b. Action occurs in a rhythmic wave pattern
2. Gastric juices
   a. Secretion of HCl (from gastric parietal cells) provides an acidic environment that is needed for enzyme action
   b. There are three phases of gastric secretion (cephalic, gastric, and intestinal) that work together in the body
   c. Destruction of stomach lining (by *Helicobacter pylori* and acid-resistant bacteria) leads to the development of ulcers that can cause further structural damage and lead to clinical manifestations
3. Gastric emptying reflex
   a. ! Clients who take medications (antibiotics, antacids, antiemetics, and antisecretory agents) that cause GI side effects or who consume alcohol or drugs can be at risk for developing additional problems that may affect absorption of nutrients
   b. ! Diabetic gastroparesis is the clinical state of decreased gastric emptying caused by hyperglycemic states and causing pain as a result of neuropathy
   c. ! Clients who undergo gastric surgical interventions may be at risk for developing gastroparesis that may be self-limiting with appropriate diet therapy and positioning to use the effects of gravity during and after meals to promote motility

d. Nutrient content of meals can influence the rate of stomach emptying

1) High fat meals remain in the stomach longer than high carbohydrate meals, which have the quickest transit time

2) Larger meals and solid meals remain in the stomach longer than smaller meals and liquids

4. Obstruction

a. Structural deformities (stenosis, mechanical and surgical intervention) place clients at risk for developing nutritional deficiencies due to impaired absorption

b. Bowel sounds must be assessed and documented each shift in order to confirm GI motility

C. Small intestine and large intestine

1. Malabsorption

! a. Occurs in the presence of clinical disease (specific enzyme deficiency, pancreatic disease, liver disease, celiac disease), medications (antacids, laxatives, and antibiotics), infectious disease (parasites), and surgical procedures (gastric/intestinal resection) leading to impaired absorption of nutrients

b. Lactose intolerance is due to a deficiency of the enzyme lactase that leads to manifestations of abdominal cramping, diarrhea, and gas due to inability to break down lactose

! c. Malabsorption of fat leads to clinical manifestation of steatorrhea (bulky, foul-smelling stool that contains unabsorbed fat)

d. The clinical condition of malnutrition can lead to development of multiple malabsorption states

! e. Celiac disease (gluten enteropathy or nontropical sprue) is a genetic autoimmune disorder; dietary gluten (protein found in wheat, rye, oats, and barley products) causes flattening of intestinal villi and clinical manifestations of malabsorption (abdominal distention, diarrhea, vomiting, steatorrhea, and muscle wasting)

1) Dietary management for clients with this condition include the use of a gluten-free diet

2) Lactose may also be restricted and medium chain triglycerides (MCTs) may be used to facilitate absorption of fat

3) The use of pancrease enzyme may be needed to support intestinal enzyme action

f. Clients who have undergone surgical procedures that result in short-bowel syndrome (decreased intestinal surface for absorption) can be prone to develop malabsorption problems

2. Irritable bowel syndrome

a. Is a motility disorder in which the client presents with altered elimination patterns (constipation/diarrhea) and chronic abdominal discomfort (pain/cramping)

! b. Diet choices that favor gas formation (carbonated beverages, vegetables, milk, and dairy products) can contribute to development of clinical symptoms

! c. Alcohol, caffeine, high fat intake, and use of fat substitutes in the diet can also contribute to development of clinical symptoms

3. Inflammatory bowel disease (IBD)
   a. Ulcerative colitis (UC) and regional enteritis (Crohn's disease) represent clinical states that are included in this category
   b. UC occurs in the large intestine; clinical manifestations include bloody diarrhea, abdominal pain and cramping, and weight loss/anorexia, which result in fluid and electrolyte losses
   c. Crohn's disease can occur at any location in the GI tract and is usually found in the ileum and colon; clinical manifestations include diarrhea, abdominal pain, weight loss, and fatigue
   d. Infections may develop due to fistula formation as a result of prolonged inflammation and ulceration of the GI tract
   e. Translocation of bacteria can further contribute to infection
   f. Rupture of the intestines can lead to the development of peritonitis
   g. Medications therapy (anti-inflammatory agents, steroids, and immunosuppressive agents) used to treat the disease state can further contribute to digestive problems
   h. Acute exacerbations of disease may result in dietary route changes (from oral to enteral or parenteral feedings) to maintain nutritional balance and adequate hydration status
4. Obstruction
   a. Can occur in the presence of ruptured diverticula leading to possible peritonitis
   b. Surgical correction for trauma related to injuries and complications of IBD may be required
5. Altered elimination patterns
   a. Diarrhea (as a symptom of disease states or due to medication therapy) contributes to fluid/electrolyte loss and places clients at risk for dehydration
   b. Constipation (as a symptom of disease states or due to medication therapy) contributes to fluid/electrolyte imbalances, abdominal pain, and gas formation

D. Rectum and anus

1. Rectum holds stool until defecation occurs and anus is the point of exit
2. Structural problems
   a. Polyps are small growths that can arise from mucous membrane surfaces throughout the body; rectal polyps can affect elimination
   b. Hemorrhoids are engorged veins in the anal or rectal area that may be present internally or externally; they can affect elimination patterns
   c. Clinical manifestations of rectal/anal structural problems are pain, bleeding, pressure and urge to defecate, and altered elimination

E. Diet-related practices that affect digestion

1. Diets that are very high in various individual nutrients (fiber, fats, protein, CHOs) can cause increased metabolic demands, leading to adverse effects on multiple body organ systems
2. Excess nutrients (CHO, protein, and fat) in the diet lead to fat deposition in the body
3. Diets that are very high in total fluid content may lead to significant fluid, electrolyte, and acid/base imbalances
4. Diets that exclude essential trace elements may lead to significant fluid and electrolyte, or acid/base imbalances and enzyme deficiencies

5. Diets that do not have adequate fluid intake place the client at risk for dehydration and altered elimination patterns
6. Diets that include megatherapy of fat-soluble vitamins in excess of recommended doses can lead to toxic symptom development
7. Adequate fiber and fluids in the diet contribute to regularity (balanced elimination pattern)
8. Poor eating habits (eating late at night and ingesting large portion sizes) can lead to development of GI symptoms and increased weight
9. The use of supplements and enzymes rather than natural food products can lead to increased metabolic stress and affect fluid, electrolyte, and acid-base balance in the body

F. Health rituals that affect digestion

1. Medications (laxatives, antidiarrheals, antacids) used to symptomatically treat GI symptoms on a day-to-day basis may cause alterations of normal digestive/elimination patterns
2. Use of enemas on a daily basis to facilitate elimination may interfere with the body's normal capacity to maintain an elimination pattern, leading to dependency on these agents to achieve elimination
3. Clients with a diagnosed GI disorder (celiac disease, Crohn's disease, UC, GERD, peptic ulcer disease, etc.) should follow the prescribed diet and take ordered medication therapy to avoid exacerbations of the disease process
4. Clients taking antibiotic therapy may require yogurt to provide *Bifidobacterium* and *lactobacillus* in the diet to maintain the necessary intestinal flora for vitamin K synthesis
5. Probiotics (supplements that are used to stimulate immune function) and prebiotics (supplements that stimulate bacterial growth) are being suggested for use to maintain normal intestinal flora and bacterial synthesis in the body
6. Daily exercise can help regulate GI elimination patterns and improve digestive actions

Practice to Pass

How does a clinical state of malabsorption affect the metabolism of nutrients in the body?

IV. CONCEPTS OF METABOLISM OF MACRONUTRIENTS

A. See Table 4–2 for a summary of catabolism and anabolism of macronutrients

B. Metabolism

1. Includes all the chemical reactions of living cells in the body that help to define body energy
2. The liver is the prime metabolic source in the body—it receives nutrients, manufactures bile, detoxifies drugs/alcohol, stores vitamins/minerals, participates in numerous chemical reactions, and aids in the synthesis of proteins needed for immune function, clotting, and transport
3. The pancreas, heart and blood vessels, and kidneys are involved in metabolic activity in the body
   a. The pancreas produces hormones such as insulin and regulates glucose levels in the body
   b. The vascular system assists in the transport of nutrients throughout the body; alterations in vascular function can impede nutrient transport and result in significant cardiac events

Table 4-2

Catabolism and Anabolism of Macronutrients

Macronutrient	Catabolism	Anabolism
Carbohydrate (4 kcal/gram)	Glycolysis (anaerobic) Acetyl-coA (aerobic) Tricarboxylic acid (TCA) Electron transport chain (ETC) Glycogenesis	Glycogenolysis Glucogenesis
Lipid* (9 kcal/gram)	Beta-oxidation Acetyl-coA (aerobic) TCA ETC	Lipogenesis Ketogenesis
Protein (4 kcal/gram)	Deamination Glucogenic, ketogenic, and direct pathways Acetyl-coA (aerobic) TCA ETC	Transamination

*Most concentrated energy source and greatest number of hydrocarbons

c. The kidneys assist in the delicate maintenance of fluid, electrolyte, and acid-base balance, as well as conversion of vitamin D to its active form

4. Thyroid hormones (T_3 and T_4) act together to balance metabolic processes throughout the body as they affect basal metabolic rate (BMR) regulation
    a. An increase in BMR can occur with height, growth, lean body mass, fever, stress, and medications
    b. A decrease in BMR can occur with fasting states, malnutrition, and during sleeping
    c. Age, temperature, and thyroid function can either increase or decrease the BMR
5. The best mix of macronutrients to meet daily energy requirements is 45–65% CHOs, 10–35% protein, and 20–35% fat

C. Anabolism

1. Anabolism refers to chemical reactions that require energy (ATP)
2. The anabolic process is a series of building up reactions
3. Examples of anabolic reactions include glycogen synthesis from glucose, triglyceride synthesis from glycerol and fatty acids, and protein synthesis from amino acids
4. Anabolic reactions are seen in response to increased body demands (growth periods, pregnancy, and following injury/illness)
5. Anabolic factors in the body include insulin, growth hormone (GH), and insulin-like growth factor 1 (IGF-1)

D. Catabolism

1. Catabolism refers to chemical reactions that release energy (ATP)
2. The mitochondria in the cells of the body represent the powerhouse of cellular respiration
3. The catabolic process is a series of breaking-down reactions

4. Examples of catabolic reactions include transfer reactions—breaking down of chemical bonds (glycogen to glucose, triglycerides to fatty acids, and glycerol and protein to amino acids) and oxidative processes

!

5. Catabolic reactions are seen in acute periods of starvation and following injuries and are involved in enzymatic reactions throughout the body
6. Catabolic factors in the body include glucagon, cortisol, cytokines, tumor necrosis factor (TNF), and interleukins

E. **Shared pathways**

1. **Acetyl-coenzyme A** (acetyl-coA)
   a. A common intermediate breakdown product in the metabolic pathway of glucose, fatty acids, and amino acids
   b. Acetyl-coA can be further broken down to enter the tricarboxylic acid (TCA) cycle to provide energy
2. TCA cycle (also called Krebs cycle or citric acid cycle [CAC])
   a. Is a series of chemical reactions involving enzymes and vitamins that lead to a release of energy through the **electron transport chain (ETC)** for all macronutrients
   b. Complete oxidation of acetyl-coA occurs in this cycle leading to formation of CO_2, H^+ ions, and energy in the presence of B vitamins that function as coenzymes
3. ETC (electron transport chain)
   a. Final pathway of the respiratory chain that releases energy due to transfer of electrons
   b. Oxidative phosphorylation involves the passage of H^+ to O_2 and energy release of ADP in a sequential series of protein enzymes
4. Vitamins
   a. The B complex vitamins niacin, folate, thiamin, and vitamin B_{12} function as coenzymes in the metabolic pathway
   b. Vitamin C also participates in the metabolism of protein in the body
   c. Vitamins participate as coenzymes during the metabolic process to provide energy release but do not themselves emit energy
5. Certain steps in the metabolic process are reversible (can move in either direction), whereas others are considered to be irreversible (e.g., pyruvate to acetyl-coA)

Practice to Pass

Compare and contrast the processes of anabolism and catabolism in the body.

V. CARBOHYDRATE METABOLISM

A. **See Table 4-3: Metabolic flow sheet for macronutrients**

B. **Anabolism**

1. **Glycogenesis** involves the buildup of CHO to be stored as glycogen in the liver and muscle cells of the body
2. **Gluconeogenesis** involves the buildup of glucose from alternate sources (amino acids, glycerol, and lactate) to maintain steady glucose levels in response to emerging needs of the body (decreased CHOs in the diet, epinephrine release due to stress, or amino acid fragments from breakdown of fatty acids)

Table 4-3

Metabolic Flow Sheet for Macronutrients

Macronutrient	Breakdown Products	Energy
Carbohydrates	Glucose stored as glycogen Glucose to pyruvate to acetyl-coA	Acetyl-coA to energy Acetyl-coA to TCA to ETC to yield energy
Lipids	Glycerol + fatty acids Glycerol to pyruvate to acetyl-coA Fatty acids reassembled and stored Fatty acid fragments to acetyl-coA	Acetyl-coA to TCA to ETC to yield energy
Protein	Amino acids to body storage Glucogenic–amino acids synthesized to glucose Ketogenic–amino acids converted directly to acetyl-coA Direct–amino acids enter TCA cycle directly	Acetyl-coA to TCA to ETC to yield energy Direct entry into TCA to ETC to yield energy

C. Catabolism

1. **Glycolysis** involves the breakdown (splitting) of glucose molecules to yield pyruvate and ATP
2. **Anaerobic metabolism** requires no oxygen (pathway of glucose to pyruvate to acetyl-coA) and leads to the formation of lactic acid in the body (increased lactate levels can occur in clients who develop shock syndromes or trauma states in response to the body's compensatory response)
3. **Aerobic metabolism** requires oxygen (TCA cycle and ETC) and leads to the release of energy
4. Glycogenolysis involves the breakdown of glycogen storage to glucose molecules
5. Blood glucose levels exert a hormonal effect on the body and the regulation of CHO metabolism helps to establish glycemic control

Practice to Pass

How is the clinical formation of ketone bodies related to carbohydrate and lipid metabolism?

D. Nutritional implications

1. B complex vitamins are needed (B_2, B_6, B_3, folate, and B_{12}) to function as co-enzymes in the TCA and ETC
2. Anaerobic versus aerobic requirements
   a. The body will revert to anaerobic metabolism if oxygen is not available in order to maintain balance
   b. If adequate glucose is not available (either by ingestion or conversion), then the body will convert pyruvate to lactic acid
   c. Anaerobic metabolism results in a buildup of lactic acid (lactic acidosis) that can cause significant clinical effects ranging from mild (nausea and cramping) to severe (death)
3. Excess CHOs are converted to fat and become deposited in the body because the liver and muscle cells have a storage limit
4. ! An incomplete breakdown of fats due to decreased CHO levels leads to the development of **ketone bodies** (acetone, acetoacetate, and β-hydroxybutyrate) that are associated with clinical manifestations of disease (diabetes, toxemia)
5. Increased level of ketones result in ketosis, which can also occur as a response to fasting, exercise, insulin levels, or intake of a low CHO diet

6. If the CHO availability is inadequate, then protein sources will be utilized (gluconeogenesis); a minimum amount of 50–100 grams/day of CHO is needed in the diet to spare protein

!

7. Blood glucose level regulation is stimulated by a complex series of hormone responses and cellular activity

VI. LIPID METABOLISM

A. See Table 4-3 for metabolic flow sheet for macronutrients

B. Anabolism

1. Lipogenesis involves the conversion/combination of glycerol and fatty acids to form triglycerides
2. Ketogenesis refers to the process whereby fats are incompletely broken down into ketone bodies

C. Catabolism

1. Triglyceride breakdown leads to the formation of glycerol, carbon fragments, and fatty acids
2. Glycerol can exchange with glucose to enter into the metabolic pathway
3. Pyruvate conversion to lactic acid can occur
4. **Beta-oxidation** (fatty acid oxidation) involves the addition of oxygen to fat molecules (to release fatty acid fragments) so that fats can enter the common metabolic pathway
5. Fatty acid fragments can convert to acetyl-coA and enter the common metabolic pathway
6. Carnitine (amino acid) acts as a stimulant for oxidation of long chain fatty acids
7. Final end products of fatty acid metabolism are CO_2 and H_2O

D. Nutritional implications

1. Ketone bodies
   - **a.** Intermediate products of acetyl-coA fragments from fatty acid degradation yield ketone bodies if CHO sources are not available (condensation of two acetyl-coA molecules)
   - **b.** Acetoacetic, acetone, and β-hydroxybutyric acid are the three ketone bodies produced in the body
   - **c.** The presence of ketone bodies suggests that the body needs an additional fuel source

!

   - **d.** Monitoring for ketone bodies and ketonuria is indicated in clients who evidence diabetes, fasting states, and low-CHO diets
   - **e.** The presence of ketone bodies leads to acidemia, decrease in appetite, metabolic rate, and lean organ mass as the body attempts to conserve and maintain energy

Practice to Pass

Why are fats not considered to be a primary energy source even though they provide 9 kcal/gram?

2. Storage and energy concerns
   - **a.** The body has a limitless capacity to store fat in the form of adipose tissue
   - **b.** Fat is not considered to be an efficient energy source due to repeated aerobic reactions that are required to produce carbon fragments that can participate in the catabolic process

c. Serum triglyceride levels are related to the ingestion of fat, CHO, and alcohol in the diet

3. Fatty acids cannot be used to make glucose
   a. Only a small portion of fats (glycerol) can participate in the conversion to glucose
   b. Due to repeated chemical reaction processing required, fats are not considered a primary source of energy

VII. PROTEIN METABOLISM

A. See Table 4-3 for metabolic flow sheet for macronutrients

B. Anabolism

1. Transamination involves the transfer of an amino group to a keto acid (vitamin B_6 is specifically required for this process)
2. The liver can synthesize nonessential amino acids in the body
3. Amino acids can be converted to fat, acetyl-coA, and glucose (gluconeogenesis)

C. Catabolism

1. Amino acids that can be used to synthesize glucose are called glucogenic
2. Amino acids that can be directly converted to acetyl-coA are called ketogenic
3. The term direct refers to amino acids that can enter the TCA cycle without undergoing chemical restructuring
4. Deamination involves the removal of an amine group from an amino acid to yield a keto acid and ammonia; this process leads to energy formation as keto acids (ketosis) become an alternate fuel source
5. The urea cycle helps to eliminate nitrogen wastes (ammonia) from the body that are a result of protein degradation

D. Nutritional implications

1. Nitrogen balance
   a. The body attempts to maintain nitrogen balance, which reflects adequate protein synthesis
   b. Stress states impose increased metabolic demands, leading to negative nitrogen balance as the body depletes stores to provide energy (less in/more out)
   c. Growth periods impose increased metabolic demands, leading to positive nitrogen balance as body builds new tissues (more in/less out)
2. Nitrogen waste elimination–urea cycle
   a. Ammonia gets converted to urea in the liver and is then excreted by the kidneys
   b. Clients with renal/liver disease have a decreased ability to get rid of waste products leading to uremia
   c. Increased levels of ammonia and urea contribute to profound fluid, electrolyte and acid-base imbalances that can have serious neurological consequences
   d. Adequate fluid levels are needed in the body to help eliminate waste products
   e. Protein levels need to be evaluated for clients who have renal/liver problems—high protein loads can further contribute to clinical manifestations because the body cannot eliminate waste products

f. Clients who have contributory disease (heart failure and diabetes) are prone to develop problems related to nitrogen waste elimination and should be closely monitored

3. B complex vitamins and vitamin C are necessary for protein metabolism
4. Storage and energy concerns
   a. Excess protein can be stored as fat in the body if it is not needed for energy or the building of body tissues
   b. Protein can be used as an energy source in the body if adequate CHO is not available

Practice to Pass

How does protein metabolism differ from the metabolism of fat and carbohydrates in the body?

VIII. IMPLICATIONS OF ALCOHOL ON NUTRIENT METABOLISM

A. Absorption pathways

1. Alcohol is absorbed directly into the bloodstream
2. Alcohol levels can be measured in the blood ranging from 0.001 to 0.50 with corresponding clinical symptoms ranging from euphoria to coma
3. There are differences in the rate of alcohol absorption, with females absorbing at a faster rate than males, and older clients being affected more readily than younger clients

B. Biochemical effects of alcohol

1. Alcohol ingestion results in a state of metabolic acidosis with an increased anion gap
2. A high ratio of NADH to NAD+ plus alcohol leads to an "altered redox state" (reduction–oxidation reaction)
3. NADH causes an acidotic shift—the amount of acetyl-coA increases and is prevented from entering the TCA cycle; this leads to the formation of fatty acids
4. Ketone bodies + fatty acids lead to an increase in triglycerides, which can lead to fatty liver infiltration, fibrosis, cirrhosis, and liver failure
5. ! Chronic alcohol use affects the pancreas and in response to elevated lipid and triglycerides levels can lead to pancreatitis
6. Chronic alcohol use can affect the cardiac muscle, leading to fibrosis, weakness, alcoholic cardiomyopathy, and congestive heart failure
7. ! Short-term or chronic alcohol use can affect the brain, leading to altered cerebellar function and differences in mood and behavior
8. Four methods of alcohol metabolism have been identified; action of alcohol dehydrogenase (liver and gastric mucosa), endoplasmic reticulum, MEOS (microsomal ethanol-oxidizing system), and fatty acids (ethyl esters)
   a. The action of alcohol dehydrogenase is dependent on the presence of NAD in the body
   b. During the metabolism of alcohol, hydrogen ions are added to NAD and NADH accumulates, resulting in significant metabolic changes (inhibits acetyl-coA from entering TCA cycle and leads to fatty acid formation with resultant liver changes)

c. Enzymatic breakdown of alcohol leads to acetaldehyde (responsible for clinical symptoms of alcohol abuse) that in turns converts to acetate to form acetyl-coA

d. Increased lactic acid formation occurs along with uric acid production

e. The MEOS enzyme system in the body responds to alcohol and increases its activity

f. The MEOS system also assists the body in detoxifying drugs; if the client has a large amount of alcohol in the system, the MEOS processes the alcohol rather than medications

! **C. Nutritional effects of alcohol**

1. Alcohol provides 7 kcal/gram but is considered to be a nonnutrient because it provides calories without nutritional benefit
2. In response to ingestion of alcohol, one usually experiences a decrease in appetite and changes in the gastric and duodenal mucosa that lead to decreased digestion and absorption of nutrients
3. Nutritional deficiencies may include deficiencies in the B complex vitamins of thiamin, folate, and vitamin B_{12}

a. A decrease in these B complex vitamins can result in a corresponding decrease of needed enzyme co-factors, an increased homocysteine level in the body, and a decrease in the production of intrinsic factor

b. The presence of nutritional anemias can be seen in response to these clinical deficiencies that will require therapeutic treatment in order to restore blood levels (refer to Chapter 3 for further discussion)

c. Associated B vitamin deficiencies can also manifest with the development of peripheral neuropathy

d. Wernicke-Korsakoff syndrome is seen in clients with alcoholism who have a severe thiamin deficiency, resulting in severe neurological impairment and psychosis

D. Alcohol and malnutrition

1. Clients with alcoholism often present as malnourished with significant depletions in potassium, magnesium, and phosphorus in addition to vitamin deficiencies previously discussed
2. Dietary patterns of clients with alcoholism are usually not well-balanced and therefore poor dietary intake further contributes to overall state of malnutrition
3. ! Since alcoholism is considered to be a disease (drug dependency addictive state), the client not only suffers from the disease process itself but also goes through the clinical symptoms of withdrawal (delirium tremors) with sudden cessation of alcohol use
4. The client needs to incorporate lifestyle changes, obtain and utilize client and family support systems, and develop beneficial health habits as an ongoing process
5. Recognition of dietary deficiencies and provision of both nutritional support and dietary education are needed to support the client in achieving life goals of maintaining sobriety

Case Study

A 58-year-old male client with a history of alcohol abuse is seen for a nutritional assessment and dietary management. Upon assessment, the client states that he "only drinks a few beers a day." Present medical history reveals an abnormal liver profile but no presence of contributory disease processes. The client states that he "doesn't understand what all the fuss is about" as he isn't having any problems.

1. What specific information would you want to confirm regarding alcohol consumption for this client?
2. Discuss the biochemical effects of alcohol consumption.
3. What effect is alcohol intake expected to have on this client's nutritional status?
4. What specific nutrient deficiencies would you expect to see in this client?
5. What methods would you utilize to improve this client's nutritional status?

For suggested responses, see page 318.

POSTTEST

1 The nurse would explain to a client who underwent gastric resection that which of the following meals is most likely to cause rapid emptying of the stomach?

1. Broiled steak and green beans
2. Fried chicken and creamed potatoes
3. Baked fish and fresh carrots
4. Pasta with broccoli and garlic bread sticks

2 The nurse is caring for a client at risk for short gut syndrome. The nurse would choose which of the following statements to explain the role of the small intestine in absorption of nutrients?

1. "Nutrients are delivered to the small intestine in a rapid manner to facilitate absorption."
2. "The acidic environment of the small intestine enhances digestive enzyme function."
3. "Increased surface area of the microvilli on the lining of the intestine favors absorption of nutrients."
4. "The small intestine is able to facilitate the absorption of dietary fibers."

3 The nurse identifies the client who has which of the following to be most at risk for malabsorption of nutrients?

1. Hypoactive bowel sounds
2. Colon resection
3. Rectal polyps
4. Gastric surgical resection

4 The nurse instructs the client who develops heartburn as a result of gastroesophageal reflux disease (GERD) to avoid which of the following foods?

1. Lettuce
2. Eggs
3. Chocolate
4. Butterscotch

5 Which of the following food items should the nurse recommend to facilitate intestinal synthesis of vitamin K for a client receiving antibiotic therapy?

1. Eggs
2. Wheat germ
3. Yogurt
4. Fish

6 Which of the following foods should the nurse remove from the lunch tray of a client diagnosed with celiac disease?

1. Butter
2. Beef barley soup
3. Fresh yellow squash
4. Coffee

7 When caring for a client with a history of alcoholism, the nurse checks laboratory values, anticipating deficiencies of which of the following micronutrients?

1. Magnesium and phosphorus
2. Sodium and potassium
3. Magnesium and chloride
4. Calcium and potassium

8 The nurse anticipates that which of the following metabolic processes will most likely occur in a client recently admitted in hypovolemic shock?

1. Gluconeogenesis
2. Anaerobic metabolism
3. Glycogenesis
4. Transamination

9 A nurse teaching a group of 13-year-old students about the role of vitamins in the metabolism of nutrients would make which of the following statements?

1. "Vitamins are needed because they provide additional energy sources."
2. "Vitamins are needed because they participate as enzymes in metabolic processes."
3. "Vitamins are needed to supply additional calories."
4. "Vitamins are needed in large quantities in order to prevent oxidation of vital nutrients."

10 A client who has a history of alcoholism is receiving intravenous therapy with 5% dextrose in 0.45% sodium chloride and a regular diet. When the client refuses the ordered thiamine supplement, the nurse should monitor for which potential complication?

1. Confusion and ataxia
2. Abdominal cramps and diarrhea
3. Headaches and nausea
4. Numbness and tingling in the extremities.

ANSWERS & RATIONALES

Pretest

1 **Answer: 1, 2, 3** Crohn's disease can occur at any location in the GI tract, and the most common clinical manifestations are diarrhea, abdominal pain, weight loss, and fatigue. The disease is not characterized by constipation or uremia. The amount of bulk or fiber in the diet is reduced during acute episodes to control the diarrhea. **Cognitive Level:** Analysis **Client Need:** Physiological Integrity: Physiological Adaptation **Integrated Process:** Nursing Process: Assessment **Content Area:** Foundational Sciences: Nutrition **Strategy:** Refer to similarities of indicators associated with the GI tract. Uremia is associated with renal disease and so cannot be a correct option. Constipation is opposite of the clinical findings in Crohn's disease and can thus be eliminated also. **Reference:** Dudek, S. (2006). *Nutritional essentials for nursing practice* (5th ed.). Philadelphia: Lippincott Williams & Wilkins, pp. 500–503.

2 **Answer: 2** The inclusion of dietary fibers helps to add fecal weight (soluble) and bulking (insoluble), which assists with elimination patterns. Option 1 is incorrect because fiber does not provide a coating effect to the gastric lining. Option 3 is incorrect because dietary fiber can affect digestion of nutrients, especially when consumed in large amounts. Option 4 is incorrect because there is no evidence to support the practice of taking mineral oil with dietary fiber to facilitate digestion, transport, and absorption. **Cognitive Level:** Application **Client Need:** Health Promotion and Maintenance **Integrated Process:** Communication and Documentation **Content Area:** Foundational Sciences: Nutrition **Strategy:** Note that each option contains the word "fiber," so read each option carefully and systematically eliminate options 1, 3, and 4 as incorrect. Choose option 2 because it is comprehensive for processes of digestion. **Reference:** Dudek, S. (2006). *Nutritional essentials for nursing practice* (5th ed.). Philadelphia: Lippincott Williams & Wilkins, pp. 22–23.

3 **Answer: 4** A client with TMJ disorder is at risk for developing swallowing problems due to pain experienced from incorrect jaw alignment. Option 1 is incorrect

because this client would have problems related to the esophagus. Option 2 is incorrect because "fast food" ingestion does not cause digestive problems. Option 3 is incorrect because a client with wisdom teeth removal may have initial discomfort and swallowing problems, but they usually resolve as healing occurs. Clients with TMJ disorder are likely to have acute exacerbations that can become problematic, affecting dietary intake and leading to a significant complication—weight loss.
Cognitive Level: Analysis **Client Need:** Physiological Integrity: Physiological Adaptation **Integrated Process:** Nursing Process: Analysis **Content Area:** Foundational Sciences: Nutrition **Strategy:** Refer to options 3 and 4, which have similarities and association to the oral cavity. Choose option 4 because it is more comprehensive. **Reference:** Rolfes, S., Pinna, K., & Whitney, E. (2006). *Understanding normal and clinical nutrition* (7th ed.). Belmont, CA: Wadsworth & Thomson Learning, p. 76.

4 **Answer: 1** Steatorrhea (bulky, foul-smelling stool) is a common finding related to malabsorption of fats. Option 2 is incorrect—gastric emptying time would be decreased as nutrients pass more quickly because they can't be absorbed. Option 3 is incorrect because diarrhea and steatorrhea are more common findings. Option 4 is a nonspecific finding that is independent of fat malabsorption and may be related to other factors such as anemia and decreased oxygenation states.
Cognitive Level: Application **Client Need:** Physiological Integrity: Physiological Adaptation **Integrated Process:** Nursing Process: Analysis **Content Area:** Foundational Sciences: Nutrition **Strategy:** The core concept is malabsorption of fat. Recall physiology of bile action on stool to direct you to option 1. If you had difficulty with the question, note similarity in ending of word "steatorrhea" and "diarrhea." **Reference:** Dudek, S. (2006). *Nutritional essentials for nursing practice* (5th ed.). Philadelphia: Lippincott Williams & Wilkins, p. 490.

5 **Answer: 2** Eating late at night can lead to development of GI symptoms as increased presence of food in the stomach leads to an increase in acid secretion. If the client lies down with a full stomach, it further causes gastric distention and aggravation of clinical symptoms. Option 1 is incorrect because use of a daily antacid can cause alterations in digestion, transport, and absorption of nutrients that can further increase GI discomfort. Option 3 is incorrect because there is nothing to indicate that this client has a problem with swallowing or dentition. Option 4 is incorrect because water and fiber are necessary in the diet to facilitate adequate elimination patterns.
Cognitive Level: Analysis **Client Need:** Health Promotion and Maintenance **Integrated Process:** Nursing Process: Evaluation **Content Area:** Foundational Sciences: Nutrition **Strategy:** Associate the client action (lying down) with definition of GERD (backflow of acidic gastric juices). **Reference:** Dudek, S. (2006). *Nutritional essentials for nursing practice* (5th ed.). Philadelphia: Lippincott Williams & Wilkins, p. 487.

6 **Answer: 4** Catabolism refers to processes involving the release of energy in order to restore body dynamics and is seen in clients undergoing acute periods of starvation and/or traumatic injury. The client in option 4 has the most severe triggering condition for catabolism. The client in option 1 would undergo catabolism, but this is a short-term event compared to option 4. The clients in options 2 and 3 are in an anabolic pattern of metabolism representing growth states and new tissue development.
Cognitive Level: Analysis **Client Need:** Physiological Integrity: Physiological Adaptation **Integrated Process:** Nursing Process: Analysis **Content Area:** Foundational Sciences: Nutrition **Strategy:** Option 4 is more comprehensive than the other options offered. **Reference:** Nix, S. (2005). *Williams' basic nutrition & diet therapy* (12th ed.). St. Louis, MO: Elsevier Mosby, p. 44.

7 **Answer: 2** Lactic acidosis is associated with anaerobic metabolism. All of the other options represent metabolic processes during which oxygen is required.
Cognitive Level: Application **Client Need:** Health Promotion and Maintenance **Integrated Process:** Nursing Process: Analysis **Content Area:** Foundational Sciences: Nutrition **Strategy:** The core issue of the question is knowledge of the nature of lactic acidosis as a bodily process. Analyze each option in terms of its use of oxygen. **Reference:** Rolfes, S., Pinna, K., & Whitney, E. (2006). *Understanding normal and clinical nutrition* (7th ed.). Belmont, CA: Wadsworth & Thomson Learning, p. 488.

8 **Answer: 1** Lactose intolerant individuals usually lack the enzyme lactase, necessary to break down milk sugars. Lack of the enzyme causes abdominal cramps, diarrhea, and gas formation. The other symptoms would not be caused by lack of lactase.
Cognitive Level: Application **Client Need:** Physiological Integrity: Physiological Adaptation **Integrated Process:** Nursing Process: Assessment **Content Area:** Foundational Sciences: Nutrition **Strategy:** Recall function of lactase to break down milk sugars and inability of this will result in formation of gas. Systematically eliminate options 1 and 3 as not due to abdominal gas formation. Eliminate option 2 since it is associated with lack of bile and pancreatic enzymes. **Reference:** Rolfes, S., Pinna, K., & Whitney, E. (2006). *Understanding normal and clinical nutrition* (7th ed.). Belmont, CA: Wadsworth & Thomson Learning, pp. 544–545.

9 **Answer: 4** Ketone bodies are formed in response to the incomplete breakdown of fatty acids, when lipids are used as an alternate energy source in response to low ingestion of CHOs, high protein or high fat intake, or

fasting states. The presence of ketone bodies is associated with acidotic states.

Cognitive Level: Analysis **Client Need:** Physiological Integrity: Reduction of Risk Potential **Integrated Process:** Nursing Process: Analysis **Content Area:** Foundational Sciences: Nutrition **Strategy:** Recall ketone bodies are formed from fatty acid breakdown and recall conditions when body does this to direct you to option 4. **Reference:** Rolfes, S., Pinna, K., & Whitney, E. (2006). *Understanding normal and clinical nutrition* (7th ed.). Belmont, CA: Wadsworth & Thomson Learning, p. 126.

10 **Answer: 3** Celiac disease is due to inability to digest gluten sources, such as found in wheat, rye, oats, and barley products. All other options have an unrelated source of gluten.

Cognitive Level: Analysis **Client Need:** Health Promotion and Maintenance **Integrated Process:** Nursing Process: Analysis **Content Area:** Foundational Sciences: Nutrition **Strategy:** Refer to the sources of gluten in option 3. **Reference:** Dudek, S. (2006). *Nutritional essentials for nursing practice* (5th ed.). Philadelphia: Lippincott Williams & Wilkins, p. 404.

Posttest

1 **Answer: 4** Meals that are high in carbohydrates, such as the meal in option 4, promote rapid gastric emptying. The other options are associated with increased transit time because they contain sources of protein or fat, and meals of these types remain in the stomach for a longer time.

Cognitive Level: Analysis **Client Need:** Health Promotion and Maintenance **Integrated Process:** Nursing Process: Analysis **Content Area:** Foundational Sciences: Nutrition **Strategy:** Recall gastric resection reduces size of stomach and review physiology of food metabolism. Note CHO will increase osmotic load, which will promote peristalsis, to choose option 4. **Reference:** Dudek, S. (2006). *Nutritional essentials for nursing practice* (5th ed.). Philadelphia: Lippincott Williams & Wilkins, p. 396.

2 **Answer: 3** The increased surface area of the microvilli on the brush border of the small intestine favors the process of absorption by increasing the surface contact area. Option 1 is incorrect—there is specialization in the GI tract that allows for specific nutrient release in order to maximize absorption. Option 2 is incorrect because the small intestine has an alkaline environment. Option 4 is incorrect because dietary fiber consists of undigested material that usually enters the large intestine for bacterial degradation and elimination as feces.

Cognitive Level: Application **Client Need:** Health Promotion and Maintenance **Integrated Process:** Teaching and Learning **Content Area:** Foundational Sciences: Nutrition **Strategy:** Note the nurse is explaining the function of the small intestine in relation to its absorption function and needs to explain it in lay terms. Eliminate options 2 and 4 as incorrect; option 1 does not provide a clear explanation. **Reference:** Rolfes, S., Pinna, K., & Whitney, E. (2006). *Understanding normal and clinical nutrition* (7th ed.). Belmont, CA: Wadsworth & Thomson Learning, pp. 555–556.

3 **Answer: 4** Gastric surgical resection can cause an alteration in the absorption of nutrients due to altered surface area, thereby delaying entry of food from the stomach to the intestines (decreasing absorption and digestion). Option 1 is incorrect because hypoactive bowel sounds may or may not affect absorption. Option 2 would affect fluid reabsorption in the large intestine, but most nutrients would have been absorbed before entering the large intestine. Option 3 may affect elimination patterns but does not affect the absorption of nutrients.

Cognitive Level: Analysis **Client Need:** Physiological Integrity: Physiological Adaptation **Integrated Process:** Nursing Process: Assessment **Content Area:** Foundational Sciences: Nutrition **Strategy:** Eliminate options 1 and 3 since these conditions would not affect nutrient absorption. Note option 4 involves the gastric area to direct you to it. **Reference:** Rolfes, S., Pinna, K., & Whitney, E. (2006). *Understanding normal and clinical nutrition* (7th ed.). Belmont, CA: Wadsworth & Thomson Learning, pp. 555–556.

4 **Answer: 3** Ingestion of chocolate can reduce lower esophageal sphincter (LES) pressure, leading to reflux and clinical symptoms of GERD. All of the other foods do not affect LES pressure.

Cognitive Level: Application **Client Need:** Health Promotion and Maintenance **Integrated Process:** Teaching and Learning **Content Area:** Foundational Sciences: Nutrition **Strategy:** The concept of the question is identification of foods that will complicate GERD. Recall the physiology of this to choose option 3. **Reference:** Rolfes, S., Pinna, K., & Whitney, E. (2006). *Understanding normal and clinical nutrition* (7th ed.). Belmont, CA: Wadsworth & Thomson Learning, pp. 459–460.

5 **Answer: 3** Antibiotic therapy can lead to destruction of normal intestinal flora that is used to synthesize vitamin K. Yogurt contains bacteria that help to promote intestinal synthesis. The other options do not contain necessary bacteria.

Cognitive Level: Application **Client Need:** Health Promotion and Maintenance **Integrated Process:** Nursing Process: Implementation **Content Area:** Foundational Sciences: Nutrition **Strategy:** Critical words are *intestinal synthesis of vitamin K* and *antibiotic therapy.* Recall yogurt is a probiotic to choose this option. **Reference:** Nix, S. (2005). *Williams' basic nutrition & diet therapy* (12th ed.). St. Louis, MO: Elsevier Mosby, pp. 95–97.

6 **Answer: 2** Celiac disease is a malabsorption disorder affecting the small intestine in which there is a problem with the ingestion of gluten, a protein normally found in grain products such as wheat, rye, oats, or barley. The other options reflect substances that do not contain gluten and should not pose problems for a client with this disorder.

Cognitive Level: Application **Client Need:** Health Promotion and Maintenance **Integrated Process:** Nursing Process: Implementation **Content Area:** Foundational Sciences: Nutrition **Strategy:** Recall knowledge of celiac disease and foods containing gluten to direct you to option 2. **Reference:** Nix, S. (2005). *Williams' basic nutrition & diet therapy* (12th ed.). St. Louis, MO: Elsevier Mosby, p. 331.

7 **Answer: 1** Because of deficient nutritional intake, the client with alcoholism frequently has deficiencies of many nutrients. Electrolytes that are particularly affected are magnesium and phosphorus, since they are utilized in maintaining energy production and numerous enzyme reactions.

Cognitive Level: Application **Client Need:** Physiological Integrity: Reduction of Risk Potential **Integrated Process:** Nursing Process: Assessment **Content Area:** Foundational Sciences: Nutrition **Strategy:** Key words are *alcoholism, lab values,* and *deficiencies.* Note all options have two answers and both must be correct for the option to be correct. Recall nutritional intake deficiencies associated with alcohol intake to direct you to option 1. **Reference:** Rolfes, S., Pinna, K., & Whitney, E. (2006). *Understanding normal and clinical nutrition* (7th ed.). Belmont, CA: Wadsworth & Thomson Learning, pp. 558–560.

8 **Answer: 2** Clients who are in shock are likely to form lactic acid as the body reverts to anaerobic metabolism in order to maintain homeostasis. Options 1 and 2 are incorrect—these represent metabolic processes that require oxygen (aerobic metabolism). Option 4 is incorrect because transamination involves the exchange of amine groups in amino acids and reflects an anabolic process.

Cognitive Level: Application **Client Need:** Physiological Integrity: Physiological Adaptation **Integrated Process:** Nursing Process: Analysis **Strategy:** Critical words are *metabolic processes* and *hypovolemic shock.* Recall concepts of shock and energy requirements to direct you to option 2. **Reference:** Rolfes, S., Pinna, K., & Whitney, E. (2006). *Understanding normal and clinical nutrition* (7th ed.). Belmont, CA: Wadsworth & Thomson Learning, pp. 542–543.

9 **Answer: 2** Vitamins function as coenzymes in many of the metabolic processes in the body to facilitate energy release. Options 1 and 3 are incorrect—by themselves vitamins do not provide energy or supply additional calories. Option 4 is incorrect—vitamins should not be consumed in large quantities because they can reach toxic levels (fat-soluble vitamins).

Cognitive Level: Application **Client Need:** Health Promotion and Maintenance **Integrated Process:** Teaching and Learning **Content Area:** Foundational Sciences: Nutrition **Strategy:** Eliminate options 1 and 3 since both are similar concepts. Eliminate option 4 since this practice would be dangerous with certain vitamins. **Reference:** Nix, S. (2005). *Williams' basic nutrition & diet therapy* (12th ed.). St. Louis, MO: Elsevier Mosby, pp. 87–88

10 **Answer: 1** Clients with alcoholism are usually deficient in thiamine, which is needed for carbohydrate metabolism. Administration of glucose solutions can precipitate symptoms of Wernicke's encephalopathy, characterized by disorientation, memory difficulties, diplopia, ataxia, and nystagmus. The other symptoms may be experienced for other reasons in the alcoholic client, but option 1 is most indicative of the thiamine deficiency.

Cognitive Level: Analysis **Client Need:** Physiological Integrity: Physiological Adaptation **Integrated Process:** Nursing Process: Assessment **Content Area:** Foundational Sciences: Nutrition **Strategy:** Critical words are *alcoholism* and *thiamine.* Recall the role of thiamine in CHO metabolism, and recognize the client is receiving a dextrose solution to associate the symptoms of option 1 to Wernicke's encephalopathy. **Reference:** Lutz, C., & Pryztulski, K. (2006). *Nutrition and diet therapy* (4th ed.). Philadelphia: F.A. Davis, pp. 110, 489.

References

Cataldo, C., DeBruyne, L., & Whitney, E. (2006). *Nutrition and diet therapy* (3rd ed.). Belmont, CA: Wadsworth, pp. 95–127.

Dudek, S. G. (2006). *Nutrition essentials for nursing practice* (5th ed.). Philadelphia: Lippincott, pp. 153–174.

Grodner, M., Anderson, A. L., & DeYoung, S. (2004). *Foundations and clinical applications of nutrition: A nursing approach* (3rd ed.). St. Louis: Mosby, pp. 12–13, 62–81, 248–254.

Kozier, B., Erb, G., Berman, A. J., & Burke, K. (2004). *Fundamentals of nursing: Concepts, process, and practice* (7th ed.). Upper Saddle River, NJ: Prentice Hall, pp. 1116–1118.

LeMone, P., & Burke, K. (2004). *Medical-surgical nursing: Critical thinking in client care* (7th ed.). Upper Saddle River, NJ: Prentice Hall, pp. 422–427, 461, 469–474, 503–504.

Lutz, C., & Przytulski, K. (2006). *Nutrition and diet therapy* (4th ed.). Philadelphia: F. A. Davis, pp. 181–198.

Nix, S. (2005). *Williams' basic nutrition & diet therapy* (12th ed.). St. Louis, MO: Elsevier Mosby, pp. 57–73, 367–391.

Rolfes, S., Pinna, K., & Whitney, E. (2006). *Understanding normal and clinical nutrition* (9th ed.). Belmont, CA: Wadsworth, pp. 73–100, 228–249.

Nutrition Needs across the Lifespan

5

Chapter Outline

Preconceptual Nutrition
Pregnancy
Infant Nutrition (0–12 months)
Childhood Nutrition (1–10 years)
Adolescent Nutrition (11–18 years)
Adult Nutrition (18–64 years)
Geriatric Nutrition (65+ years)

Objectives

- Explain the importance of preconceptual nutrition for the client of childbearing age.
- Describe nutritional requirements for the pregnant and lactating client.
- Explain nutritional concerns for the pregnant client with preexisting disease or encountering health problems during the course of the pregnancy.
- Describe nutritional requirements for the infant, child, and adolescent client.
- Describe nutritional requirements for the adult client.
- Describe nutritional requirements for the geriatric client.
- Explain the importance of meeting increased nutritional demands during the life span as the client develops and matures.
- Explain how developmental needs, cultural diversity, and financial concerns can influence nutritional status during the lifespan of the client.

NCLEX-RN® Test Prep

Use the CD-ROM enclosed with this book to access additional practice opportunities.

Review at a Glance

critical periods time periods during the development of tissues and organ systems in which cell division and differentiation are most rapid; these tissues and organs have increased susceptibility to injurious substances at this time, hence the term critical period

failure to thrive (FTT) inadequate growth pattern during infancy that results in a documented weight and/or height that is significantly below expected standards of growth

gestational diabetes emergence of altered glucose metabolism during the term of pregnancy in a client with no clinical history of diabetes

hyperemesis gravidarum (HG) severe nausea and vomiting associated with pregnancy accompanied by severe fluid and electrolyte depletion that can adversely affect maternal well-being and compromise nutritional status if the client is not restored to proper hydration balance

maximum heart rate a number calculated by taking 220 minus the age in years; used to calculate target heart rates

nursing bottle syndrome state of dental disease and decay resulting from prolonged exposure to substances high in glucose content

nutritional stores substances needed to support life processes and the developing fetus

physiological anemia of pregnancy expected consequence during pregnancy that arises from an increase in blood volume that results in hemodilution

target heart rate a range of percentages, usually 50–90%, into which an individual's heart rate should fall during aerobic exercise; percentage depends on level of fitness; range calculated by taking each percentage times the maximum heart rate

teratogen any agent that can cause development of abnormal structures in developing embryo/fetus

TORCH an acronym used to identify infectious disease that can cause serious harm to the developing fetus; diseases include toxoplasmosis, rubella, cytomegalovirus, and herpes simplex

PRETEST

1 As prophylaxis against neural tube defects (NTD), the nurse should recommend that a client planning to conceive for the first time should take in how many milligrams of folic acid daily? Provide a numerical response.

Answer: ________________________

2 A new breastfeeding client is having difficulty with sore nipples. The nurse assesses the client for which of the following since it is the most probable cause of this problem?

1. Infection of the nipples
2. Infant is poorly positioned
3. Not cleansing breasts after feeding
4. Allowing breast milk to dry on nipples

3 A pregnant client is at the first prenatal visit. The nurse determines the client's body mass index (BMI) is 27.5. The nurse identifies the recommended weight gain for this client is:

1. Less than or equal to 15 lbs.
2. 15-25 lbs.
3. 25-35 lbs.
4. 28-40 lbs.

4 An elderly client states that fruits in any form cause diarrhea. Which of the following foods would the nurse suggest to be the most appropriate alternative to ensure the client receives adequate vitamin C?

1. Spinach
2. Corn
3. Sweet potatoes
4. Celery

5 A new postpartum client has been told that her baby infant has phenylketonuria (PKU). Which of the following instructions should the nurse provide to the mother to ensure adequate nutritional management for this newborn?

1. "Feed the baby a wide variety of foods when she starts eating solid foods."
2. "A special PKU diet will be necessary during the first year."
3. "Your baby must follow a diet that restricts the amount of phenylalanine."
4. "Your baby will grow out of this and can be managed using standard nutritional support."

6 The nurse is teaching a client how to introduce solids to an infant. Which of the following statements by the client indicates that the client has correct understanding?

1. "I can puree whatever the family is eating each night and offer it to my baby."
2. "I can stop the formula now that solids are being given."
3. "I can add cereal to my infant's bottle several times each day until he starts to eat finger foods."
4. "I'll introduce one pureed food at a time and keep feeding it for several days before trying a new one."

7 The nurse is caring for a client who suffered major trauma in an auto accident and has been having difficulty healing wounds. The nurse encourages the client to increase foods high in which of the following vitamins?

1. Vitamin C
2. Vitamin B_1
3. Vitamin B_{12}
4. Vitamin K

8 A pregnant client with a glycosylated hemoglobin (HbA_{1c}) level of 12% asks the nurse what this level indicates. The nurse explains:

1. "You have been consuming inadequate calories and carbohydrates."
2. "You have been maintaining your glucose levels well during past 24 hours."
3. "You must be started on insulin; your glucose levels are out of control."
4. "You have had poor glucose control during the last 4–8 weeks."

9 An elderly client complains of difficulty swallowing foods such as bread. The nurse plans to assess for which of the following normal age-related physiological changes as the most likely explanation for the problem?

1. Jaw bone deterioration
2. Decreased peristalsis
3. Periodontal disease
4. Decreased saliva

10 The nurse has instructed a client with constipation about ways to increase fiber in the diet. Which of the following food selections by the client indicates teaching has been successful?

1. White bread
2. Pureed spinach
3. Kidney beans
4. Spaghetti

See pages 151–152 for Answers and Rationales.

I. PRECONCEPTUAL NUTRITION

A. Definition

1. This is the nutritional status of a woman before conception and pregnancy
2. An optimal level of nutrition during preconceptual period ensures that a woman begins pregnancy with all the necessary nutritional stores to produce substances required to maintain a healthy pregnancy and support the developing embryo/fetus

B. Preconception planning

1. Overview
    - **a.** Course of pregnancy and outcome are profoundly affected by nutritional status
    - **b.** Women who enter pregnancy in optimal nutritional state are more likely to have an uneventful pregnancy and deliver a healthy infant; consumption of a nutritious diet is essential for women considering pregnancy
2. Components of preconceptual planning
    - **a.** Comprehensive assessment of current nutritional status

!

b. Identification of nutritional alterations that may impact pregnancy and developing embryo/fetus
   1) Consumption of restrictive diets such as strict vegetarian or lactose intolerant may result in inadequate intake of essential nutrients
   2) Weight alteration: underweight women may lack **nutritional stores** (substances that support life processes and the developing fetus) needed to support pregnancy and developing fetus; pre-pregnancy weight is linked to birthweight of the infant; overweight women may also suffer from nutrient deficiencies
   3) History of eating disorder (anorexia nervosa, bulimia): individuals may have depletions of nutritional stores, low weight, and may be unable to consume an adequate diet
   4) History of pica (ingestion of nonnutrient substances) and other unusual food practices or cravings: ingestion of nonfood items replaces essential nutrients and interferes with processing
   5) History of alcohol or drug abuse: may have depletions of nutritional stores, affecting consumption of an adequate diet, and/or lack resources to purchase nutrient-rich foods
   6) Cultural, ethnic, and religious practices related to nutrition

c. Development of comprehensive individualized nutrition plan based on current nutritional status

d. Incorporation of exercise program during the pregnancy period based on prior exercise experience and client's overall functional ability

3. Nursing considerations during the preconceptual period

!

a. Assessment
   1) Obtain baseline weight; compare against ideal weight standards based on height, weight, and body mass index (BMI)
   2) Obtain comprehensive health history including personal, social, cultural, family, medical and reproductive data, use of prescription and nonprescription medications and use of herbal remedies (see Box 5-1)
   3) Using MyPyramid and client's dietary recall, assess adequacy of current diet particularly intake of protein, folic acid, magnesium, iron, calcium, vitamin C, and B complex vitamins (refer to Table 5-1 for a listing of recommended nutrients for preconception and pregnancy)
   4) Perform comprehensive physical exam; assess for potential signs of malnutrition or nutrient deficiencies that could have impact on pregnancy state
   5) Assess laboratory results including urinalysis, complete blood count, complete lymphocyte count, serum proteins (albumin, prealbumin, transferrin), urine urea nitrogen, and urinary creatinine
   6) If nutritional alterations are noted, identify potential causes: lack of knowledge, incorrect understanding of information, lack of financial resources, poor access, and cultural or religious issues

b. Priority nursing diagnoses: Imbalanced nutrition: more than body requirements; Imbalanced nutrition: less than body requirements

c. Planning and implementation
   1) Review health history data; identify factors that place client at risk for alterations in nutritional status

Box 5-1

Components of Comprehensive Health History during Preconceptual Planning

I. Gynecologic and Reproductive History
- Gynecological problems (e.g., infections, surgeries), pregnancies (history and outcomes)

II. Current and Past Medical History
- Presence of chronic illness (e.g., diabetes, congenital heart, seizures, asthma), past illness and surgeries, prescription medicines, blood type, Rh factor, allergies

III. Family Medical History
- Partner's presence of chronic illness (e.g., diabetes, congenital heart, seizures, asthma), past illness and surgeries, familial history of genetic disorders, blood type, Rh factor, allergies
- Family chronic illnesses, reproductive histories, and genetic disorders

IV. Psychosocial History
- Support systems, occupation (work conditions, exposure to hazardous substances or organisms), financial resources, healthcare resources (e.g., insurance), housing accommodations

V. Cultural and Religious Considerations
- Childbearing and childrearing beliefs, practices, and concerns related to cultural and religious preference

VI. Health Promotion History
- Usual meal pattern, consumption of micro- and macronutrient supplements, use of herbs, consumption of alcohol, caffeine, tobacco, illicit drugs, over-the-counter drug use, participation in exercise (aerobic, strength, and stretching), immunizations, dental care, routine medical care, changes in weight or eating patterns during last year (include reasons for changes)

Table 5-1

Recommended Intake of Micro- and Macronutrients for Preconception and Pregnancy (Healthy Clients)

		Pregnancy		
Nutrient	**Preconception**	***≤18 yrs.***	***19–30 yrs.***	***31–50 yrs.***
Calories	2,200	*	1st: + 0 2nd: + 300 3rd: + 300	1st: + 0 2nd: + 300 3rd: + 300
Protein	46 grams	*	70 grams	60 grams
Calcium	1,000 mg	1,300 mg/day	1,000 mg/day	1,000 mg/day
Iron	15 mg/day	27 mg/day	27 mg/day	27 mg/day
Magnesium	320 mg/day	400 mg/day	350 mg/day	360 mg/day
Vitamin C	75 mg	80 mg/day	85 mg/day	85 mg/day
Thiamine (Vitamin B_1)	1.1 mg/day	1.4 mg/day	1.4 mg/day	1.4 mg/day
Riboflavin (Vitamin B_2)	1.3 mg/day	1.4 mg/day	1.4 mg/day	1.4 mg/day
Vitamin B_6	1.3–1.5 mg/day	1.9 mg/day	1.9 mg/day	1.9 mg/day
Vitamin B_{12}	2.4 mcg/day	2.6 mcg/day	2.6 mcg/day	2.6 mcg/day
Folic Acid	400 mcg/day	600 mcg/day	600 mcg/day	600 mcg/day

*Based on gynecological age and individual needs

Adapted and reprinted with permission from: Dietary Reference Intakes: Food and Nutrition Board, Institute of Medicine—National Academy of Sciences, Recommended Levels for Individual Intake. Courtesy of National Academy Press, Washington DC. Retrieved October 8, 2005 from *http://www.nap.edu.*

2) Increased metabolic state of pregnancy will lead to positive nitrogen balance requiring a greater intake of protein, calories, and other nutrients in order to maintain optimal nutritional state

3) Using MyPyramid as a teaching guide and in collaboration with client, plan a diet that meets individual needs for all essential macronutrients and micronutrients, falls within limits of caloric restraints, and is sensitive to the client's cultural, ethnic, and social needs; assist client in proper selection of food items that will help meet dietary goals

! 4) The use of prenatal vitamins is recommended for all pregnant clients in order to provide a nutritional base during the pregnancy state; specific formulations include greater amounts of folate, iron, and calcium that are required for prevention of neural tube defects; iron is included in prenatal vitamins and client should be advised of potential gastrointestinal (GI) effects and elimination patterns (darkened stools) as a result of vitamin therapy; clients who experience nausea may have to adjust the timing of prenatal vitamin dose to prevent adverse GI symptoms; use reduces risk of preterm delivery, low infant birth weights, and birth defects

5) Discuss with client causes of nutrition alterations; provide additional information, clarify misconceptions, identify resources for financial concerns and refer as needed, suggest interventions to reduce discomforts, and develop strategies to maintain nutrition within constraints of cultural or religious beliefs (refer to Table 5-2 for a perspective on cultural nutritional concerns)

Practice to Pass

Why is preconceptual nutrition so important in providing a nutritional baseline for both the mother and developing fetus?

6) Plan exercise regime that will include aerobic activity for a minimum of 30 minutes most days of week, strength training at least two times per week, and stretching exercises at least three times per week

d. Evaluation

! 1) Monitor weight; compare against initial baseline weight

! 2) Monitor adequacy of nutrient intake using food intake tool

! 3) Monitor client for signs of nutrient deficiencies

! 4) Monitor client for compliance with prenatal vitamin therapy

5) Determine client's level of understanding of teaching through verbalization or return demonstration

II. PREGNANCY

A. Placental development and function

1. Overview

a. Is an organ of exchange for nutrients and metabolic products between developing embryo/fetus and mother

b. Is comprised of maternal and fetal component; accounts for 1.5 lbs of pregnancy weight (see Box 5-2)

c. Development of placenta begins during the third week of embryonic development with metabolic exchanges between mother and fetus beginning at 4 weeks

d. Consumption of adequate nutrients and calories essential to support development and maintenance of placenta

Table 5-2

Cultural and Religious Issues and Practices Influencing Nutritional Status*

Cultural or Religious Group	Practices/Issues
African American	"Traditional foods" are high in fat, cholesterol, sodium, low in calcium Frying and adding fat to food common Obesity, cardiovascular disease, diabetes common
Asian	"Traditional diet" is plant-based. Low in fat, saturated fat, and cholesterol; rich in fiber and nutrients; may be high in sodium High risk for osteoporosis
Native American	Diet varies with region Some use corn and other cultivated crops as staples; many attempt to live off land Widespread poverty and use of food assistance programs (food stamps, food distribution on reservations) Diabetes, obesity common
Hispanic (Mexican origin)	Traditional diet is vegetarian. High in complex carbohydrates such as corn, beans, and squash High in calories, fats (saturated in particular), and sugar Use fat in food preparation or use fatty methods Obesity, diabetes, and high triglycerides common
Islam	No pork or birds of prey No alcohol, tea, or coffee Fast during certain religious holidays/times
Christianity	Catholics—no meat on Ash Wednesday or Fridays in Lent; fasting on some religious days Eastern Orthodox—some fasting Mormons—no coffee, tea, alcohol, or tobacco Seventh Day Adventists—most are lacto-ovo-vegetarians No coffee, tea, alcohol, or strong seasonings At least 4–5 hours between meals and no snacking
Judaism (those following strict dietary rules)	Consume only kosher meat and poultry No pork, shellfish, or fishlike mammals Cannot consume milk or dairy at same meal with meat or poultry; require separate utensils for preparing/serving meat and dairy

*Although identified by a specific ethnic/religious group, practices vary with area of origin and sect. Not all individuals within these groups follow these practices or have these issues.

Box 5-2

Average Distribution of Weight Gain in Pounds (lbs.) during Pregnancy

Infant birth weight	7.5
Placenta	1.5
Maternal blood volume increase	4
Maternal fluid volume increase	4
Uterine size increase	2
Breast size increase	2–3
Amniotic fluid	2
Maternal fat stores	7–10

2. Metabolic
   a. Production of glycogen, cholesterol, and fatty acids for use by developing fetus and for production of hormones
   b. Increases storage of glycogen and iron
   c. Breaks down complex organic compounds such as proteins
   d. Produces fetoplacental transfer enzymes
3. Transfer
   a. Through processes of simple diffusion, facilitated diffusion, active transport, pinocytosis, osmosis, and hydrostatic pressure, substances are transferred between fetal and maternal circulations
   b. Factors affecting placental transfer rates include size of molecules, electrical charge of substance, lipid solubility, area of placenta, maternal/fetal/placental blood flow, saturation of substances, and fetal/maternal metabolism
4. Endocrine
   a. Production of human chorionic gonadotropin (hCG)
      1) Detectable in maternal blood serum at 8–10 days after fertilization; levels peak at 50–70 days gestation, decreasing thereafter
      2) Maintains corpus luteum
      3) Stimulates corpus luteum to increase secretion of progesterone and estrogen; essential for proliferation of cells in breast and uterus; uterus supplies nutrients to developing embryo/fetus and secretes hormones to maintain pregnancy
      4) Promotes production of testosterone in male fetuses through interstitial cell stimulation of testes
   b. Production of human placental lactogen (hPL)
      1) Detected in maternal serum at approximately 4 weeks
      2) Stimulates maternal metabolic processes whereby fetus receives more protein, glucose, and minerals
   c. Production of estrogen and progesterone
      1) Stimulate proliferation of cells in maternal uterus and breast (estrogen)
      2) Increases maternal vascularity and vasodilation (estrogen)
      3) Increases secretions in fallopian tubes and uterus supplying nutrients to developing embryo (progesterone)
      4) Promotes development of decidual cells of uterine endometrium to facilitate implantation (progesterone)
      5) Decreases contractility of uterine smooth muscle preventing spontaneous abortion (progesterone)

B. Fetal growth and development

1. Pre-embryonic
   a. Constitutes first 14 days of human development starting with fertilization
   b. Fertilized ovum or zygote travels thorough fallopian tubes toward uterus undergoing cellular multiplication
   c. Zygote develops into solid mass of cells called a blastocyst; nourishment for blastocyst supplied by uterine glands secreting lipids, mucopolysaccharides, and glycogen

d. Blastocyst embeds itself into uterine endometrium; endometrium covers blastocyst completely

e. Blastocysts form three primary germ layers (ectoderm, mesoderm, endoderm) from which all tissues, organs, and organ systems develop

f. Consumption of adequate nutrients by pregnant women is essential to supply substances required to nourish blastocyst

2. Embryonic

a. Begins at day 15 until approximately 8 weeks gestation when embryo is about 3 cm in length

b. Period of high susceptibility to **teratogens** (substances that can cause significant damage resulting in structural deformity, genetic abnormalities, and even death in the developing fetus) and other factors such as radiation exposure, maternal infection, drugs, chemicals, and other maternal conditions that can affect the developing embryo or fetus

c. Development and circulation of placenta occurs during this time

d. Essential organs and main external features develop, including heart, brain, ears, eyes, nose, and limbs

e. All major organs are formed by end of embryonic period

! f. During embryonic phase, consumption of adequate nutrients is essential; however, mother must avoid ingestion of substances that may harm developing embryo/fetus

3. Fetal

a. Starts with ninth week of gestation; is a period of rapid growth and maturation of all organs, organ systems, and external structures

b. Fetal heart tones are audible with ultrasound at 8–12 weeks

c. Fetus is considered full term at 38 weeks gestation

d. As fetus increases in size, metabolic and nutritional demands upon pregnant woman increase, including increased caloric requirements and increased need for some micro/macronutrients

C. Gestational age and trimesters

1. Gestational age is defined as number of complete days of fetal development starting with first day of last normal menstrual cycle (or LMP)

a. Prenatal estimates of gestational age using last menstrual period are 75–85% accurate

b. During second trimester gestational age is estimated by measuring fetal biparietal diameter, femur length, abdominal circumference, and head circumference via ultrasound; average of these measurements provides most accurate estimation of gestational age

c. At birth infant's gestational age is established within first 4 hours of birth using external physical characteristics and neurological development evaluations (such as Brazelton assessment)

2. Trimester is a term used to describe the gestational period of pregnancy; the entire period is divided into 3 equal time periods of 3 months each, called trimesters

a. Each trimester is characterized by specific changes in the pregnant woman and developing embryo/fetus

b. Nutritional requirements change during each trimester in response to fetal growth patterns and maternal metabolic changes

D. Concept of critical periods

1. Teratogen exposure

a. All tissues and organ systems have period of time, called **critical periods,** when cell division and differentiation are most rapid; at this time tissues and organ systems have increased susceptibility to injurious substances

b. Any agent that can cause development of abnormal structures in the developing embryo/fetus is called a teratogen

c. Teratogens include drugs, viruses, chemicals, radiation, and others

d. Damage produced by a teratogen is determined in part by the period of embryonic/fetal development in which exposure occurs

e. Pregnant women must be cautioned about ingestion of potentially harmful substances and must use caution when preparing food to reduce risk of exposure to potential teratogens

2. TORCH Studies

a. TORCH is an acronym (for toxoplasmosis, rubella, cytomegalovirus, and herpes simplex) used to identify infectious diseases that can cause serious harm to developing fetus

b. If exposed to these infectious agents during first 12 weeks of gestation, there is an increased risk for development of anomalies in infant

1) Toxoplasmosis

a) Is an infection caused by the protozoan *Toxoplasma gondii*

b) Common modes of contraction include consumption of poorly cooked meat, unpasteurized goats' milk, unwashed fruits and vegetables, and contact with the feces of cats

c) Clean fruits and vegetables thoroughly before consumption, cook meats thoroughly, and refrain from drinking unpasteurized milk

d) As a preventive measure, do not have pregnant clients clean cat litter boxes

2) Rubella

a) Is an infection caused by the rubella virus

b) Teratogenic effects of organism are greatest during first trimester but are also possible during second trimester, particularly first 2 months

3) Cytomegalovirus

a) Is an infection caused by a virus belonging to herpes simplex group

b) Is the most common viral source of intrauterine infection

c) Is transmitted by close human contact

d) May cross the placenta and enter the uterus from the cervix

4) Herpes simplex

a) Is an infection caused by herpes simplex virus (HSV-I or HSV-II)

b) Painful blister-like lesions on the genitalia characterize the primary infection; lesions may also be present on vaginal walls, cervix, urethra, and anus

c) After the primary infection, the virus lies dormant in the nerve ganglia of the affected area

d) The frequency of the reoccurrence of the infection seems related to the severity of the initial infection; a pregnant woman has increased recurrence rates particularly in later months of gestation

! e) The risk to the developing fetus depends on whether the infection is primary or recurring and the onset of labor during an acute phase may necessitate a C-section

E. Terminology

1. Prenatal period
   a. Time period from conception to birth
   b. Consists of three phases: germinal (conception–2 weeks), embryonic (2–8 weeks), and fetal (8 weeks–birth)
2. Neonatal period
   a. A period of time from birth through 28th day of life
   b. Major emphasis is upon time immediately after birth and while hospitalized; period of transition from uterine to extrauterine life
   c. Infant must make transition to external nutrient supply (breastfeeding/bottlefeeding)

F. Maternal weight factors

1. Baseline measurements
   ! a. Weight is monitored throughout pregnancy
   b. Weight at first prenatal visit provides baseline measurement
2. Reasonable weight gains
   ! a. Adequate weight gain essential for fetal growth and ultimately affects infant's birth weight
   ! b. Desired weight gain is based upon prepregnancy weight using Body Mass Index (BMI) criteria and preconceptual nutritional status of client
      1) Underweight clients (BMI less than 19.8) should gain 28 to 40 lbs
      2) Normal-weight clients (BMI 19.8 to 25) should gain 25 to 35 lbs
      3) Overweight clients (BMI 26 to 29) should gain 15 to 25 lbs
      4) Obese clients (BMI 30 and greater) should gain 15 lbs or less
   c. Women falling outside recommendations for ideal body weight at the start of the pregnancy are advised to adjust their weight gain during pregnancy accordingly
      1) Underweight women are advised to gain more weight during pregnancy
      2) Overweight women are advised to limit weight gain during pregnancy; however, pregnancy should not be used as a time for weight loss
3. Exercise and activity
   a. Mild to moderate exercise and activity is beneficial to overall well-being
   b. Exercise can help maintain cardiovascular fitness and muscle tone as well as relieve pregnancy-related discomforts such as constipation and insomnia
   c. Before beginning an exercise program during pregnancy, a woman should consult with her healthcare provider
      1) Most sports and exercises are permitted; however, pregnancy is not the time to engage in a new or strenuous sport
      2) When engaged in aerobic activities, the **target heart rate** should not exceed 70% of **maximum heart rate** (adjusted for age and weight—see Box 5-3)

Box 5-3

Calculation of Target Heart Rate for Exercise during Pregnancy

Step One: Calculate maximum heart rate (beats per minute)

220 − age in years = ____ (maximum heart rate)

Step Two: Calculate target heart rate

0.70 × ____ (maximum heart rate) = ____ (target heart rate)

3) There is less oxygen available for aerobic activity during pregnancy; therefore, it is important to recognize signs of fatigue and refrain from exercising to exhaustion

! 4) Warning signs of overexertion include back pain, absent fetal movement, dizziness, tachycardia, pubic pain, shortness of breath, contractions, vaginal bleeding, and fluid loss

5) Consume adequate calories to maintain weight, drink adequate fluids for hydration, and wear clothing that facilitates dissipation of heat

! **d.** Contraindications to exercise during pregnancy include high-risk conditions related to pregnancy (such as preterm rupture of membranes, gestational hypertension, incompetent cervix, persistent second and third trimester bleeding, and preterm labor) and a prior history of preterm labor or intrauterine growth retardation (IUGR) in previous pregnancies

! **e.** Clients who have contributory disease (independent of pregnancy) may require regulation and adjustment of exercise programs to account for increased metabolic state of pregnancy; even though pregnancy is considered a healthy state, many clients have underlying disease processes (such as cardiac, respiratory, oncologic, endocrine, and autoimmune) that can affect pregnancy state and ability to exercise

! **f.** Scuba diving is contraindicated because of increased risk for hyperoxia, hypoxia, hypercapnia, asphyxia, and decompression sickness

G. Nutritional concerns for the pregnant client

1. Increased metabolic needs

a. There are significant changes in both rate and character of metabolic activity during pregnancy

b. During second trimester, metabolic rate increases by 15%, peaking at 20% at term

c. Insulin efficiency decreases during latter part of pregnancy

d. Due to the physiological changes in pregnant woman's body and demands of growing fetus, several alterations in intake of micro/macronutrients and calories must be made by the pregnant woman

2. Common symptoms

a. Nausea and vomiting

1) Are most common during first trimester

2) Probable causes include decreased gastric emptying with resultant gastric distention, relaxation of lower esophageal sphincter (LES) from increased gastric pressure and hormonal changes, hypoglycemia, and anxiety

3) Interventions to alleviate symptoms: consume carbohydrates before getting out of bed in AM; eat small frequent meals; avoid foods with offensive

odors; refrain from drinking fluids with meals; avoid coffee/tea/ spicy foods; limit high-fat foods

b. Heartburn

1) Caused by increased levels of progesterone, causing relaxation of LES with rise of gastric secretions into esophagus, and increased fetal size where fetus places pressure on stomach, pushing gastric secretions into esophagus

2) Interventions to alleviate heartburn: consume small frequent meals; avoid drinking liquids immediately before or during meals; avoid coffee, high-fat or spicy foods; wait at least one hour before reclining after a meal

c. Physiological anemia of pregnancy

1) During pregnancy blood volume increases by approximately 50%

2) Total red blood cell (RBC) count increases approximately 18% without iron supplementation and approximately 30% with iron supplementation

! **3)** Blood volume increases more than RBC volume, hematocrit (HCT) of pregnant woman decreases slightly, called "physiologic anemia of pregnancy"; usual acceptable range 37–47%; condition is not considered pathological unless the HCT falls below 35%; iron requirements increase from 300 mg to 1,000 mg; iron is an essential component in prenatal vitamin formulations

d. Cravings and aversions

1) The client may experience cravings for certain foods and possibly nonnutritive substances

2) Craving for nonnutritive substances, called pica, occurs in all cultures; some cultures believe if a woman does not ingest these substances, harm will come to developing embryo/fetus; substances commonly consumed include dirt and clay

3) Encourage clients to refrain from ingesting nonnutritive substances; they replace essential nutrients and may interfere with their absorption

4) Clients may experience cravings for various foods that may result in intake of excessive calories or failure to consume required essential nutrients

5) Clients may experience aversions to certain foods or aromas that can result in an increase of nausea or alteration of food intake patterns

6) It is important to recognize that aversions are usually self-limiting and may even resolve during the pregnancy; however, avoidance may be warranted as long as the client has these feelings

e. Altered bowel patterns

1) Constipation is common during second and third trimester

2) Causes of constipation: iron in prenatal vitamins, enlarging uterus, decreased bowel motility, decreases in physical activity, and inadequate fluid or fiber intake

! **3)** Interventions to alleviate: Consume at least eight 8 oz. glasses of water per day; increase consumption of whole grains; and increase activity levels

f. Fluid retention

1) Enlarging uterus places pressure on abdominal blood vessels impairing venous return from the lower extremities; vessels in lower extremities become congested, resulting in fluid shifts into interstitial spaces that cause ankle edema; hormonal changes increase sodium retention, which causes further fluid retention

2) Interventions to reduce edema: elevate feet and legs; avoid restrictive clothing, encourage side-lying position when sleeping or resting; encourage walking and performing ankle exercises

3. Change in status from "normal" to high-risk

a. A high-risk pregnancy is one in which there is potential for a negative outcome for either the pregnant woman or fetus

b. Many risk factors can be identified during first prenatal visit; a normal pregnancy can become high-risk at any time

c. Gestational onset conditions that can change a pregnant woman's risk status include hypertension, alterations in amniotic fluid (hydramnios or oligohydramnios), alterations in placental placement (placenta previa, placenta abruptia), alterations in blood (isoimmunization—Rh sensitization and ABO incompatibility), **hyperemesis gravidarum, gestational diabetes,** and TORCH infection

d. Although the potential adverse physiological and psychological effects on the fetus or pregnant woman are of primary importance in high-risk pregnancies, significant nutritional aberrations may occur in some conditions

H. Nutritional concerns for the high-risk client

1. Preexisting maternal disease

a. Cardiac history

1) Heart disease results in difficulty meeting the increased workload demands imposed on the heart by pregnancy

2) Treatment will depend upon functional capacity in relation to daily activities

3) The most common heart disease encountered is congenital heart disease; other frequent diseases include rheumatic heart disease and peripartum cardiomyopathy

! 4) Nutrition-related interventions include caffeine restrictions, a diet high in protein and iron but not high in sodium, and greater intake of B vitamins (important for fetal neurological development)

5) Due to an increase in technology and transplant medicine, there are heart transplant clients who become pregnant and require intensive monitoring and follow-up during the childbearing process

b. Respiratory history

1) As pregnancy progresses, volume for lung expansion in thoracic space decreases due to the enlarging uterus; upper respiratory passages may become edematous as estrogen levels rise

2) Common respiratory conditions include asthma, cystic fibrosis, pulmonary infections, and pulmonary edema

3) Nutritional interventions that may be utilized include increased calories for increased metabolic states and additional supplementation of micronutrients such as vitamin B_{12}

4) Precipitation of respiratory attacks during the pregnancy period requires intensive monitoring and follow-up during the childbearing process

c. Immune history

1) Immune diseases encountered include systemic lupus erythematosus (SLE) and acquired immunodeficiency syndrome (AIDS)

2) Both SLE and AIDS are associated with impairment of the immune system

3) Ingestion of a nutritious diet that is adequate in protein is imperative to maintain immune function

4) Dietary intake must be closely monitored to ensure all essential nutrient requirements are being met; supplements of micro/macronutrients may be required

5) AIDS and SLE are treated with drug regimes that may cause hematologic changes such as anemia; closely monitor for anemia

d. Neurological history

1) Common preexisting neurological conditions include seizure disorders and migraine headaches

2) Pregnancy-related nutritional concerns for a client with seizure disorder centers around folic acid and vitamin K; folate might interfere with uptake of some anticonvulsant medications, increasing likelihood of seizures; despite difficulty, folic acid supplementation is still recommended to prevent neural tube defects; vitamin K production may be inhibited by some anticonvulsants

3) Migraine headaches may be triggered by food substances; common triggers that have been identified include alcohol, hypoglycemia, cured meats, and monosodium glutamate (MSG); avoid ingestion of these substances

2. Development of maternal disease

a. Gestational diabetes

1) Gestational diabetes (GD) is defined as emergence of altered glucose metabolism during the pregnancy period in a client who has had no previous history of diabetes

2) High-risk factors for development of GD are marked obesity, personal history of GD, glycosuria, strong family history of diabetes mellitus, and age > 35 years

3) Potential etiological factors in development of GD: undiagnosed preexisting disease, stress of pregnancy revealing metabolic abnormality, and altered maternal metabolism

4) GD places the client at greater higher risk for developing high-risk conditions such as hydramnios, hypertension, and dystocia

5) Risks for the fetus/infant include increased congenital anomalies, macrosomia, intrauterine growth restriction, respiratory distress syndrome, hyperbilirubinemia, and hypocalcemia

6) GD is screened with plasma glucose (126 mg/dL fasting or 200 mg/dL nonfasting), and glucose challenge test (50 gram challenge at 24 to 28 weeks); diagnosis is by glucose tolerance test or GTT (100 gram challenge after fasting glucose drawn; further measurements drawn at 1, 2, and 3 hours); two or more values must be high for diagnosis

a) GTT ≥ 95 mg/dL fasting

b) GTT ≥ 180 mg/dL at 1-hr draw

c) GTT ≥ 155 mg/dL at 2-hr draw

d) GTT ≥ 140 mg/dl at 3-hr draw

7) GD is treated primarily with diet; insulin therapy may be required if adequate glucose control is not achieved with diet; moderate exercise is recommended unless there are medical or obstetrical complications

8) Glucose levels are monitored frequently; fasting and 1- or 2-hour postprandial levels measured; self-monitored blood glucose levels by client at home is preferred over intermittent monitoring; glycosolated hemoglobin (HbA_{1c}) levels may be monitored to assess overall glucose control; HbA_{1c} levels of >10% pose significant risk for delivering an infant with malformations

9) Monitor fetal growth and correlate with maternal condition; due date may change leading to induction and/or C-section delivery based on maximum functioning of placenta, fetus, and maternal condition

10) GD is treated by use of a diabetic diet; if this is not successful, then insulin is the drug of choice during the pregnancy period; client education and teaching is necessary to assist the client with dietary changes, monitoring expectations, and use of treatment modalities

b. Hypertension of pregnancy

1) Four types of hypertensive disorders are associated with pregnancy: transient hypertension, gestational proteinuria, preeclampsia, and eclampsia; the most common are preeclampsia and eclampsia

2) Preeclampsia affects multiple maternal organ systems causing decreased organ perfusion; if disease progresses, seizures may develop and client is said to have eclampsia

3) Although underlying etiology and pathology for preeclampsia is not fully understood, it is known that maternal vasospasm and vascular endothelial damage occur

4) Potential adverse maternal effects from preeclampsia include hyperreflexia, headache, seizure, retinal detachment, intracerebral hemorrhage, acute tubular necrosis, pulmonary edema, thrombocytopenia, abruptio placentae, and subcapsula hematoma of liver

5) Potential adverse fetal/infant effects from preeclampsia include small gestational age, prematurity, sedation at birth, hypermagnesemia at birth, and death

6) Treatment for preeclampsia varies with the severity of the disease progression; dietary management for the client with mild and severe preeclampsia is a well-balanced diet with moderate to high protein (1.5 gram/kg/day) and sodium ingestion not to exceed 6 gram/day; if client is nauseous or shows signs of impending seizure, then diet is withheld

7) The only therapeutic treatment that will stop hypertension is delivery of the infant; if the client is progressing to seizure development (eclampsia), then aggressive medical management will be instituted (intravenous [IV] magnesium sulfate)

c. Hyperemesis gravidarum (HG)

1) This condition is characterized by excessive vomiting during pregnancy, resulting in profound fluid and electrolyte loss and possible organ damage

2) It may result in dehydration, electrolyte imbalances, acidosis, weight loss, ketonuria, hepatic damage, and renal damage

3) Treatment goals: control emesis, correct dehydration, correct electrolyte imbalances, and restore/maintain nutrition

4) Initial treatment includes IV Lactated Ringers solution with 100 mg vitamin B_6 per liter; if ineffective, make client NPO, continue IV fluids with

added potassium, and supplement thiamine, folic acid, and other B vitamins as needed; institute total parenteral nutrition (TPN) if still no effect; upon improvement, progress oral intake slowly; often Dramamine is added to the treatment regimen in order to minimize clinical symptoms and provide immediate relief; gastric tube feedings have been successfully used to treat HG

3. Prior obstetrical risk event
   a. Infertility issue
      1) Numerous reproductive technologies are available for difficulty with conception; these include artificial insemination, in vitro fertilization, gamete intrafallopian transfer, and zygote intrafallopian transfer
      2) Multiple birth pregnancies are often associated with use of reproductive technologies due to fertilization of multiple ova
      3) Multiple pregnancies are associated with increased prenatal risk
      4) Severe malnutrition can reduce fertility; women develop amenorrhea and men have fewer viable sperm
      5) Pharmacologic agents administered when using reproductive technologies may produce side effects such as nausea, vomiting, and bloating; nutritional status of the client must be closely monitored
   b. Pregnancy issues
      1) Previous history of abortion, preterm birth, uterine anomaly, and diethylstilbestrol (DES) exposure place the client at increased risk for preterm birth; multiparity >3 places client at increased risk for preeclampsia
      2) Numerous causes for spontaneous abortions and preterm births include embryo/fetal malformation, placenta malformation, or dysfunction
      3) Adequate nutritional stores are required to support development and maintenance of the placenta and to support the embryo/fetus; loss of nutritional stores through an inadequate diet may result in fetal malformation or placental malformation/dysfunction
   c. Delivery issues
      ! 1) Clients weighing under 45.5 kg (100 lbs) are at increased risk for cephalopelvic disproportion and prolonged labor
      ! 2) Clients weighing over 91 kg (200 lbs) are at increased risk for hypertension and cephalopelvic disproportion
      3) It is important to attain an ideal weight before conception; nutritious dietary patterns must be maintained throughout the weight management program to ensure that nutritional stores are maintained
4. Habits that place the client at risk
   a. Smoking
      1) Smoking one or more packs per day has profound negative effects on both the pregnant client and developing embryo/fetus
      2) Smoking eases hunger and may be used as a substitute for food, placing smoker at risk for nutritional deficiencies
      3) Vitamin C metabolism is increased in smokers, creating an increased need for this nutrient
      4) Lower intakes of fiber, vitamin A, beta-carotene, folate, and vitamin C have been found in smokers

5) Adverse maternal effects include: decreased appetite, infertility, increased risk for hypertension, placenta previa, abruptio placentae, and premature rupture of membranes

6) Adverse embryo/fetal infant risks include: decreased perfusion to placenta resulting in decreased oxygen and nutrients, low birth weight, intrauterine growth retardation, preterm birth, and (recently noted) higher incidence of sudden infant death syndrome (SIDS) than general population

! 7) Clients must be advised to stop smoking

! 8) Nutritional status of the smoking client must be closely assessed early in pregnancy; deficits must be addressed as soon as possible; continued evaluation of nutritional status including weight gain must continue throughout pregnancy

! 9) Fetal growth must be closely monitored throughout the pregnancy

b. Alcohol consumption

1) Alcohol consumption has been associated with significant risks for both pregnant client and developing embryo/fetus

2) Maternal adverse effects include poor nutritional state and possible hepatic dysfunction or failure

3) Embryo/fetal adverse effects include increased risk for fetal alcohol syndrome

! 4) Alcohol may replace other nutrients in diet; alcohol has been associated with alterations in the way nutrients are absorbed and metabolized; consumption is not recommended in pregnancy

c. Drugs

1) Over-the-counter, prescription, and illicit drugs can have deleterious effects on both the pregnant client and developing embryo/fetus; it is recommended that all drugs be avoided unless medical need outweighs risks

2) Ingestion of addicting drugs is associated with poor maternal nutrition, maternal infection, maternal-infant attachment complications, fetal anomalies, low infant birthweight, preterm birth, and stillbirth

3) Clients abusing drugs are at risk for poor nutrition for numerous reasons that include use of financial resources for the purchase of drugs versus food, loss of appetite, loss of interest in food from drug effects, and increased nutritional needs resulting from infections associated with drug use

5. Fetal risk event

a. Congenital issues

1) Folic acid deficiency has been identified as an etiological factor in development of neural tube defects

! 2) Folic acid should be administered to all pregnant women and those considering pregnancy

b. Pregnancy issues

1) Adequate maternal nutritional stores are essential to provide necessary substances for fetal growth and to support pregnancy

2) Poor maternal nutrition affects fetal weight gain most significantly in third trimester; poor maternal nutrition has been associated with preterm birth

3) Gestational diabetes increases fetal weight gain, resulting in infants that are large for gestational age, making delivery more difficult and possibly increasing risk for postpartum hemorrhage

c. Delivery issues

1) Excessive weight gain is associated with increased weight gain in developing fetus

2) The large for gestational age infant is at risk for cesarean delivery and birth trauma and due to cephalopelvic disproportion; hypoglycemia, polycythemia, and hyperviscosity may also occur

! 3) Monitor weight closely to prevent excess weight gain; clients may require dietary teaching to identify foods that will supply adequate nutrients without excess calories

I. Nursing considerations during the pregnancy period

1. Assessment

a. Using MyPyramid and client's dietary recall, assess adequacy of current diet particularly the intake of protein, folic acid, magnesium, iron, calcium, vitamin C, and B complex vitamins

! b. Perform comprehensive physical exam; assess for signs of nutrient deficiencies

c. Weigh client and compare with weight gain goals set at initial visit

! d. Assess for intake of alcohol, caffeine, and drugs, and for tobacco use

e. If nutritional alterations noted, identify potential causes: lack of knowledge, incorrect understanding of information, lack of financial resources, poor access, presence of pregnancy-related discomforts, cultural or religious issues

! f. Assess fetal growth: mother's weight gain, ultrasound for biparietal diameter, head/abdomen ratio, and fetal weight

2. Priority nursing diagnoses: Imbalanced nutrition: more than body requirements; Imbalanced nutrition: less than body requirements; Risk for imbalanced nutrition: more than body requirements; Risk for impaired fetal growth and development

3. Planning and implementation

a. In collaboration with the client, determine alterations needed in intake of calories and/or nutrients due to actual/potential deficiencies or excesses

b. Using MyPyramid as teaching guide and in collaboration with client, plan a diet that meets individual needs for all essential micro/macronutrients, falls within limits of caloric restraints, and is sensitive to the client's cultural, ethnic, and social needs; assist client in identifying foods rich in micronutrients

! c. Encourage the use of prescribed prenatal vitamins during the pregnancy period

d. Discuss with client the causes of nutrition alterations; provide additional information, clarify misconceptions, identify resources for financial concerns, and refer appropriately; suggest interventions to reduce discomforts and develop strategies to maintain nutrition within parameters of cultural or religious beliefs

e. Discuss the client's plan for providing infant nutrition (breast or bottle); discuss advantages and disadvantages of both methods (see Tables 5-3 and 5-4); support client's decision; provide teaching related to method selected

1) Breastfeeding (nipple preparation, breastfeeding techniques, potential problems/corrections, and nutritional needs during lactation—maternal and infant)

2) Bottlefeeding (formula types, preparation/storage, techniques, and meeting infant's nutritional needs)

Practice to Pass

A breastfeeding working client must go out of town for four days on business. The client would like to continue breastfeeding. What suggestions could the nurse make?

Table 5-3 Advantages and Disadvantages of Breastfeeding

Advantages	Disadvantages
Maternal 1. No additional expense 2. Readily available, no mixing, etc. 3. Promotes uterine contractions, decreases incidence of postpartum hemorrhage, and facilitates return to pre-pregnant size 4. Promotes bonding 5. Help mobilize fat stores for postpartum weight loss 6. Conserves iron stores because of amenorrhea 7. May protect against breast and ovarian cancer	1. Irregular ovulation and menses 2. False sense of security and nonuse of contraceptives 3. Increased nutritional requirements 4. Father cannot participate in early feeding experience 5. Initially mother may have discomfort and be uncertain infant is getting adequate milk
Infant 1. Milk contains optimal amounts of nutrients that are easily tolerated and digested; has unique nutrient, enzyme, and hormone content 2. Receives maternal antibodies 3. Decreased incidence of otitis media, vomiting, diarrhea 4. Promotes bonding 5. Promotes better tooth and jaw development 6. Less chance of overfeeding 7. Protects against food allergies 8. Improves cognitive development	1. Potential transmission of pollutants 2. Potential interruptions of breastfeeding (e.g., mother taking medication, which passes through milk and is potentially injurious to infant)

!

4. Evaluation
   - **a.** Monitor weight; compare against initial baseline weight
   - **b.** Monitor adequacy of nutrient intake using food intake tool
   - **c.** Monitor client for signs of nutrient deficiencies
   - **d.** Monitor client for compliance with prenatal vitamin therapy
   - **e.** Determine client's understanding of teaching through verbalization or return demonstration

Table 5-4 Advantages and Disadvantages of Bottlefeeding

Advantages	Disadvantages
Maternal 1. Regular ovulation and menses (easier for birth control) 2. Promotes bonding of entire family because all can participate in feeding 3. Can objectively measure how much milk infant is receiving; builds mother's confidence in caring for infant 4. More freedom for mother; others can feed infant in her absence	1. Extra expense (formula, bottles, nipples) 2. Preparation time; safe storage issues 3. Does not promote uterine contractions; may require medication 4. Does not help mobilize fat stores; may be more difficult to lose pregnancy weight
Infant 1. Less risk of transmission of pollutants 2. No interruptions when mother taking medication, etc. 3. Promotes bonding of entire family because all can participate in feeding	1. Does not receive as many maternal antibodies; may be at risk for increased infection 2. Chance of overfeeding; obesity

III. INFANT NUTRITION (0–12 MONTHS)

A. Breastfeeding

1. Increased metabolic needs
   a. During first year of life, infant grows more rapidly than in any other developmental period
   b. Metabolic processes proportionally higher in comparison with other periods
2. Maternal requirements
   a. Nutritional requirements for lactation are higher than at any other time in life; increases in calories, protein, fluids, vitamins, and minerals are required to prevent loss of maternal stores during milk production (review Table 5-5)
   b. Clients with diets deficient in protein, carbohydrate, fat, folate, and most minerals still produce high-quality milk, but do so by depleting maternal nutrient stores; if diet continues to be inadequate, maternal tissues will be robbed of essential nutrients; vitamin content in breast milk will decline with continued consumption of inadequate diet by mother
3. Infant requirements
   a. Infants require approximately 100–108 kcal/kg/day and 2.2 grams/kg/day protein
   b. Requirements for micro- and macronutrients change as the infant develops during the first 12 months of life (see Table 5-6)

B. Breast milk characteristics

1. Colostrum
   a. Is produced first several days postpartum; is thick with a cream or yellow color

Table 5-5

Recommended Intake of Micro- and Macronutrients for Lactation (Healthy Clients)

	Lactation		
Nutrient	***≤ 18 yrs***	***19–30 yrs***	***31–50 yrs***
Calories	+ 500*	+ 500*	+ 500*
Protein	71 grams	71 grams	71 grams
Calcium	1,300 mg/day	1,000 mg/day	1,000 mg/day
Iron	10 mg/day	9 mg/day	9 mg/day
Magnesium	2.6 mg/day	2.6 mg/day	2.6 mg/day
Vitamin C	115 mg/day	120 mg/day	120 mg/day
Thiamine (Vitamin B_1)	1.4 mg/day	1.4 mg/day	1.4 mg/day
Riboflavin (Vitamin B_2)	1.6 mg/day	1.6 mg/day	1.6 mg/day
Vitamin B_6	2 mg/day	2 mg/day	2 mg/day
Vitamin B_{12}	2.8 mcg/day	2.8 mcg/day	2.8 mcg/day
Folic Acid	500 mcg/day	500 mcg/day	500 mcg/day

*Above normal requirements

Adapted and reprinted with permission from: Dietary Reference Intakes: Food and Nutrition Board, Institute of Medicine—National Academy of Sciences, Recommended Levels for Individual Intake. Courtesy of National Academy Press, Washington DC. Retrieved October 9, 2005 from *http://www.nap.edu/*.

Table 5-6 Recommended Intake of Micro- and Macronutrients for Infants and Children

					Older Children and Adolescents			
	Infants		Children		*Male*		*Female*	
Nutrient	*0–6 months*	*6–12 months*	*1–3 years*	*4–8 years*	*9 to 13*	*14 to 18*	*9 to 13*	*14 to 18*
Protein	13 grams	14 grams	16 grams	24–28 grams	45 grams	59 grams	46 grams	44 grams
Calcium	210 mg	270 mg	500 mg	800 mg	1,300 mg	1,300 mg	1,300 mg	1,300 mg
Iron	0.27 mg	11 mg	7 mg	10 mg	8 mg	11 mg	8 mg	15 mg
Magnesium	30 mg	75 mg	80 mg	130 mg	240 mg	410 mg	240 mg	360 mg
Vitamin C	40 mg	50 mg	15 mg	25 mg	45 mg	75 mg	45 mg	65 mg
Vitamin A	400 mcg	500 mcg	300 mcg	400 mcg	600 mcg	900 mcg	600 mcg	700 mcg
Vitamin D	5 mcg	5 mcg	5 mcg	5 mcg	5 mcg	5 mcg	5 mcg	5 mcg
Thiamin (Vitamin B_1)	0.2 mg	0.3 mg	0.5 mg	0.6 mg	0.9 mg	1.2 mg	1.0 mg	1.0 mg
Riboflavin (Vitamin B_2)	0.3 mg	0.4 mg	0.5 mg	0.6 mg	0.9 mg	1.3 mg	0.9 mg	1.0 mg
Vitamin B_6	0.1 mg	0.3 mg	0.5 mg	0.6 mg	1 mg	1.3 mg	1.0 mg	1.2 mg
Vitamin B_{12}	0.4 mcg	0.5 mcg	0.9 mcg	1.2 mcg	1.8 mcg	2.4 mcg	1.8 mcg	2.4 mcg

Adapted and reprinted with permission from: Dietary Reference Intakes: Food and Nutrition Board, Institute of Medicine—National Academy of Sciences, Recommended Levels for Individual Intake. Courtesy of National Academy Press, Washington, DC. Retrieved October 9, 2005 from *http://www.nap.edu/*

b. It contains maternal antibodies and other anti-infective agents that protect infant from infection

c. Contains proportionally more protein, minerals, fat soluble vitamins, and sodium than mature milk

2. Transitional milk

a. Is produced approximately 3–6 days postpartum

b. Has a higher concentration of fat, lactose, water-soluble vitamins, and calories but less protein than colostrum

3. Mature milk

a. Contains approximately 10% solids and 90% water and provides 20 kcal/oz

b. Exact composition varies with time during feeding; early milk called foremilk, later called hindmilk; foremilk has higher fat content

c. Human milk has unique composition ideal for a growing infant

1) Protein content 4–5%; high whey concentration; easily digested

2) Carbohydrate content approximately 35–45%; lactase promotes growth of GI normal flora and promotes calcium absorption

3) Fat comprises approximately 50% of calories; easily digested due to presence of enzyme for fat digestion

4) Adequate vitamins and minerals except vitamin D

d. Breastfed infants should be fed on demand; during the first month of life they may feed 8–12 times per day

4. Quality versus quantity

a. There is a misconception that quantity implies quality in relation to breast milk; a woman can have an adequate supply (quantity) of breast milk production, but if the infant does not gain weight (assessment of milk quality), then supplemental feedings and/or dietary measures may need to be initiated in order to maintain infant weight gain

b. Recognition of dietary maternal intake (adequate calories and fluid) and selection of food items (evaluation for flatus potential in the infant) are important assessment factors that may require focus during client teaching in order to meet nutritional goals

C. Bottlefeeding

1. Formula preparations

a. Three major types of commercial formula: cow's-milk-based, soy-protein-based, and specialized therapeutic

b. Protein concentration varies between 1.45 and 1.6 grams/dL; caloric value is 20 kcal/oz

c. Cow's-milk-based formulas composed of nonfat cow's milk, whey, vegetable oil, and lactose

d. Soy-based formulas replace cow's milk with soy protein, glucose replaces lactose, and vegetable oil contributes fat; infants with primary lactase deficiencies or galactosemia are often given soy-based formulas

e. Specialized and therapeutic formulas have hydrolyzed protein to facilitate digestion; products are indicated for infant with severe allergies to milk and soy protein or malabsorption due to GI or liver disease

2. Types of formulas

a. Standard commercial formulas are distributed in ready-to-feed, concentrated liquid, and dry powder formulations

b. Concentrated liquids and dry powders must be prepared according to manufacturer directions; improper preparation may overtax the infant's immature renal system or decrease the amount of nutrients the infant receives

! c. Care must be taken to avoid overfeeding the formula-fed infant; number of feedings, amount per feeding, and total formula volume per day varies as the infant ages (see Table 5-7)

D. Infant physiology

1. Carbohydrate (CHO) metabolism

Table 5-7

General Parameters for Formula Feeding

Age	Number of Feedings in 24 Hours	Amount per Feeding (oz)	Amount Per Day (oz)
1 wk–1 month	6–8	4–5	21–24
1–3 months	5–6	5–7	24–32
3–6 months	4–5	6–7	24–32
6–12 months	3–4	6–8	16–24

a. Simple CHOs (monosaccharides, disaccharides) are digested well
b. Complex CHO digestion is impaired due to limited production of pancreatic amylase
c. Amylase levels become sufficient for digestion of complex CHOs between 3 and 6 months

2. Lipid metabolism
a. Decreased production of pancreatic lipase impairs fat absorption
b. Limited bile production affects fat absorption; bile production does not approach normal levels until approximately 6 months

3. Protein metabolism
a. Kidney function is immature at birth resulting in impaired ability to concentrate urine; urine-concentrating ability approaches adult-like levels at 4 to 6 weeks
b. Excessive intake of protein can stress kidney function, causing dehydration
c. Deaminization of amino acids by the liver remains somewhat immature during the first year of life
d. Sufficient amounts of trypsin are available to break down protein into polypeptides and some amino acids at birth

E. Measuring nutritional outcomes

1. Weight gains
a. Weight doubles in first 4–6 months of life; triples by one year
b. Formula-fed infants tend to gain weight faster than breastfed infants due to higher concentration of protein in formula and larger volumes of intake

2. Elimination patterns
a. In general, breastfed newborns have more frequent stools than formula-fed infants; stool is yellow and thinner
b. With maturity, frequency of bowel movements varies considerably in both breast- and formula-fed infants
c. Newborns void 5–25 times per day for a total 24-hour volume of 25 mL/kg; as they mature most infants have 6–8 wet diapers per day
d. Infants require 150 mL/kg of fluids in 24 hours

3. Developmental growth charts
! a. Assessment of an infant's growth one of the best measures of infant nutrition
! b. Measure height and weight at each visit; compare values with age- and gender-appropriate percentile growth charts

F. Developmental expectations

1. Coordination of muscle and reflex development
a. Reflexes involved in ingestion of food and fluids develop gradually during the first year of life
b. At birth, infantile or visceral swallowing reflex is present; food bolus is passively moved down tongue by gravity, posterior wall of pharynx moves forward, displacing soft palate and propelling bolus into esophagus, peristalsis moves bolus into the stomach; process is only effective for fluids
c. Mature or somatic swallow reflex is developed at approximately 6 months; at this time, infant's tongue has become smaller; food boluses move into pharynx by the action of tongue against hard palate

d. At approximately 6–7 months, fine motor skills are developed sufficiently for infant to hold bottle

e. Between 9–12 months, fine motor skill development permits infants to feed themselves using finger foods

2. Meeting developmental milestones

a. In addition to height and weight measurements, achievement of developmental milestones is an excellent indicator of infant growth and development

b. Development must be assessed thoroughly at each well-child checkup; standardized developmental screening tests such as the Denver Developmental Screening test may be used; only trained professionals should administer them

c. Results of screening tests alone must not be used as the sole indicator of the infant's development; data from the comprehensive health history, family history, and developmental screen must be taken into consideration

d. Numerous specific milestones during the first year of life are associated with feeding

3. Failure to thrive (FTT)

a. Is defined as inadequate growth caused by the inability to obtain or use calories for growth; the infant usually falls below the 5th percentile on a growth chart

b. Is classified as organic FTT and nonorganic FTT

c. Common causes of organic FTT include congenital heart disease, cystic fibrosis, acquired human immunodeficiency syndrome, gastroesophageal reflux, malabsorption syndromes, neurological disease, and developmental anomalies

d. Numerous etiological factors have been implicated in nonorganic FTT and include poverty, health beliefs, inadequate knowledge, stress, feeding resistance, and insufficient breast milk

e. Treatments focus upon increasing the nutrient intake to allow for "catch-up" growth and promotion of continued growth and resolving the underlying problem when possible

G. Feeding behaviors to avoid

! 1. Giving cow's milk during the first year

a. Whole milk, goat's milk, skim milk, 1–2% fat milk, and evaporated milk are *not* advised during first 1–2 years of life

b. Whole milk is deficient in essential fatty acids, iron, zinc, vitamin E, and vitamin C

c. Ingestion of whole milk before 1 year of age has been associated with iron deficiency anemia due to the low concentration and poor bioavailability of iron in cow's milk; some studies have implicated that GI blood loss occurs with milk ingestion

d. Increased protein, sodium, potassium, and chloride levels in cow's milk increase renal solute load for immature infant kidneys; may cause dehydration

2. Adding cereal to the bottle

! a. *Do not* add dry cereal to bottles of formula as it can increase the aspiration potential due to increased swallowing pressure exerted by the infant to swallow the solution

! b. Too often, the nipple size of the bottle is increased by the parent in order to compensate for the increased thickness of the solution; this can lead to a further risk for aspiration

c. Mix cereal with formula then introduce with a spoon; this facilitates development of chewing muscles and coordination

3. Nursing bottle syndrome

   a. Nursing bottle syndrome or nursing bottle caries are caused by ingestion of milk, juice, soda pop, or other sweetened beverage by bottle at night or during naps; it is also found in infants who use a bottle as a pacifier, breastfed infants with frequent nocturnal feeds, and infants using pacifiers coated with sweet substances

   b. Dental caries, dental decay, and erosion are due to bacterial action resulting from food substances remaining on dental enamel

   c. To prevent nursing bottle syndrome: no infant should be put to bed with a bottle, replace sweet substances with water, avoid using bottles as pacifiers, and avoid adding sweet coatings to pacifiers

H. Progression of diet guidelines

1. Starting solid foods

   a. Do not introduce solids until 4–6 months of age; introduction before this time is inappropriate because of immature GI system

   b. Early feeding exposes infants to food allergens; this may result in development of food allergies

   c. Presence of primitive reflexes such as extrusion reflex early in infant life may make oral feeding difficult; limited motor development such as poor head control makes feeding solids difficult

   d. Infants who have a family history of food allergy should not receive solids until 6 months of age

2. Sequencing of food

   a. Infant cereals (rice) often are the first solid of choice because of increased iron and energy provided; single grain, precooked, partially hydrolyzed cereal is well tolerated by infant

   b. Sequencing then leads to vegetables or fruits with meats being added last; because infants develop preference for sweets, vegetables should be given before fruits

3. Introduction of new foods

   a. To identify food allergies, introduce new foods one at a time

   b. Offer a new food for 4–7 days before trying another

   c. May be homemade or commercially prepared

   d. Offer one to two teaspoons of solid food initially; increase amount over time

   e. As amount of solid food increases, decrease the amount of formula

   f. This type of introductory pattern helps to identify potential allergy development and how the infant is tolerating the food item

4. Safety aspects

   a. At ages less than 4 years, there is increased risk for choking

   b. Preventive measures include:

      1) Cook foods well; cut into small pieces

      2) Never leave infant unsupervised when eating

      3) Avoid hard round foods not easily dissolved in saliva such as grapes, raw vegetables, popcorn, and hot dogs

4) Do not permit an infant to eat or drink when lying down
5) Carefully observe infants who have been given teething medications that may anesthesize the posterior pharynx
6) Do not add cereal to bottle or increase bottle nipple size—this can increase risk for aspiration

! c. Avoid use of regular canned fruit or vegetables because they are not designed for infants due to excessive sodium and/or sugar content; fruit canned in its own juice is allowable

! d. Refrain from using honey in foods or fluids due to risk for infant botulism

I. Nutritional concerns for the high-risk infant

1. Prematurity issues
   a. Infants are classified according to gestational age and size that has been found to correlate with mortality (e.g., premature, low birthweight, fetal death)
   b. The most rapid rate of growth occurs during 26–36 weeks gestation; infants born prematurely have not experienced this growth
   c. Both prematurity and low birth weight cause profound impact on nutritional status—they often accompany each other in the clinical setting
   d. Premature infants require proportionally more calories, protein, and other nutrients than full-term infants yet lack mature kidneys to excrete byproducts of protein metabolism (see Table 5-8)
   e. Fat and glycogen stores are limited; the limited amounts and potency of fat enzymes impairs fat digestion and causes malabsorption of calories and nutrients; the infant is at risk for vitamin E deficiency from impaired fat absorption; vitamin E deficiency may cause hemolytic anemia
   f. There is increased risk for osteopenia due to decreased bone mineralization; bone mineralization usually occurs in utero during third trimester

Table 5-8

Recommended Intake in Clinically Stable Preterm Infants

Nutrients per 100 kcal	< 1,000 grams	> 1,000 grams
Energy, kcal	100	100
Protein, gram	3–3.16	2.5–3.0
Calcium, mg	100–192	100–192
Iron, mg	1.67	1.67
Magnesium, mg	6.6–12.5	6.6–12.5
Vitamin E, IU	5–10	5–10
Vitamin K, mcg	6.66–8.33	6.66–8.33
Vitamin A, IU	583–1,250	583–1,250
	with lung disease 2,250–2,333	with lung disease 2,250–2,333
Vitamin D, IU	125–333	125–333
Thiamine (Vitamin B_1), mg	150–200	150–200
Riboflavin (Vitamin B_2), mcg	200–300	200–300
Vitamin B_6, mcg	125–175	125–175
Vitamin B_{12}, mcg	0.25	0.25

g. Conditions related to organ immaturity such as respiratory distress syndrome, necrotizing enterocolitis, and bronchopulmonary dysplasia may require alternative feedings techniques and alterations in nutrients

2. Structural issues

a. Oral neuromuscular development (such as breathe/suck/swallow and coordination) are delayed, making oral feeding difficult

b. Muscle weakness causes infant to tire during feeding

c. Decreased stomach capacity affects oral feeding; poor muscle tone of lower esophageal sphincter causes regurgitation

d. Presence of congenital anomalies such as tracheoesophageal fistula, cleft lip/palate, congenital diaphragmatic hernia, biliary atresia, and abdominal wall defects may require alternative feeding techniques and alterations in nutrients

3. Alternate feeding placements

a. The route for administration of feedings is determined by the infant's ability to coordinate sucking, swallowing, and breathing; coordination of these behaviors usually occurs at approximately 32–34 weeks gestation, and is not fully synchronized until 36–37 weeks

b. Alert infants born at 32–34 weeks gestation are fed by nipple; may supplement nipple feedings with enteral feedings if intake is too low

c. Younger infants are fed enterally with nasogastric, orogastric, or gastrostomy tube; feedings may be via intermittent bolus or continuous using a pump

d. Infants with delayed gastric emptying, apnea associated with feeding, or who are at risk for aspiration may be fed through tube placed into duodenum or jejunum

e. Parenteral feedings are reserved for acutely ill infants unable to accept enteral feedings and very small infants (< 1,500 grams) to supplement enteral feedings until adequate volumes are achieved

f. Infants fed by nonoral routes are at risk for feeding resistance; nonnutritive oral stimulation must be initiated to decrease incidence (see Box 5-4)

4. Inborn errors of metabolism

a. Congenital hypothyroidism

1) Deficiency of thyroid hormones present at birth

2) Potential early signs present at birth: poor feeding, lethargy, prolonged jaundice, respiratory difficulties, cyanosis, constipation, and bradycardia

3) Classic signs do not appear until 6 weeks or later: atypical facies, thick/dry/mottled/cool skin, coarse/dry/lusterless hair, abdominal distention, hyporeflexia, hypothermia, bradycardia, hypotension with narrow pulse pressure, wide cranial sutures, and anemia

4) Retarded bone age and delayed development of the nervous system are serious consequences of disorder

! 5) Lifelong thyroid hormone replacement is treatment (see Box 5-5 for related nursing considerations)

b. Galactosemia

1) Is an autosomal-recessive disorder; an enzyme required to covert galactose into glucose is missing; if untreated, infant will die

2) Clinical manifestations are jaundice, splenomegaly, portal hypertension, cataracts, lethargy, hypotonia, vomiting, and weight loss

Box 5-4

Prevention and Treatment of Feeding Resistance

1. Assess infant for vigorous suck, coordination of sucking and swallowing, intact gag reflex, sucking on tubes/hands/pacifier, rooting, wakefulness before and sleepiness after feeds, these indicate readiness to feed.
2. Talk to infant and position face-to-face to increase interaction during feeding.
3. Use tactile stimulation and move gradually toward mouth.
4. Encourage exploration by infant using infant's mouth, lips, tongue.
5. Provide pacifier as a means of encouraging nonnutritive sucking.
6. If enterally fed, stimulate infant during feed by holding infant face-to-face and giving oral stimulation.

3) Is treated by eliminating all milk and lactose-containing foods; use lactose-free formula in infants

c. Phenylketonuria

1) Is an autosomal recessive genetic disorder; an enzyme needed to metabolize the essential amino acid phenylalanine into tyrosine is missing

2) Clinical manifestations are failure to thrive, frequent vomiting, irritability, hyperactivity, and unpredictable, erratic behavior

3) If not treated, mental retardation will develop

! 4) Is treated by dietary management; phenylalanine is found in all proteins; cannot remove entirely from diet; 20–30 mg per day of phenylalanine is usual level of restriction per day; goals are to provide adequate nutrients for growing infant/child and keep phenylalanine levels within safe range; diet can prevent mental retardation but cannot correct neurological damage that has already occurred; when diet can be stopped is a source of controversy; most recommend following diet through adolescence; Nutrasweet contains phenylalanine and has a warning label attesting to this fact

! 5) Because PKU has been identified (by mandatory heel stick testing at birth) and managed with diet therapy, women who have PKU are now having babies themselves; this may require additional monitoring of the pregnant client

5. Disease states: general considerations

a. During acute illness, infants may experience decreases in appetite, decreases in nutritional intake, alterations in digestion and absorption of nutrients, increases in need for various nutrients and increased loss of nutrients; in a high-risk infant, alterations may be more pronounced due to poor nutritional stores at onset of illness; nutritional alterations are minimized during acute illness

Box 5-5

Nursing Considerations for Infant Receiving Thyroid Replacement Therapy

1. Family must understand treatment is lifelong and drug must be given as directed to achieve normal growth and development.
2. Drug has no taste and may be given with formula, food, or water.
3. If dose is missed, a double dose should be given the next day.
4. Inform family of signs of inadequate treatment (too low dose)—fatigue, sleepiness, decreased appetite, and constipation.
5. Inform family of signs of overdose: rapid pulse, dyspnea, irritability, insomnia, fever, diaphoresis, and weight loss; family should know how to count pulse; physician should give family parameters as to when to withhold dose (i.e., certain pulse rate).

b. Continue breast, formula, or enteral feeding as tolerated during acute illness; if solids have been introduced, offer a variety of foods as tolerated; increase fluids to replace losses in infants presenting with vomiting, diarrhea, or fever

c. A chronically ill infant is at even a greater risk for nutritional problems than the acutely ill infant; as with acute illness, similar factors result in nutrition alterations; chronically there may also be losses from medication side effects

d. Nutritional regime for the chronically ill infant must allow for progression of normal growth and development, promote catch-up growth as indicated, and improve disease outcomes; improved outcomes can best be achieved through early nutritional interventions

J. Nursing considerations during the infancy period

! 1. Assessment

a. Obtain height and weight; compare with gender and gestational-age appropriate percentile growth charts

b. Perform comprehensive physical exam including dentition; assess for signs of malnutrition or nutrient deficiencies

c. Assess for causes of alterations in nutrition: difficulties with breastfeeding (see Table 5-9), bottlefeeding, and food introduction; access/transportation is-

Table 5-9

Common Problems with Breastfeeding

Common Problems	Causes	Solutions
Sore nipples	1. Infant poorly positioned. 2. Infant chews on nipple. 3. Infant overeager to nurse. 4. Nipples not allowed to dry. 5. Milk sticks to bra/pads.	1. Position baby near breast and insert nipple. 2. Get infant on breast with rooting reflex. Remove infant from breast by breaking suction with finger. 3. Pre-express to enhance letdown reflex. Feed more often. 4. Air-dry after nursing; change pads frequently. 5. Moisten pad before removal.
Breast engorgement	1. Missed or infrequent feedings. 2. Incomplete emptying after feeding. 3. Poor letdown reflex. 4. Infant sleepy or not eager to nurse.	1. Feed every 1.5 hours. Express/pump when feedings missed. 2. Nurse 10–15 minutes per breast. Express milk if infant unable to empty breast. 3. Massage breasts before feeding. Take warm shower and let water run over breasts and shoulders. Use relaxation techniques. 4. Rouse infant (unwrap blanket, change diaper). Pre-express milk and place on nipple or infant's lips.
Poor letdown	1. Letdown reflex not well established. 2. Mother overtired. 3. Mother anxious/tense.	1. Allow infant at least 15 minutes per side. Massage breasts before nursing. Drink noncaffeine fluids before and during nursing. 2. Rest when infant does. Lie down when nursing. Simplify chores. 3. Allow more rest time. Identify source of tension and eliminate.

Practice to Pass

A preterm infant receiving enteral feeding has been demonstrating behaviors associated with feeding resistance. What measures could the nurse implement to reduce the likelihood of this problem developing?

sues, knowledge deficits, incorrect understanding of information, lack of financial resources, and cultural or religious issues

d. Assess for achievement of developmental milestones

2. Nursing diagnoses: Imbalanced nutrition: more than body requirements; Imbalanced nutrition: less than body requirements; Risk for imbalanced nutrition: more than body requirements; Risk for impaired infant growth and development
3. Planning and implementation
   - **a.** Determine alterations needed in intake of calories and/or nutrients due to actual/potential deficiencies or excesses present
   - ! **b.** Administer infant vitamins; instruct caregiver on correct administration and common side effects
   - **c.** Discuss with caregiver causes of nutrition alterations; provide additional information, clarify misconceptions, identify resources for financial concerns, and refer as appropriate
4. ! Evaluation
   - **a.** Monitor weight and track weight gain as client ages
   - **b.** Monitor adequacy of nutrient intake via food intake recall per caretaker
   - **c.** Monitor for signs of nutrient deficiencies
   - **d.** Determine caregiver's understanding of teaching through verbalization or return demonstration

IV. CHILDHOOD NUTRITION (1–10 YEARS)

A. Metabolic needs according to age

1. Needs differ considerably among toddlers, preschoolers, and school-age children; total energy needs increase with age, but calories per kilogram of weight decrease
2. Individual energy requirements depend on the child's growth and physical activity
3. Specific requirements for micro- and macronutrients change as the child ages
4. Toddler growth slows in comparison with infancy; birth weight quadruples by age 2.5 years; height increases approximately 3 inches per year
5. Preschool and school-age growth averages 2–3 kg per year and 6–8 cm (2.5–3.5 inches) per year
6. In older school-age children, nutritional stores are laid down for puberty growth spurt

B. Preschool age (1–5 years)

1. Children typically display erratic and ritualistic eating patterns, placing them at risk for nutritional deficiencies; many are picky eaters with strong food preferences; isolated foods may be consumed voraciously for several days only to be refused subsequently; mealtimes may be stressful due to disruptive behavior
2. Young preschoolers are still at risk for choking; cut food into small pieces; avoid round hard foods that do not easily dissolve in saliva that may cause choking
3. Use MyPyramid as reference for planning young child's meals but alter proportion size; younger school-age children may eat fewer servings within each group
4. ! Numerous techniques may be useful in facilitating nutrient intake in young child (do not force child to eat, maintain relaxed mealtime atmosphere, offer one new

food along with a favorite food, use child-sized portions, serve foods with mild flavor, and serve finger foods)

5. Early eating patterns influence lifelong dietary habits; continue to offer a variety of nutrient-rich foods from all food groups

C. School age (6–10 years)

1. Energy needs are proportionally less in early school-age child
2. Nutrient stores for puberty being laid
3. Use MyPyramid to plan meals for school-age child

D. Growth and development issues

1. Performance in school is linked to the consumption of adequate nutrients particularly at breakfast; encourage regular meal patterns; utilize school breakfast and lunch programs that provide free or reduced price meals for low-income children
2. Access to fast foods puts school-age children at risk for consumption of high-calorie and high-fat diet; select healthy snacks that augment other selections from MyPyramid (popcorn, fresh fruit or vegetables, peanut butter, cheese, nuts, eggs, and yogurt)

E. Special nutritional concerns

1. Eating disorders
   a. Obesity
      1) Clinical research has established a definite link between development of obesity as a child and presence of obesity in adulthood
      2) Risk factors for obesity include a positive family history, decreased activity, poverty (lower income family is at increased risk), and ethnicity (Hispanics, Native Americans, and African Americans have increased risk)
      3) Obesity in children is associated with an increased risk for cardiovascular disease, joint problems, decreased respiratory function, impaired immune function, early puberty, dysmennorhea, and diabetes mellitus
      4) Childhood obesity is also associated with poorer academic performance, social isolation, depression, low self-esteem, and discrimination
      5) Treat with a comprehensive plan including dietary changes, increased activity, and psychosocial support; use nonpunitive attitude; when possible, maintain child's weight as a growth spurt occurs so child in essence grows into weight
      6) Monitor child's weight at well-child visits particularly if at risk for obesity; employ strategies to prevent obesity (decrease TV time, increase activity, don't force child to eat or "clean plate," limit high-calorie foods in household, do not use food as a reward, and limit fat to 30% in diet)
   b. Failure to thrive (FTT)
      1) Infants who have been diagnosed with FTT require assistance in meeting individualized nutritional goals
      2) Continued monitoring of client is needed, paying attention to weight gain, intake of nutrients and fluids, and correlation with growth and height curves to determine whether nutritional goals have been achieved
   c. Meal omissions
      1) Breakfast is the most commonly skipped meal due to time constraints
      2) Provide nutritious easily portable foods to encourage intake

d. Clients who have diagnosed eating disorders (anorexia or bulimia) are subject to nutritional deficiencies with a multisystem presentation

2. Outside influences

a. School and peer group influence eating patterns during school-age period

b. Schools may play an active role in reinforcement of nutrition education

3. Disease states

Practice to Pass

A mother reports that her toddler has not been eating well and she is concerned about the child's nutritional state. How would the nurse respond?

a. Acute disease places a child at increased risk for nutritional alterations: decreased appetite, decreased nutritional intake, altered digestion and absorption of nutrients, increased needs for various nutrients and increased loss of nutrients

b. Offer a variety of foods as tolerated during illness; increase fluids to replace losses in a child presenting with vomiting, diarrhea, or fever; resume regular diet as soon as possible

F. Nursing considerations during the childhood period

! 1. Assessment

a. Obtain height and weight; compare with gender- and age-appropriate percentile growth charts

b. Perform comprehensive physical exam including dentition; assess for signs of nutrient deficiencies

c. Assess for causes of alterations in nutrition: development-related eating patterns (ritualistic/erratic), psychosocial issues, peer pressure, complex schedules, knowledge deficits, incorrect understanding of information, and lack of financial resources

2. Nursing diagnoses: Imbalanced nutrition: more than body requirements; Imbalanced nutrition: less than body requirements; Risk for imbalanced nutrition: more than body requirements; Risk for impaired child growth and development

3. Planning and implementation

a. In collaboration with child and caretaker, determine alterations needed in intake of calories and/or nutrients due to actual/potential deficiencies or excesses present

Practice to Pass

Clients report that their school-age child has been gaining excessive weight during the last year. How would the nurse respond?

b. Administer vitamin supplements as needed; instruct client and caregiver on correct administration and common side effects

c. Discuss causes of nutritional alterations with client and caregiver; provide additional information, clarify misconceptions, and identify resources for psychosocial concerns

! 4. Evaluation

a. Monitor height and weight; track trends in growth

b. Monitor adequacy of nutrient intake via food intake recall per client caregiver

c. Monitor for signs of nutrient deficiencies

d. Determine client and caregiver's understanding of teaching through verbalization or return demonstration

V. ADOLESCENT NUTRITION (11–18 YEARS)

A. Metabolic needs according to age

1. Is a period of rapid growth; male needs are greater than female needs because of the increased muscle mass, lean body tissue, and bone development in males

2. There is an increase in body fat in females
3. Individual needs vary depending on rate of appetite, growth, body size, and physical activity level

B. Adolescent age

1. There are significant increased requirements for numerous micro- and macronutrients
2. MyPyramid may be used to plan dietary intake with age/developmentally appropriate alterations

C. Growth and development issues

1. The male adolescent growth spurt begins at 12–13 years, peaks at 14, and continues until approximately 19 years
2. The female adolescent growth spurt begins at 10–11 years, peaks at 12, and continues until approximately 15 years
3. Adolescents frequently consume inadequate amounts of vitamins A, C, B_6, iron, calcium, zinc, and magnesium
4. They may have increased consumption of carbonated beverages, coffee, tea, and alcohol, replacing consumption of nutrient-dense fluids such as milk and fruit juice
5. They frequently engage in dieting; adhere to fad or restrictive diets; skip meals; snack on high caloric, fat, or sugar foods; and eat more meals outside home (particularly fast foods)

D. Outside influences

1. Motivation for an adolescent's dietary alterations include negative body image, peer pressure, independence, busy schedules, resistance to current values, and self-identification
2. There is increased exposure to alcohol, drugs, and tobacco; these may cause profound alterations in nutritional status
3. An increased number of meals eaten away from home or missed due to social activities, school, and work places adolescents at risk for caloric and nutrient deficiencies

E. Special nutritional concerns

1. Pregnancy
   a. Contributing factors to adolescent pregnancy: peer pressure for sexual activity, inconsistent use of contraception, troubled family relationships
   b. There is increased incidence in the poor or near-poor adolescent
   c. There is increased risk of complications: pregnancy-induced hypertension, cephalopelvic disproportion, preterm labor, low birth weight infant, and prematurity
   d. Nutrient stores are often inadequate for pregnancy due to fetal needs superimposed upon the adolescent's growth and development needs; younger adolescents are at greatest risk for nutritional deficits
   e. Common alterations in eating patterns found in adolescence (such as meal skipping, dieting, and increased intake of fast foods or soda pop) create increased nutritional concerns
   f. They are often resistant to weight gain during pregnancy due to concerns over body image
   g. They require increased nutrients in comparison with pregnant adults

2. Obesity
   a. A large percentage of adolescents are overweight or obese; the incidence of overweight among adolescents has tripled since 1980 with increases in asthma and Type 2 diabetes in children
   b. There are gender-specific obesity BMI scales for adolescents
      1) BMI for obese 12- to 14-year-old males is ≥ 23 and for females is ≥ 23.4
      2) BMI for obese 15- to 17-year-old males is ≥ 25.8 and for females is ≥ 24.8
      3) BMI for obese 18- to 19-year-old males is ≥ 26.8 and for females is ≥ 25.7
   c. Risk factors for obesity in adolescents are similar to all children
   d. A comprehensive nutritional regime is imperative with attention focused on acceptable weight limits and establishment of good eating habits
3. Eating disorders (refer to Box 5-6 for clinical manifestations)
   a. Anorexia nervosa (AN)
      1) Impact of AN (refusal to eat not attributable to physical causes) can lead to significant physical and emotional changes that can have long-term consequences for the adolescent client
      2) Even though this eating disorder is associated with adolescence, clinical evidence is now supporting that emergence of altered eating patterns can occur prior to adolescence; therefore, all children (regardless of age) should be assessed for presence of eating disorders if symptoms develop or if there is expressed concern
      3) It is more common in females with a peak onset between 12–13 or 18–19 years; however, this does not preclude the presentation of males with this type of eating disorder or even the presence arising at different ages
      4) It is important to keep the lines of communication open between parent and child and offer support to the adolescent client during periods of stress
   b. Bulimia nervosa (BN)
      1) Is a disorder in which the individual engages in binge eating (consumption of large amount of high calorie/fat food in a short period of time) followed by purging behaviors; measures include self-induced vomiting, abuse of laxatives or diuretics, and excessive exercise
      2) Etiological/risk factors similar to anorexia nervosa, yet this eating disorder can often go undetected as client's physical status may prevent further inspection of eating pattern behaviors

Box 5-6

Potential Clinical Manifestations of Eating Disorders

- Tooth enamel damage
- Edema in feet and legs
- Wasted appearance
- Alopecia or thin hair
- Lanugo
- Hypotension, bradycardia
- Puffy cheeks
- Weight change
- Possible amenorrhea in older teens

3) The presence of bulimia has been primarily associated with females; nevertheless, it can present in male clients

4) The presence of BN can lead to a lifelong cyclical pattern of altered eating behaviors that can have long-term metabolic and emotional consequences for the adolescent client

4. Sports

a. Most exercise requires consumption of a well-balanced diet with increases in water and calories; proportion of increase depends on type of exercise (sprint vs. endurance); endurance exercises > 90 minutes (such as long distance running), sprint under 90 minutes (such as football); endurance nutritional requirements are greater

b. Nutrient and fluid distribution will vary according to phase of exercise cycle (i.e., training, pre-exercise, during exercise, and after exercise) (see Table 5-10)

c. Athletes may be at risk for calcium and iron deficiencies due to decreased intake of dairy products, increased needs related to bone growth and blood volume increases, and menses; supplementation may be required

d. Athletes desiring increased muscle mass must be cautioned to avoid using drugs, hormones, and nutrient supplements; the preferred method for increasing muscle mass is increased strength training with an increase in calories; weight gain should not exceed 1–2 lbs. per week

5. Disease states

a. General considerations

1) Acute disease places an adolescent at increased risk for nutritional alterations: decreased appetite, decreased nutritional intake, altered digestion and absorption of nutrients, increased needs for various nutrients and increased loss of nutrients; aberrations may be more profound during periods of most rapid growth

2) Offer a variety of foods as tolerated during illness; increase fluids to replace losses in an adolescent presenting with vomiting, diarrhea, or fever; resume regular diet as soon as possible

b. Mononucleosis

1) Infection of the B-lymphocytes commonly caused by the Epstein-Barr virus

2) Is common in adolescents living in group settings

3) Clinical manifestations: enlarged lymphatic tissue, sore throat, fever, malaise, and headache; severe cases may present with splenomegaly, hepatomegaly, and jaundice

Table 5-10

Fluid and Nutrient Recommendations for Adolescent Athlete

Training	55–75% carbohydrate 25–30 % fat 15–20 % protein
Pre-exercise (or competition)	2–4 hrs before—low fat, low protein, high carbohydrate diet
During exercise (or competition)	4–8 oz fluid every 15 minutes; fluid may be water or electrolyte/carbohydrate drink
After exercise (or competition)	16 oz fluid for every pound lost during exercise; fluid may be water or electrolyte/carbohydrate drink

4) Dietary management during acute phase: foods easy to swallow that maintain adequate calories and nutrient intake; during convalescence ingest adequate calories and nutrients to maintain intact immune system and prevent secondary infection

F. Nutritional considerations during the adolescent period

!

1. Assessment
   a. Obtain height and weight; compare with gender- and age-appropriate percentile growth charts
   b. Perform comprehensive physical exam including dentition; assess for signs of nutrient deficiencies; assess for signs of eating disorders
   c. Assess for causes of alterations in nutrition: peer pressure, body image, complex schedules, knowledge deficits, incorrect understanding of information, lack of financial resources, familial relationship issues, resistance to current values, and self-identification
2. Nursing diagnoses: Imbalanced nutrition: more than body requirements; Imbalanced nutrition: less than body requirements; Risk for imbalanced nutrition: more than body requirements; Risk for impaired adolescent growth and development
3. Planning and implementation
   a. Determine alterations needed in intake of calories and/or nutrients due to actual/potential deficiencies or excesses present
   b. Administer supplements as needed; instruct client about correct administration, common side effects, adverse reactions, and food interactions
   c. Discuss with client and caregiver causes of nutrition alterations; provide additional information, clarify misconceptions, identify resources for psychosocial concerns
4. Evaluation

!

   a. Monitor height and weight; track trends of growth
   b. Monitor adequacy of nutrient intake via food intake recall per client or caregiver
   c. Monitor for signs of nutrient deficiencies
   d. Monitor for potential complications related to possible use of nutritional supplements
   e. Determine client and caregiver's understanding of teaching through verbalization or return demonstration

Practice to Pass

A normal-weight teen is going to college and has expressed concern about gaining weight. How should the nurse respond?

VI. ADULT NUTRITION (18–64 YEARS)

A. Metabolic needs according to age

1. There is significant variation in metabolic needs due to differing age, weight, height, and physical activity; as an adult ages, overall energy needs usually decrease but requirements in selected nutrients may increase
2. Total caloric expenditure is estimated by adding the basal metabolic rate (BMR), calories expended during physical activity and the thermic effect of foods (energy needed for digestion, utilization, and storage of nutrients, usually about 10% of daily calories)

3. BMR is influenced by body composition, hormones, fever, body size, environmental temperature, starvation/fasting/malnutrition, stress, and medications
   a. Individuals with higher lean body mass have higher metabolic rates; men usually have higher rates than women due to increased muscle mass
   b. Thyroid hormones, T_3 and T_4, increase metabolic rates when levels are increased; decreases in T_3 and T_4 levels cause decreases in metabolic rates
   c. Metabolic rate will increase by 7% for each degree Fahrenheit above 98.6
   d. Severe nutritional deprivation such as starvation, fasting, and malnutrition decreases the metabolic rate
   e. Stress hormones such as catecholamines, glucocorticoids, and glucagons increase the metabolic rate
   f. Barbiturates, opioids, and muscle relaxants decrease the metabolic rate
4. Consumption of adequate micro/macronutrients and calories is essential to avoid deficiencies and to maintain metabolic processes necessary for optimal health (refer to Table 5-11) for recommended intake levels
   a. Due to an increase in nutritional misinformation, clients are at risk for over- or underconsumption of macro- and micronutrients; reliable nutrition resources and reference guides must be utilized by adults

Table 5-11 Recommended Intake of Micro- and Macronutrients for Adults (Healthy Clients)

	19–30 years		31–50 years		51–70 years		> 71 years	
Nutrient	***Male***	***Female***	***Male***	***Female***	***Male***	***Female***	***Male***	***Female***
Protein	56 grams	46 grams	56 grams	46 grams	56 grams	46 grams	56 grams	46 grams
Calcium	1,000 mg	1,000 mg	1,000 mg	1,000 mg	1,200 mg	1,200 mg	1,200 mg	1,200 mg
Iron	8 mg	18 mg	8 mg	18 mg	8 mg	8 mg	8 mg	8 mg
Magnesium	400 mg	310 mg	420 mg	320 mg	420 mg	320 mg	420 mg	320 mg
Vitamin C	90 mg	75 mg	90 mg	75 mg	90 mg	75 mg	90 mg	75 mg
Vitamin A	900 mcg	700 mcg	900 mcg	700 mcg	900 mcg	700 mcg	900 mcg	700 mcg
Vitamin K	120 mcg/day	90 mcg/day	120 mcg/day	90 mcg/day	120 mcg/day	90 mcg/day	120 mcg/day	90 mcg/day
Vitamin D	5 mcg	5 mcg	5 mcg	5 mcg	10 mcg	10 mcg	15 mcg	15 mcg
Folate	400 mcg	400 mcg	400 mcg	400 mcg	400 mcg	400 mcg	400 mcg	400 mcg
Thiamine (Vitamin B_1)	1.2 mg	1.1 mg	1.2 mg	1.1 mg	1.2 mg	1.1 mg	1.2 mg	1.2 mg
Riboflavin (Vitamin B_2)	1.3 mg	1.1 mg	1.3 mg	1.1 mg	1.3 mg	1.1 mg	1.3 mg	1.1 mg
Vitamin B_6	1.3 mg	1.3 mg	1.3 mg	1.3 mg	1.7 mg	1.5 mg	1.7 mg	1.5 mg
Vitamin B_{12}	2.4 mcg	2.4 mcg	2.4 mcg	2.4 mcg	2.4 mcg	2.4 mcg	2.4 mcg	2.4 mcg

Adapted and reprinted with permission from: Dietary Reference Intakes: Food and Nutrition Board, Institute of Medicine—National Academy of Sciences, Recommended Levels for Individual Intake. Courtesy of National Academy Press, Washington DC. Retrieved October 9, 2005 from *http://www.nap.edu/.*

b. Consumption of micronutrients in excess of recommendations can result in adverse reactions and toxicities

c. Consumption of insufficient calories may result in nutrient deficiencies and excess weight loss; excess calories may result in excess weight gain

d. Because risk for development of chronic illness increases during adulthood, consumption of a healthy diet is imperative to facilitate prevention of chronic illness

B. Maintaining and achieving ideal body weight (IBW)

1. Maintenance of ideal body weight is essential to optimal health and prevention of obesity-associated chronic illnesses; as an adult ages, the tendency to decrease physical activity, increase weight, and lose lean body mass increases; an increased central fat distribution is related to Type 2 diabetes

2. The most effective method to achieve IBW is a comprehensive plan

a. Consume a diet adequate in micro- and macronutrients

1) Use the MyPyramid for selection of foods and quantities

2) Choose a variety of foods from each group in the MyPyramid; over- or underconsumption of specific foods may result in nutrient deficiencies

3) Consider client's cultural, ethnic, and religious preferences when planning diet (refer to Table 5-2)

4) Determine age-appropriate intake for specific nutrients using nutrition reference guides such as the Daily Reference Intakes (DRI), Recommended Dietary Allowances (RDA), Estimated Average Requirements (EAR), Adequate Intake (AI), and Tolerable Upper Intake Limit (UL)

b. Maintain a caloric intake appropriate for height and weight

! 1) Use standardized height/weight tables and BMI tables to determine healthy weight

! 2) Calculate client's total caloric expenditure

3) Alter MyPyramid guidelines to reflect caloric and nutrient needs

C. Special nutritional concerns

1. Stress

a. Stress is a condition in which humans respond to change in a normal balanced state; results from internal, external, developmental, and situational stressors

! b. Physiological conditions associated with stress responses and hypermetabolism include chronic obstructive pulmonary disease (COPD), burns, trauma, major infections, and surgery

c. Regardless of the etiology, stress produces significant changes in biopsychosocial and nutritional states

1) Common biophysical changes: release of mineralocorticoids, glucocortocoids, and catecholamines causing sodium retention, protein anabolism, protein catabolism, decreased renal blood flow, increased myocardial contractility, and increased blood clotting

2) Common psychosocial changes include anxiety, fear, anger, and depression

3) Common changes affecting nutritional state include gluconeogenesis, hypermetabolism, loss of nitrogen and potassium in urine, increased fat mobilization, hyperglycemia, protein anabolism, and protein catabolism; with prolonged stress, essential stores of protein, glucose, and other nutrients

are lost, impairing body's ability to adapt to future stress and increasing likelihood of complications such as infection

d. With life-threatening stress such as major traumatic injuries, the first goal is support of vital functions to save the client's life; after stabilization, nutritional treatment focuses upon provision of calories, protein, fluids, and micronutrients

1) Calories promote healing and replace lost nutritional stores; determine energy (calorie) needs with adjustment for stress and activity

2) Proteins replace lost stores, lessen protein catabolism, and maintain an intact immune system

3) Fluid replacement is determined by amount lost through blood loss, fever, GI fluids, wound drainage, and diuresis

4) Numerous micronutrients may be administered, including B vitamins, vitamin C, vitamin K, vitamin A, iron, and zinc; these micronutrients facilitate wound healing, blood clotting, blood cell synthesis and maturation, tissue synthesis, and promote immune function

5) Clients taking anticoagulants must be monitored carefully for potential complications, accurate dosing and administration and dietary compliance with therapy (warfarin and vitamin K levels)

e. During acute stress phase, GI function may be impaired, requiring parenteral administration of fluids and nutrition; when peristalsis returns to small intestine, begin enteral feeding to stimulate intestinal blood flow and function, stimulate gut-associated lymphoid tissue, and potentially reduce hypermetabolism and subsequent refeeding syndrome; resume regular diet as soon as possible and progress from clear liquids to regular diet; nutrient and/or caloric supplements may be provided until client is able to consume adequate calories by mouth

2. Occupational influences

a. The amount of time spent away from home influences dietary intake; this usually is associated with more convenience foods and restaurant foods; potential for increased calories, fat, and sugar in the diet occurs

b. Increased stress levels may be associated with job performance

c. Alterations in nutritional intake and stress may increase the likelihood of chronic illness (cardiovascular disease, diabetes mellitus) further altering nutritional status

d. Some occupations expose the client to hazardous substances or organisms; exposure may result in disease processes that lead to nutritional alterations

3. Lifetime dietary habits

a. Previous nutritional habits affect health maintenance through adulthood; poor nutritional habits may contribute to the development of chronic diseases such as cardiovascular disease, diabetes mellitus, cancer, and obesity; numerous nutritional alterations may occur as a result of the disease or its treatment

1) Cardiovascular problems (e.g., coronary heart disease, hypertension) often require low-fat, low-cholesterol, or sodium-restricted diets

2) Cancer treatments may profoundly affect nutritional states; common alterations include anorexia, nutrient losses, and altered digestion and metabolism of nutrients; high-fat diets, consumption of red meat, and excess caloric intake have also been implicated in the development of cancer

3) Diabetes mellitus requires significant changes in the composition of meals and their timing; specific recommendations are given for consumption of proteins, fats, and carbohydrates; pharmacological support is often required in conjunction with dietary management

4) Obesity requires a comprehensive plan of weight reduction and exercise; most traditional plans include reduction of caloric and fat intake

b. Culture affects food preferences, preparation, number and timing of meals, health beliefs related to food, food's meaning, and use; characteristic dietary patterns/preferences are associated with various subcultures

4. Exercise and activity requirements

a. Aerobic exercise for a minimum of 30 minutes of low to moderate physical activity should be done most days

1) Moderate activity: walking at 3–4 mph, swimming, canoeing, and ice skating

2) Activity duration, intensity, and frequency should increase over time; more vigorous activities include brisker walking, cycling, and running

b. Strength training exercises should be done 2 times per week and stretching exercises 3 times per week minimum

1) Perform 8–10 strength training exercises that work the major muscle groups; 8–12 repetitions of same exercise

2) Increase weight over time; maintain proper form and breathing throughout weight lifts

3) Select stretching exercises that maintain posture; hold stretch for 30 seconds and repeat 3–5 times

D. Nursing considerations during the period of adulthood

1. Assessment

a. Using MyPyramid and client's dietary recall, assess adequacy of current diet

b. Perform comprehensive physical exam; assess for signs of nutrient deficiencies and chronic illnesses

c. If nutritional alterations are noted, identify potential causes: lack of knowledge, incorrect understanding of information, lack of financial resources, poor access, presence of chronic illness related dietary constraints, and cultural or religious issues

d. Determine level of activity; assess adequacy and toleration

2. Nursing diagnoses: Imbalanced nutrition: more than body requirements; Imbalanced nutrition: less than body requirements; Risk for imbalanced nutrition: more than body requirements

3. Planning and implementation

a. In collaboration with client, determine alterations needed in intake of calories and/or nutrients due to actual/potential deficiencies or excesses present; use MyPyramid as a teaching guide

b. Develop a meal plan reflecting needed alterations; assist client to identify appropriate sources of micro- and macronutrients

c. Administer supplements as needed; instruct client about correct administration, common side effects, adverse reactions, and food interactions

d. Instruct female clients about the relationship between reduced estrogen and loss of bone mass as aging occurs; provide specific information to perimenopausal females about the need for calcium and vitamin D supplements (refer back to Chapter 3 and refer to Chapter 7)

Practice to Pass

An adult client wants to know why he keeps gaining weight when, as a young man, he had no problem with weight control. What factors could affect the state of weight control in an otherwise healthy adult client?

e. Discuss with client causes of nutrition alterations; provide additional information, clarify misconceptions, identify resources for financial concerns and refer as appropriate, suggest interventions to reduce constraints and discomforts, and develop strategies to maintain nutrition within constraints of cultural or religious beliefs

f. In collaboration with client, determine alterations needed in activity level

! 4. Evaluation

a. Monitor weight; compare against initial baseline weight

b. Monitor adequacy of nutrient intake using food intake tool

c. Monitor client for signs of nutrient deficiencies

d. Monitor client for signs of adverse reactions from supplements

e. Assess efficacy of nonnutritional interventions to reduce nutritional alterations

f. Determine client's understanding of teaching through verbalization or return demonstration

VII. GERIATRIC NUTRITION (65+ YEARS)

A. Metabolic needs according to age

1. By age 90, there is a 20% decrease in Resting Energy Expenditure (REE) caused by decreased muscle mass; changes result in decreased muscle tone, decreased strength, and decreased aerobic capacity that may cause decreased physical activity; vicious cycle of further loss of muscle tone, strength, and aerobic capacity may result
2. Onset and progression of REE decrease vary significantly among individuals
3. Caloric requirements decrease as result of REE changes; specific recommendations from the Food and Nutrition Board are based on height, weight, and activity level
4. Alterations in glucose tolerance related to decreased insulin secretion and decreased insulin sensitivity may occur

B. Nutrient absorption with aging

1. Chewing difficulties can result from periodontal disease, loss of teeth, or dysphagia due to stroke or neuromuscular disease, leading to reduced intake; decreased saliva from aging or medication effect also contributes to this
2. Decreased peristalsis contributes to reduced absorption of nutrients and constipation; atrophic gastritis affects one-third of those over age 60, with resulting inflamed stomach, bacterial growth, reduced hydrochloric acid and intrinsic factor
3. Decreased digestive enzymes, GI motility, and vitamin absorption are also of concern

C. Maintaining ideal body weight (IBW)

1. Numerous physiological and functional changes may impair the geriatric client's ability to maintain ideal body weight
2. Chronic illnesses and treatment regimes such as medications and therapeutic diets may affect the client's ability to maintain IBW

a. Common medication-related side effects that may result in nutritional alterations include: nausea and vomiting, diarrhea, constipation, decreased absorption of nutrients, increased excretion of nutrients, oral mucosal changes, anorexia, malabsorption, and inactivation of nutrients

b. Restrictive therapeutic diets (such as low sodium) may result in decreased caloric intake, decreased nutrient intake, and intake of foods not within diet guidelines

D. Special nutritional concerns

1. Outside influences

   a. The loss of friends and family may result in decreased socialization and loss of opportunities for social eating

   b. Clients who must rely on others to gain access to food procurement or assist with food preparation are at risk for nutritional alterations

2. Lifetime dietary habits

   a. Previous nutritional habits affect health maintenance through older adulthood; poor nutritional habits may have contributed to the development of chronic disease with resultant medical treatments causing significant system impact

      1) The elderly client often has a multiple medication profile and is therefore at risk to develop complications (both nutritionally and physiologically) as a result of concurrent therapies

      2) Normal changes associated with the aging process can lead to altered nutritional states because thirst response decreases and the body's ability to handle fluid and electrolyte balance becomes less sensitive

   b. The elderly client may have gone through significant losses due to death of spouse and family members that can affect eating patterns and socialization levels; clients who now have no one to eat with, or no one to help them prepare food, often encounter nutritional alterations

   c. Culture, religion, and ethnic background influence dietary choices but may be affected by a change in living arrangements as when elderly clients are placed in assisted living facilities and nursing homes; it is important to recognize the impact of these influences on clients' continuing to meet nutritional needs

3. Exercise and activity requirements

   a. By age 90, there is a 20% decrease in resting energy expenditure (REE)

   b. Strength training exercises can improve muscle mass, which will improve muscle tone and increase strength; the client will be able to engage in physical activity more effectively

   c. Aerobic activity can improve aerobic capacity; cardiopulmonary function will improve

4. Decreasing physiological ability

   a. GI changes alter client's perception of food's palatability, impair ability to chew, ingest, and process food

      1) Tooth loss, dental caries, and periodontal disease

      2) Decreased gastric secretions and pancreatic/intestinal enzymes due to decreased blood flow to/from villae and decreased mucosal mass

      3) Decreased salivation and taste perception due to decreased taste buds and papillae; sweet and salty taste buds deteriorate first; bitter and sour later

      4) Decreased gastrointestinal processes of digestion, absorption, peristalsis, and metabolism

b. Sensory changes can impair the client's ability to sense the palatability of food; others may cause a client to become uncomfortable eating in social situations
   1) Decreased visual acuity and hearing loss
   2) Increased odor threshold, decreased perceived odor intensity, decreased ability to identify odors
   3) Decreased sensation of thirst
c. Nervous system changes may impair the client's ability to purchase, prepare, and consume food; others may cause a client to become uncomfortable eating in social situations; common changes include:
   1) Tremors and decreased reaction times
   2) Cognitive and personality changes such as short-term memory loss, depression, and dementia
d. Common nutrient deficiencies found in the elderly include protein, fiber, iron, calcium, magnesium, and vitamins D, B_{12}, and B_6
   1) Gradually increase fiber-rich foods in diet (fruit, whole grains, beans, and vegetables); these often provide the other nutrients that the elderly client lacks
   2) Techniques to increase caloric density if needed include adding milk powder to liquid milk, replacing water with milk in recipes, and increasing high-calorie snacks

5. Financial concerns
   a. Fixed incomes may result in decreased resources available to purchase food or food with high nutritional value
   b. Presence of chronic disease may further usurp limited resources due to purchases of medications and care products; with decreasing dollars available for food, client may choose cheaper, less nutrient-dense foods

E. Nursing considerations during the geriatric period

1. Assessment
   a. Using MyPyramid and client's dietary recall assess adequacy of current diet
   b. Perform comprehensive physical exam; assess for signs of nutrient deficiencies and chronic illnesses
   c. If nutritional alterations are noted, identify potential causes: lack of knowledge, incorrect understanding of information, lack of financial resources, poor access, presence of chronic illness–related dietary constraints, functional constraints, and cultural or religious issues
   d. Determine level of activity; assess adequacy and toleration
2. Nursing diagnoses: Imbalanced nutrition: more than body requirements; Imbalanced nutrition: less than body requirements; Risk for imbalanced nutrition: more than body requirements
3. Planning and implementation
   a. In collaboration with client, determine alterations needed in intake of calories and/or nutrients due to actual/potential deficiencies or excesses present; use MyPyramid as a teaching guide
   b. Develop a meal plan reflecting needed alterations; assist client in identification of appropriate sources of micronutrients
   c. Administer supplements as needed; instruct client about correct administration, common side effects, adverse reactions, and food interactions

Practice to Pass

How can the nurse support the elderly client in meeting nutritional goals?

d. The U.S. government funds the Elderly Nutrition Program; identify resources for congregate meals or home-delivered meals

e. Discuss with client causes of nutrition alterations; provide additional information, clarify misconceptions, identify resources for financial concerns and refer as appropriate, suggest interventions to reduce constraints/discomforts, and develop strategies to maintain nutrition within constraints of cultural or religious beliefs

f. In collaboration with client, determine alterations needed in activity level, giving special consideration to limitations posed by chronic disease (cardiovascular, respiratory as examples)

! 4. Evaluation

a. Monitor weight; compare against initial baseline weight

b. Monitor adequacy of nutrient intake using food intake tool

c. Monitor client for signs of nutrient deficiencies

d. Monitor client for signs of adverse reactions from supplements

e. Assess efficacy of nonnutritional interventions to reduce nutritional alterations

f. Determine client's understanding of teaching through verbalization or return demonstration

Case Study

A 40-year-old male client reports that he is "out of shape," overweight, and has a strong family history of Type 2 diabetes mellitus and heart disease. He would like to make lifestyle changes to improve his health. Develop a comprehensive plan for this client.

1. What assessment information do you need?
2. How would you calculate his daily caloric needs?
3. What ethnic, cultural, and religious considerations must be included in the planning?
4. What type of exercise would be appropriate? What information is needed to determine a safe level of exercise?

For suggested responses, see pages 318–319.

POSTTEST

POSTTEST

1 A moderately overweight client who is 4 weeks pregnant is at the first prenatal visit. The nurse should give highest priority to which of the following nutritional information during teaching?

1. "Add an additional 300 calories to your daily diet now to ensure adequate nutrients are available to support your developing fetus."
2. "You will need to follow a weight reduction diet, no lower than 1200 calories and adequate in essential nutrients."
3. "As long as your diet is well balanced in all nutrients, a vitamin/mineral supplement will not be required."
4. "You must eat a nutritionally sound diet. Pregnancy is not the time to lose weight."

2 A 2-day postpartum client informs the nurse, "Something is wrong with my milk; it is yellow." Which of the following statements by the nurse is most appropriate?

1. "You probably have a breast infection and will need to stop breastfeeding.
2. "You are most likely dehydrated. Increase your consumption of caffeine-free fluids so the milk will not be so thick."
3. "The yellow fluid is normal and is called colostrum, a precursor to milk. It is full of nutrients and wonderful for the baby to drink."
4. "What foods have you been eating? Some foods can discolor the milk."

3 The nurse has completed client teaching about introducing solid foods to an infant. The nurse determines teaching has been effective when the mother identifies the first solid food she will introduce is:

1. Pureed canned squash
2. Pureed apples
3. Yogurt
4. Infant rice cereal

4 When caring for a pregnant client with congenital heart disease, the nurse plans for which alterations in the client's diet during pregnancy?

1. Reduced calories and reduced fat
2. Caffeine and sodium restrictions
3. Decreased protein and increased complex carbohydrates
4. Fluid restriction and reduced calories

5 An adult female client has been treated for iron deficiency anemia. To evaluate the effectiveness of the treatment, the nurse would assess for resolution of which of the following symptoms?

1. Dermatitis
2. Pale conjunctiva
3. Bleeding gums
4. Hair pigment changes

6 An infant with congenital hypothyroidism is placed on thyroid replacement therapy. Which of the following information is the most essential information for the nurse to include in discharge teaching with the parents?

1. The supplement may be mixed with formula.
2. Notify the physician if the infant continues to be excessively sleepy.
3. This replacement must be taken for the child's entire life to ensure normal growth and development.
4. Notify the physician if the child becomes excessively irritable and diaphoretic.

7 The nurse interprets that a premature infant is at greatest risk for inadequate intake of which of the following vitamins because of alterations in fat absorption?

1. B complex
2. Vitamin C
3. Vitamin E
4. Folic acid

8 An adult client being started on sodium warfarin (Coumadin) had previously been taking over-the-counter vitamin K supplements. The nurse teaches the client to do which of the following at this time?

1. Discontinue taking the supplements.
2. Increase the intake of dietary sources of vitamin K so no additional supplementation will be needed.
3. Take vitamin K supplements every other day while on anticoagulant therapy.
4. Discuss this issue with the healthcare provider at the next scheduled appointment.

9 A regular diet has been resumed for a client following a major traumatic injury. The nurse selects from the diet menu which of the following meals that would be most appropriate for the client?

1. Vegetable lasagna, bibb lettuce with dressing, white roll, slice of pound cake
2. Chicken breast, brown rice, broccoli, fresh orange slices
3. Fried codfish fillet, macaroni and cheese, peas, jello
4. Roast beef, mashed potatoes, corn, and ice cream

10 The nurse has completed a comprehensive health history on an 80-year-old recently widowed client who lost 15 pounds in 2 months. The nurse anticipates which of the following is the most likely explanation?

1. Reliance on fixed income
2. Depression and sense of loss over spouse's death
3. Use of limited funds for medications
4. Limited opportunities for social eating

See pages 152–154 for Answers and Rationales.

ANSWERS & RATIONALES

Pretest

1 **Answer: 0.4 mg/day** Due to strong correlation between NTD and folic acid deficiency, a 0.4 mg/day supplement is recommended for client considering pregnancy. Note that a dose of 0.6 mg/day is recommended for pregnant women; 4 mg/day is recommended for short-term dosing for women with past history of pregnancy with NTD. **Cognitive Level:** Application **Client Need:** Health Promotion and Maintenance **Integrated Process:** Nursing Process: Implementation **Content Area:** Foundational Sciences: Nutrition **Strategy:** Note the question addresses the recommended dose for someone trying to conceive, which may be different than for someone already pregnant. Recall specific knowledge of folate requirements to provide the correct response. **Reference:** Rolfes, S., Pinna, K., & Whitney, E. (2006). *Understanding normal and clinical nutrition* (7th ed.). Belmont, CA: Wadsworth & Thomson Learning, p. 336.

2 **Answer: 2** A poorly positioned infant can cause trauma to the nipple. Although nipples can become infected, it is not most common cause; breasts should be cleansed after feeding; letting breast milk dry on nipples has been an effective treatment for sore nipples due to high fat content and anti-infective substances in breast milk. **Cognitive Level:** Analysis **Client Need:** Health Promotion and Maintenance **Integrated Process:** Nursing Process: Assessment **Content Area:** Maternal-Newborn **Strategy:** A critical word in the question is *most,* indicating all or some of the options may be correct, but one choice is the best. Eliminate option 1 since this is not frequently seen. Eliminate options 3 and 4 since they are also not a likely cause. **Reference:** Nix, S. (2005). *Williams' basic nutrition & diet therapy* (12th ed.). St. Louis, MO: Elsevier Mosby, p. 187.

3 **Answer: 2** According to BMI criteria, the client would be considered "overweight" and advised to maintain weight gain between 15-25 lbs. A less than 15 lb. gain is the restriction for "obese" clients; weight gains of 25 lbs. or greater are for clients of normal weight or who are underweight. **Cognitive Level:** Analysis **Client Need:** Health Promotion and Maintenance **Integrated Process:** Nursing Process: Planning **Content Area:** Foundational Sciences: Nutrition **Strategy:** Critical words are *prenatal* and *BMI* of *27.5.* Recognize this BMI is high to direct you to option 2. **Reference:** Nix, S. (2005). *Williams' basic nutrition & diet therapy* (12th ed.). St. Louis, MO: Elsevier Mosby, p. 179.

4 **Answer: 1** Dark, leafy vegetables like spinach are an alternative source of vitamin C. Corn is a good source of fiber but not vitamin C; sweet potatoes are rich in vitamin A; celery provides water and fiber. **Cognitive Level:** Application **Client Need:** Health Promotion and Maintenance **Integrated Process:** Nursing Process: Implementation **Content Area:** Foundational Sciences: Nutrition. **Strategy:** Critical words are *most appropriate, alternative,* and *vitamin C.* Note all options are vegetables and recall those with a high vitamin C content to choose option 1. **Reference:** Nix, S. (2005). *Williams' basic nutrition & diet therapy* (12th ed.). St. Louis, MO: Elsevier Mosby, p. 104.

5 **Answer: 3** PKU is a genetic disorder that reflects a problem with the metabolism of phenylalanine (amino acid). A special diet should be followed that restricts/limits the intake of this amino acid in order to avoid potential metabolic complications. The other options do not acknowledge that this inborn error of metabolism has lifelong consequences. **Cognitive Level:** Application **Client Need:** Health Promotion and Maintenance **Integrated Process:** Teaching and Learning **Content Area:** Foundational Sciences: Nutrition **Strategy:** A critical phrase is *adequate nutritional management.* Recall knowledge of PKU and need for lifelong therapy to direct you to option 3. **Reference:** Nix, S. (2005). *Williams' basic nutrition & diet therapy* (12th ed.). St. Louis, MO: Elsevier Mosby, pp. 338–339.

6 **Answer: 4** Foods should be introduced singly to identify allergies if they occur. Combination foods, such as those that would be served to the family, are not advised due to difficulty identifying allergies, and some table foods may have high-sodium substances not tolerated well by

an infant. Cereal should not be placed in bottle because it deprives the infant of an opportunity to develop chewing muscles. Formula should not be stopped all at once; it should be gradually weaned as the amount of solids increases to prevent weight and nutrient loss. **Cognitive Level:** Analysis **Client Need:** Health Promotion and Maintenance **Integrated Process:** Nursing Process: Evaluation **Content Area:** Foundational Sciences: Nutrition **Strategy:** Read each option carefully and systematically eliminate options 1, 2, and 3 since they do not answer the question or give incorrect advice. **Reference:** Nix, S. (2005). *Williams' basic nutrition & diet therapy* (12th ed.). St. Louis, MO: Elsevier Mosby, p. 201.

7 **Answer: 1** Vitamin C promotes collagen formation and hence wound healing. Vitamins B_1 and B_{12} are involved primarily with the neurological system; vitamin K is involved with the blood coagulation cascade.
Cognitive Level: Application **Client Need:** Health Promotion and Maintenance **Integrated Process:** Nursing Process: Implementation **Content Area:** Foundational Sciences: Nutrition **Strategy:** The core concept is difficulty with wound healing. Recall that ascorbic acid aids in tissue repair to choose option 1. **Reference:** Nix, S. (2005). *Williams' basic nutrition & diet therapy* (12th ed.). St. Louis, MO: Elsevier Mosby, p. 102.

8 **Answer: 4** Glycosylated hemoglobin (HbA_{1c}) levels are indicators of longer term glucose control (last 4-8 weeks); 12% indicates poor control, not good control. To determine cause and best treatment, a comprehensive evaluation of diet and so on would be indicated. One value of 12% would not necessitate insulin administration.
Cognitive Level: Application **Client Need:** Physiological Integrity: Reduction of Risk Potential **Integrated Process:** Teaching and Learning **Content Area:** Foundational Sciences: Nutrition **Strategy:** The core concept of the question addresses interpretation of glycosylated hemoglobin levels, with this being a high level. Systematically eliminate incorrect options 1 and 2. Note option 3 may be correct but cannot be told to client with absolute certainty and choose option 4. **Reference:** Rolfes, S., Pinna, K., & Whitney, E. (2006). *Understanding normal and clinical nutrition* (7th ed.). Belmont, CA: Wadsworth & Thomson Learning, p. 799.

9 **Answer: 4** Decreased saliva makes it difficult to moisten the food bolus so that it can be swallowed. Periodontal disease and jaw deterioration affect chewing. Decreased peristalsis affects passage of bolus once in esophagus.
Cognitive Level: Application **Client Need:** Health Promotion and Maintenance **Integrated Process:** Nursing Process: Assessment **Content Area:** Foundational Sciences: Nutrition **Strategy:** Critical words are *elderly,* and *difficulty swallowing.* Eliminate option 2 since it does not involve chewing and swallowing. Recall physiological changes of aging to choose option 4. **Reference:** Nix, S. (2005). *Williams' basic nutrition & diet therapy* (12th ed.). St. Louis, MO: Elsevier Mosby, p. 217.

10 **Answer: 3** Kidney beans are legumes and contain 5.6 grams of insoluble fiber per 1/2 cup. The other foods are not fiber rich.
Cognitive Level: Analysis **Client Need:** Health Promotion and Maintenance **Integrated Process:** Nursing Process: Evaluation **Content Area:** Foundational Sciences: Nutrition **Strategy:** Recall knowledge of fiber content of foods. Eliminate options 1 and 4 as incorrect. Note spinach is creamed to eliminate it as well. **Reference:** Nix, S. (2005). *Williams' basic nutrition & diet therapy* (12th ed.). St. Louis, MO: Elsevier Mosby, pp. 21–22.

Posttest

1 **Answer: 4** Weight reduction is never indicated during pregnancy. Moderate weight gains of 15-25 pounds are recommended for overweight clients. Option 1 is incorrect—an increase in calories in the first trimester is not indicated, whereas in the second trimester and third, caloric needs are increased by 300. Option 2 is incorrect—weight reduction is not indicated during pregnancy. Option 3 is incorrect—all pregnant women receive supplements (prenatal vitamins) to ensure adequate folic acid is obtained, regardless of dietary intake.
Cognitive Level: Application **Client Need:** Health Promotion and Maintenance **Integrated Process:** Teaching and Learning **Content Area:** Foundational Sciences: Nutrition **Strategy:** Critical words are *overweight, 4 weeks pregnant,* and *highest priority.* Recall concepts of nutritional needs in the first trimester of pregnancy to choose option 4. **Reference:** Nix, S. (2005). *Williams' basic nutrition & diet therapy* (12th ed.). St. Louis, MO: Elsevier Mosby, p. 179.

2 **Answer: 3** Colostrum is produced before milk until about 4 days postpartum. It is yellow, rich in nutrients, and should be consumed by the baby. Option 1 is incorrect—there is nothing to suggest that the client has a breast infection (temperature or breast soreness). Option 2 is incorrect—dehydration may be associated with letdown of milk, not color. Option 4 is incorrect—foods do not affect color but may alter taste.
Cognitive Level: Application **Client Need:** Health Promotion and Maintenance **Integrated Process:** Communication and Documentation **Content Area:** Maternal Newborn **Strategy:** Note that the client is only 2 days post partum. Recall colostrum is secreted in the first few days to direct you to option 3. **Reference:** Nix, S. (2005). *Williams' basic nu-*

trition & diet therapy (12th ed.). St. Louis, MO: Elsevier Mosby, pp. 186–189.

3 **Answer: 4** Single-grain infant cereals are recommended first because they are easily digestible and have added iron content. Option 3 is incorrect because yogurt is a milk product, and introduction should be delayed until 12 months because of the risk of milk allergy. Options 1 and 2 are incorrect because fruits and vegetables are usually given following the introduction of cereals.
Cognitive Level: Application **Client Need:** Health Promotion and Maintenance **Integrated Process:** Nursing Process: Evaluation **Content Area:** Foundational Sciences: Nutrition. **Strategy:** Recall need to begin solid food introduction with a cereal to choose option 4. **Reference:** Nix, S. (2005). *Williams' basic nutrition & diet therapy* (12th ed.). St. Louis, MO: Elsevier Mosby, p. 201.

4 **Answer: 2** Caffeine may increase heart rate that is already stressed due to pregnancy. Sodium may cause fluid retention. Both may need to be restricted. The other answers are incorrect because calories, fat, and protein are not usually decreased due to the risk of nutrient deficiencies.
Cognitive Level: Application **Client Need:** Health Promotion and Maintenance **Integrated Process:** Nursing Process: Planning **Content Area:** Foundational Sciences: Nutrition **Strategy:** The critical words are *heart disease.* Recall the significance of caffeine and sodium on cardiac function to direct you to option 2. **Reference:** Nix, S. (2005). *Williams' basic nutrition & diet therapy* (12th ed.). St. Louis, MO: Elsevier Mosby, pp. 182–185.

5 **Answer: 2** A sign of anemia is pale conjunctiva. If resolved, the conjunctiva should be pinker. The other symptoms are not specific to iron deficiency and are usually associated with other vitamin or mineral deficiencies.
Cognitive Level: Application **Client Need:** Physiological Integrity: Physiological Adaptation **Integrated Process:** Nursing Process: Evaluation **Content Area:** Foundational Sciences: Nutrition **Strategy:** Critical words are *iron deficiency* and *effectiveness.* Recall symptoms of anemia to direct you to option 2. **Reference:** Rolfes, S., Pinna, K., & Whitney, E. (2006). *Understanding normal and clinical nutrition* (7th ed.). Belmont, CA: Wadsworth & Thomson Learning, p. 443.

6 **Answer: 3** At the beginning of therapy, it is essential that parents understand its importance. Other information is less of a priority. The other options contain information about administration, assessing effectiveness, and side effects, which can be explained next.
Cognitive Level: Analysis **Client Need:** Health Promotion and Maintenance **Integrated Process:** Nursing Process: Planning **Content Area:** Pharmacology **Strategy:** Critical words are *most essential,* indicating some or all of the options are correct, but one is much more important. Note the condition is congenital, indicating it will be life long to direct you to option 3. **Reference:** Adams, M., Josephson, D., & Holland, L. (2005). *Pharmacology for nurses: A pathophysiologic approach.* Upper Saddle River, NJ: Pearson/Education, pp. 574–575.

7 **Answer: 3** Vitamin E is a fat-soluble vitamin, and the infant is at greatest risk of deficiencies due to impaired fat absorption. The other nutrients are also at risk for deficiency but usually because of inadequate stores. All of the other options represent water-soluble vitamins.
Cognitive Level: Analysis **Client Need:** Health Promotion and Maintenance **Integrated Process:** Nursing Process: Analysis **Content Area:** Foundational Sciences: Nutrition **Strategy:** The core issue of the question is the ability to discriminate between fat-soluble and water-soluble vitamins. Note correlation of altered fat absorption in question to the only option that is a fat-soluble vitamin. **Reference:** Rolfes, S., Pinna, K., & Whitney, E. (2006). *Understanding normal and clinical nutrition* (7th ed.). Belmont, CA: Wadsworth & Thomson Learning, p. 516.

8 **Answer: 1** A client receiving anticoagulant therapy should not take additional supplementation of vitamin K, either through dietary intake or supplemental therapies, because vitamin K antagonizes sodium warfarin (Coumadin). Option 2 is not advised because increased dietary intake can also influence this drug, resulting in altered clotting times. Option 3 is incorrect for the reasons stated above. While it is important to discuss any supplemental therapy with the healthcare provider (option 4), the time delay would place the client at risk for complications related to anticoagulant therapy.
Cognitive Level: Application **Client Need:** Physiological Integrity: Reduction of Risk Potential **Integrated Process:** Teaching and Learning **Content Area:** Foundational Sciences: Nutrition **Strategy:** The core issue of the question is an interaction between oral anticoagulant therapy and vitamin K. Recall correlation of vitamin K to clotting to direct you to option 1. **Reference:** Rolfes, S., Pinna, K., & Whitney, E. (2006). *Understanding normal and clinical nutrition* (7th ed.). Belmont, CA: Wadsworth & Thomson Learning, pp. 382–384.

9 **Answer: 2** Nutrient stores exhausted during major trauma include protein, B complex vitamins, zinc, and vitamins A and C. Option 2 is rich in all these nutrients. All of the other options reflect a lack of specific nutrients needed to replenish stores.
Cognitive Level: Analysis **Client Need:** Health Promotion and Maintenance **Integrated Process:** Nursing Process:

Implementation **Content Area:** Foundational Sciences: Nutrition **Strategy:** Critical words are *major traumatic injury* and *replenish nutrients.* Recall significance of protein and vitamins for wound healing to direct you to option 2. **Reference:** Nix, S. (2005). *Williams' basic nutrition & diet therapy* (12th ed.). St. Louis, MO: Elsevier Mosby, pp. 413–415.

10 **Answer: 2** The most likely explanation is the death of the spouse. All of the other choices reflect factors that would have been present previously; the client had no problems until the spouse died. Depression and loneliness have been documented as major causes of nutrient alterations in the elderly. **Cognitive Level:** Analysis **Client Need:** Psychosocial Integrity **Integrated Process:** Nursing Process: Analysis **Content Area:** Foundational Sciences: Nutrition **Strategy:** Critical words are *recently widowed.* Recognize all options contain factors contributing to poor dietary habits of the elderly, but option 2 has a connection to the loss of spouse. **Reference:** Nix, S. (2005). *Williams' basic nutrition & diet therapy* (12th ed.). St. Louis, MO: Elsevier Mosby, p. 213.

References

Adams, M., Josephson, D., & Holland, L. (2005). *Pharmacology for nurses: A pathophysiologic approach.* Upper Saddle River, NJ: Pearson Education, pp. 574–575.

Cataldo, C. B., DeBruyne, L. K., & Whitney, E. N. (2006). *Nutrition and diet therapy* (7th ed.). Belmont, CA: Wadsworth & Thomson Learning, pp. 199–203.

Dudek, S. G. (2006). *Nutrition essentials for nursing practice* (5th ed.). Philadelphia: Lippincott, Williams & Wilkins, pp. 344–367.

Kozier, B., Erb., G., Berman, A. J., & Burke, K. (2004). *Fundamentals of nursing: Concepts, process, and practice* (7th ed.). Upper Saddle River, NJ: Prentice Hall.

LeMone, P., & Burke, K. (2004). *Medical-surgical nursing: Critical thinking in client care* (3rd ed.). Upper Saddle River, NJ: Prentice Hall.

Nix, S. (2005). *Williams' basic nutrition & diet therapy* (12th ed.). St. Louis: Elsevier Mosby.

Rolfes, S., Pinna, K., & Whitney, E. (2006). *Understanding normal and clinical nutrition* (7th ed.). Belmont, CA: Wadsworth & Thomson Learning, pp. 474–571.

Nutrition Therapy for Eating Disorders, Burns, and Cardiac, Endocrine, and Gastrointestinal Disorders

6

Chapter Outline

The Client with an Eating Disorder

The Client with Burns

The Client with a Cardiac Disorder

The Client with an Endocrine Disorder

The Client with a Gastrointestinal (GI) Disorder

Objectives

- Review basic physiological principles relevant to clients with selected cardiac, metabolic, endocrine, or gastrointestinal disorders.
- Identify specific nutritional therapies that can be used to treat clients with selected cardiac, metabolic, endocrine, or gastrointestinal disorders.
- Discuss the importance of adequate nutritional monitoring of clients with selected cardiac, metabolic, endocrine, or gastrointestinal disorders to prevent further complications.
- Review dietary measures used to treat clients with selected cardiac, metabolic, endocrine, or gastrointestinal disorders.
- Discuss the impact of selected cardiac, metabolic, endocrine, or gastrointestinal disease states on the nutritional well-being of a client.

NCLEX-RN® Test Prep

Use the CD-ROM enclosed with this book to access additional practice opportunities.

Review at a Glance

15-15 rule treatment of hypoglycemia: if blood glucose < 60 mg/dL, consume 15 g carbohydrate (2–3 glucose tablets; 6–10 Lifesavers candies; 4–6 ounces juice), recheck blood glucose in 15 minutes, repeat if needed

anorexia eating disorder characterized by excessive weight loss and refusal to maintain appropriate weight for normal age and height that results in altered body image and multisystem abnormalities

bulimia eating disorder characterized by repeated cycling behaviors of bingeing and purging that result in altered body image and multisystem abnormalities

Curreri formula formula used to determine kilocalorie (kcal) requirements after a burn injury: adult: (25 kcal × kilogram (kg) preburn body weight) + (40 kcal × % of body burned); child (< 12 years): (60 kcal × kg preburn bodyweight) + (35 kcal × % of body burned)

dumping syndrome can occur when two-thirds or more of the stomach is removed and intake of concentrated liquid leads to hyperperistalsis, diarrhea, abdominal pain, and vomiting 30–60 minutes after eating

dyslipidemia abnormal lipid profile in the clinical setting

gastric bypass diet postoperative diet that focuses on food consistency and volume in restoring normal nutritional status; diet is adequate in protein and nutrient density to promote healing

gastroparesis delayed emptying time and decreased GI motility that can occur as a surgical complication or as a complication of a disease process (e.g., diabetic gastroparesis)

glycosylated hemoglobin (Hemoglobin A_{1c}) test that measures degree of glucose control over the previous three months

high-density lipoproteins (HDLs) substances that carry lipids away from arteries to liver for metabolism; decreased level = increased risk of coronary artery disease; level increased with exercise and estrogen

homocysteine amino acid produced by breakdown of essential amino acids found in dietary proteins that correlates with increased incidence of heart disease and decreased levels of B vitamins

hypermetabolic response increased energy and metabolism requirements due to stress, trauma, burns, or disease states

low-density lipoproteins (LDLs) substances that have affinity for artery walls; increased level = increased coronary artery disease

omega-3 fatty acids most unsaturated form of fat; decreases triglyceride levels, inflammation, clotting time, and heart arrhythmias; found in coldwater fish (mackerel, albacore tuna, salmon, sardines, lake trout, shellfish) and flaxseed

Parkland formula formula used to determine fluid replacement needs after a burn injury: 4 mL Lactated Ringer's solution × kilogram (kg) preburn body weight × % of body burned; 1/2 total given over first 8 hours; 1/4 total given over second 8 hours; 1/4 total given over third 8 hours

Russell's sign clinical evidence of self-induced vomiting characterized by abrasions on the dorsal surface of the hand

sodium sensitivity excessive sodium intake related to increased BP, fluid retention, volume, and SVR

very low-density lipoproteins (VLDLs) substances that carry lipids from liver to tissues for use and storage; direct correlation to coronary artery disease uncertain

PRETEST

1 A client newly diagnosed with anorexia nervosa refuses to eat. Which of the following interventions by the nurse would be most appropriate?

1. Have the client's mother come to the nursing unit during meals.
2. Sit with the client and offer gentle encouragement.
3. Leave the client alone to eat in privacy.
4. Obtain an order to place a feeding tube.

2 When planning for the nutritional needs of a client with partial- and full-thickness burns, the nurse calculates the total kilocalories needs in relation to which of the following?

1. Preburn height and weight
2. Extent of the burn
3. Cause of the burn
4. Location of the burn

3 A client with a colostomy has been experiencing increased flatus for the past 3 days. Which client information provided during assessment would lead the nurse to suspect an etiology for this occurrence?

1. The client has been eating pasta for the past 3 days.
2. The client has been eating cereal and milk for breakfast each morning.
3. The client has been eating at a salad bar for lunch for the past 3 days.
4. The client has been drinking more fluids for the past 3 days.

4 The nurse is assisting a client who has a newly created ileostomy with menu selection. In order to offset the potential electrolyte losses from the ileostomy, the nurse suggests the following foods? Select all that apply.

1. Asparagus
2. Potatoes
3. An orange
4. A chicken breast
5. Tomato juice

5 The nurse is counseling a 14-year-old diabetic client about diet and insulin. The client has soccer practice every day after school. Because the blood glucose records indicate daily levels are between 120 and 140 mg/dL before practice, the nurse provides which instruction to the client?

1. No additional food is needed before practice.
2. Decrease carbohydrate (CHO) intake by 15 grams before practice.
3. Increase CHO intake by 15 grams before practice.
4. Increase regular insulin injection by 2 units.

6 The nurse has reviewed the American Diabetes Association Exchange Lists with a diabetic client. The nurse concludes that instruction is effective when the client chooses which food pairs as an equivalent allowable exchange?

1. 1 tablespoon peanut butter = 1 ounce ground beef
2. 1 cup milk = 1 cup yogurt
3. 1/2 cup carrots = 1/2 grapefruit
4. 1/2 bagel = 1/2 cup eggplant

7 A client newly diagnosed with irritable bowel syndrome asks the nurse how future attacks can be prevented. What is the nurse's best response?

1. Include seltzer water with each meal.
2. Use a stimulant laxative once a day.
3. Reduce the amount of fiber in the diet.
4. Identify and reduce emotional stressors.

8 In order to reduce the development of dumping syndrome in a post-gastric resection client, the nurse encourages the client to:

1. Increase fluid intake with meals to decrease nausea.
2. Provide a diet that is low in complex carbohydrates and high in fat and protein.
3. Eat several small meals throughout the day.
4. Have milk with every meal to coat the stomach lining.

9 A client is diagnosed with hypercholesterolemia. The nurse would instruct the client to limit intake of which of the following favorite foods in the client's diet? Select all that apply.

1. Yogurt
2. Liver
3. Chicken
4. Eggs
5. Carrots

10 The nurse has just admitted a client who has bulimia and has been abusing laxatives and diet pills. The nurse places highest priority on which of the following goals of care?

1. Promote adequate nutrition and retention of food.
2. Promote the acceptance of self and body.
3. Promote the development of insight into the behaviors.
4. Promote the development of realistic dieting expectations.

See pages 183–185 for Answers and Rationales.

I. THE CLIENT WITH AN EATING DISORDER

A. Anorexia

1. Description
   a. This is a DSM-IV diagnosis that consists of a disturbance in body perception, level of denial, and refusal to maintain body weight that is characteristic of developmental age and height
   b. It is accompanied by amenorrhea related to altered hormonal state of at least 3 consecutive cycles or primary amenorrhea

c. Clients with anorexia are prone to develop severe osteopenia (decrease in bone mineral density)

d. Clients with anorexia can exhibit binge eating or purge type behavior; overall, anorexia is referred to as a restrictive type of eating disorder

! e. Personal characteristics of clients with anorexia include the following: high achiever, perfectionism, obsessive-compulsive behavior, social isolation, compliancy, dependency, feeling of self-worth tied to weight, shape, or thinness, distorted body image

f. Parental issues may include rigid parental control, failure to separate from mother, fear of growing up

2. Associated nutritional problems

! a. There are refusal behaviors associated with eating that are correlated with an intense fear of gaining weight or becoming fat

b. There is a weight loss of at least 25% of original body weight

! c. Bizarre eating habits/rituals are present: cutting foods into tiny pieces, refusal to eat certain types of foods, eating very slowly, delaying eating by arranging and rearranging food on the plate, eating only specific quantities of food (e.g., 6 carrots, 2 tablespoons yogurt), and secretly disposing of food

d. There is a focus on control issues related to food/weight intake that range from daily weighing and measuring of body parts, counting calories and fat grams in all foods, to excessive exercise to burn off calories consumed

e. Vitamin deficiencies (vitamin B complex) affect brain functioning and judgment, and cause lethargy, confusion, delirium, and insomnia

f. Protein-energy malnutrition (PEM) is present, which can alter growth and development and slow the basal metabolic rate; it is characterized by low albumin level, low hemoglobin and hematocrit levels, dry scaly skin, and alopecia

! g. There may be an acute starvation state characterized by electrolyte imbalance (may cause heart rhythm disturbances that can be fatal) and depressed immune system (infections can be life threatening)

h. A decreased fluid volume contributes to electrolyte deficiencies

i. Multisystem effects of the disease process can lead to serious outcomes that can include death

3. Dietary measures used as treatment

a. Multidisciplinary approach: physicians, nurses, psychiatrists, family therapists, and dietitians

! b. Goals: stop weight loss, establish regular eating patterns, and correct malnutrition and cachexia (general ill health, weakness, and emaciation)

c. See Box 6-1 for nutritional guidelines for treatment of anorexia

d. Provide guidance on nutrition and exercise

4. Nutritional monitoring

a. Teamwork, consistency, and trust are essential for success

b. Supervise mealtimes as needed to ensure eating

c. Record food intake and exercise/activity

d. Use behavior modification: reward food intake, not weight gain

e. Minimize emphasis on food; never force client to eat

! f. The following are indicators of successful treatment: slow weight gain (1–2 pounds per week); no signs of malnutrition (normal lab values, resumption of

Box 6-1

Nutritional Guidelines for Treatment of Anorexia

- Restore hydration and correct electrolyte imbalance.
- Individualize diet plan.
- Increase food intake gradually (200 kilocalories/week).
- Include foods from each of the food groups.
- May allow exclusion of 2 or 3 individual foods from diet plan, but not entire food groups.
- Include additional calcium to restore bone mineralization.
- Provide small frequent meals.
- Offer finger foods and snacks at room or cold temperatures (decreases satiety).
- Reduce caffeine intake.
- Include high-fiber and low-sodium foods (decreases constipation and fluid retention).
- Offer juice or milk, which provide for a high energy or kcal intake.
- Include multivitamin and mineral supplements.
- Provide IV nutritional support or nasogastric tube feedings for severe cases of malnutrition and wasting (never as punishment).
- Teach a new approach to food choices, emphasizing nutrients and quality of food.
- Gradually reintroduce formerly avoided or forbidden foods.

menses); tolerance of fat and sodium in diet (no GI upset or bloating; no fluid retention); compliance with diet and follow-up counseling; change in eating habits and attitudes toward food and weight

g. Baseline labs such as serum chemistry, electrolytes, urea nitrogen (BUN), creatinine, thyroid function, complete blood count (CBC), and urinalysis (UA) are needed to validate client status and direct treatment methods

h. A target weight goal of within 10% of a healthy weight range for the individual client should be determined and projected as an outcome

i. Multivitamins, vitamin D, and calcium should be included in the diet

5. Disease impact

a. It is most commonly seen in females in adolescence through young adulthood; however, other age groups and males do present with this type of eating disorder and should not be overlooked during the assessment phase

b. Treatment requires a long-term, family-based approach

c. Many clients with anorexia have lifelong issues with this disease process and have recurrent symptoms and relapses

d. Anorexia is a serious disease that can result in death as a consequence of starvation, electrolyte imbalance, or psychological disorders that result in suicide

e. There is an increased mortality rate associated with this disease process due to the multisystem effects that can result

B. Bulimia

1. Description

a. This is a DSM-IV diagnosis that identifies recurrent binge eating with purging that prevents weight gain in the individual client; this behavior extends for a timeframe of 3 months with at least 2 episodes per week; psychological manifestations of this disease include a distorted body image and a decreased self-esteem that further perpetuate the cyclic behavior

b. Bulimic behavior exists in purging type (regular self-induced vomiting, laxative abuse, or diuretic use) and nonpurging type (severe dietary restriction [fasting] or excessive exercise)

c. Personal characteristics include the following: low self-esteem, perfectionism, impulsive/compulsive behavior, social isolation, sets high unrealistic goals, fear of becoming obese, obsession over body shape and weight, depression, and substance abuse

2. Associated nutritional problems

   a. There is a sense of loss of control over eating; food is consumed for emotional value, not nutrition

   b. There are recurrent episodes of bingeing/gorging (eating large amounts of food in a discrete amount of time, such as 2 hours)

   c. Frequent purging occurs (self-induced vomiting, laxative abuse, or use of diuretics) and excessive exercise to prevent weight gain

   ! d. Electrolyte imbalance occurs secondary to vomiting, laxative and diuretic use; this can lead to cardiac dysrhythmias and injury to kidneys

   e. Laxative overdose can lead to serious complications, such as cathartic colon syndrome (use of stimulant laxatives leads to deteriorating function of the colon)

   f. Excessive emesis depletes potassium and leads to death by heart failure

   g. Binge-fasting cycle can occur (eating is accelerated by the intense hunger that follows a rigid period of dieting)

   h. The client may consume thousands of kilocalories of easy-to-eat, low fiber, high fat, or high carbohydrate foods (e.g., cookies, ice cream, doughnuts, sweets)

   i. The behavior can be secretive in nature, and many bulimic clients will present with normal body weight at times

   j. Dental erosion, caries, and gum disease as well as parotid gland and submandibular gland enlargement can be seen as a consequence of self-induced vomiting

   k. **Russell's sign** (abrasions found on the dorsal hand surface) may be evident due to self-induced vomiting behaviors

3. Dietary measures used as treatment

   ! a. Multidisciplinary approach: physicians, nurses, psychiatrists, family therapists, and dietitians

   b. Goal: weight maintenance and decreased frequency of binge-purge behavior

   c. Develop structured plan for meals and snacks

   d. See Box 6-2 for nutritional guidelines for treatment of bulimia

4. Nutritional monitoring

   a. Teamwork, consistency, and trust are essential for success

   b. Supervise mealtimes as needed to discourage bingeing-purging

   c. Record food intake and exercise activity

   d. Weigh at scheduled intervals only

   e. Don't use food as a reward

   f. Normalize eating pattern (decrease bulimic activity) and maintain weight

Box 6-2

Nutritional Guidelines for Treatment of Bulimia

- Correct electrolyte imbalances.
- Allow to eat enough to satisfy hunger (at least 1,600 kilocalories per day).
- Prolong eating time with fruits, vegetables, and salads.
- Require sitting down and use of utensils to eat; no finger foods.
- Serve foods at warm temperature (increases satiety).
- Include whole-grain, high-fiber foods (increases bulk).
- Include complex carbohydrates (increases satiety) and some fat (slows gastric emptying).
- Use foods in "ready-made" portions (e.g., yogurt, frozen dinners, precut chicken or meat).
- Maintain regular mealtimes.

5. Disease impact
   a. It is most commonly seen in females in adolescence through young adulthood; however, other age groups and males do present with this type of eating disorder and should not be overlooked during the assessment phase
   b. Many clients with bulimia continue to experience relapses throughout their lives
   c. Stressors and other life changes can exacerbate eating behavior patterns
   d. Many experience deterioration of tooth enamel and swelling of salivary glands
   e. There may be increased mortality due to cardiac arrest secondary to electrolyte imbalance
   f. Many clients suffer loss of normal bowel function secondary to laxative abuse

Practice to Pass

What psychosocial assessment data would be relevant to a client with a distorted body image?

II. THE CLIENT WITH BURNS

A. Description

1. Contact between tissue and an energy source such as heat, chemicals, electric current, or radiation results in tissue destruction and loss of fluids and electrolytes (fluid shifting during hypovolemic and diuretic phases)
2. A **hypermetabolic response** (increased energy expenditure) occurs that is proportional to the size and extent of the injury
3. Lowered resistance to disease and infection occur as cellular integrity is altered
4. Restoration of capillary permeability occurs as the body attempts to maintain balance

B. Associated nutritional problems

1. ! An elevated metabolic rate (above 100%) continues until most of the wound is healed or grafted
2. Negative nitrogen balance occurs related to loss of protein through burned skin and the use of body proteins for energy production
3. Fat reserves are depleted
4. There is loss of fluids and electrolytes
   a. Hyponatremia: sodium is lost in interstitial fluid
   b. Hyperkalemia: potassium moves from injured cells into bloodstream

5. Paralytic ileus can occur (absence of peristalsis, accumulation of gas, and distention of the bowel) usually within the first 48–72 hours postburn
6. A poor appetite and weakened state results in reduced caloric intake and weight loss
7. There is an increased risk of aspiration and a risk of development of Curling's ulcer (stress ulcer); a nasogastric tube is inserted and histamine receptor blocking drugs are given to minimize development of these potential effects
8. Inhalation injury can lead to problems with swallowing due to edema, inflammation and bruising; alternate feeding routes may have to be used to prevent further complications

C. Dietary measures used as treatment

1. The initial priority is fluid and electrolyte replacement
    a. **Parkland formula:** 4 mL Lactated Ringer's solution kilogram (kg) preburn body weight × % of body burned; ½ total is given over first 8 hours; ¼ total is given over second 8 hours; ¼ total is given over third 8 hours
    b. IV fluid therapy should produce 30–50 mL urine output per hour
2. Goals: positive nitrogen balance, wound healing, and prevention of weight loss
3. A nasogastric tube will be inserted and attached to low intermittent suction until gastrointestinal (GI) function returns
4. The client is given a high kilocalorie, high protein diet as soon as GI function returns and client is stabilized
5. Determine kilocalorie (kcal) requirements: **Curreri formula**
    a. Adult: (25 kcal × kilogram [kg] preburn body weight) + (40 kcal × % of body burned)
    b. Child (<12 years): (60 kcal × kg preburn body weight) + (35 kcal × % of body burned)
    c. The Curreri formula often exceeds actual energy needs; another formula is the Harris-Benedict equation (BEE × activity factor × injury factor) × 1.5–2.0
    d. If possible, measure actual energy needs using indirect calorimetry
6. Determine protein requirements: 1.5–2.0 grams of protein per kg of body weight per day; 20% of total calories); children need 2.0–2.5 grams per kg per day; utilize liquid supplements as needed
7. Utilize vitamin and mineral supplements for wound healing (zinc, vitamin C, vitamin A, and a multivitamin)
8. The oral route is preferred; nasogastric or nasointestinal tube feedings are utilized to ensure intake of prescribed number of kilocalories; total parenteral nutrition (TPN) may be initiated to provide >1,000 kcal/24 hours with protein, glucose, vitamins, and minerals; TPN is indicated if there is >10% loss of preburn body weight, inadequate enteral intake, malnutrition, or debilitated state prior to burn injury
9. Consider supplemental glutamine and arginine (nonessential amino acids) to support nutritional needs and improve wound healing

D. Nutritional monitoring

1. Measure daily weight: maintain weight within 10% of preburn body weight
2. Keep daily kilocalorie counts: keep within prescribed number (overfeeding can also be detrimental due to body's hypermetabolic state)
3. Carefully record intake and output (I & O)

4. Provide constant encouragement to eat: ask family/friends to bring in favorite foods
5. Continue high protein intake until all wounds are healed
6. Taper total calories as healing occurs (to prevent excessive weight gain)
7. Utilize services of clinical dietitian to coordinate care, establish dietary goals, and educate client and family members for the treatment and rehabilitation phase

E. Disease impact

1. Burn injuries account for a large proportion of accidental deaths in the United States and the care/treatment of burn victims requires extensive resources and financial funding
2. Burn injuries affect all age groups, cultures, and family members
3. Burn injuries have a major impact on quality of life with changes in physical abilities, social status, psychological well-being, and employment status
4. Functional as well as residual damage (scarring) can lead to profound changes in both physical and psychological dynamics for the client and family members
5. Increased mortality associated with major burns is due to development of sepsis during the postburn phases
6. Preburn nutritional status and contributory medical history also impact on the client's ability to heal and respond to treatment

Practice to Pass

A 185-pound client has sustained a 45% total body surface area burn. What fluid replacement do you anticipate for this client? What kilocalorie requirements will this client have?

III. THE CLIENT WITH A CARDIAC DISORDER

A. Hypertension and coronary artery disease

1. Description
   a. Coronary artery disease (CAD): damage that occurs when blood vessels become narrowed and occluded
      1) Related to atherosclerosis: deposit of cholesterol and lipids (plaque) along the inner walls of arteries
      2) ! Nonmodifiable risk factors: age, male gender (although females have increased risk after menopause), African American race, family history
      3) ! Modifiable risk factors: hypertension, obesity, cigarette smoking, increased serum lipids, physical inactivity, diabetes mellitus, stressful lifestyle
   b. Hypertension: sustained blood pressure (BP) > 140/90
      1) Related to increased cardiac output (CO) or increased systemic vascular resistance (SVR)
      2) ! Risk factors: same as for CAD plus excess sodium diet, excessive alcohol use, and low socioeconomic status
      3) Increased BP puts constant stress on arterial walls, which accelerates the atherosclerosis process
2. Associated nutritional problems
   a. CAD
      1) Elevated serum lipids: cholesterol and triglycerides > 200 mg/dL
      2) Decreased **high-density lipoproteins (HDLs),** which carry lipids away from arteries to liver for metabolism, leading to an increased risk for CAD; HDL levels increase in response to exercise and estrogen; there is a minimum amount of HDL needed for cardioprotection in the body
      3) Elevated **low-density lipoproteins (LDLs),** which have affinity for arterial walls and lead to an increased risk for development of CAD; trans fats

raise LDL cholesterol (sources: baked goods, crackers, French fries, some soft margarines, and others)

4) Elevated **very low-density lipoproteins (VLDLs),** which carry lipids from liver to tissues for use and storage; have some impact on CAD development but exact mechanism is still uncertain

5) Elevated **homocysteine** (amino acid derived from dietary protein) levels, which correlate with increased incidence of heart disease and decreased levels of B vitamins (vitamin B_6, B_{12}, and folate)

6) Obesity (BMI ≥ 30) that leads to increases in heart size, myocardial oxygen consumption, and mortality rate

7) Diabetes mellitus type 2: characterized by insulin resistance (body cells resistant to action of insulin), which leads to hyperinsulinemia that alters the lining of blood vessels to promote plaque deposits; also associated with alterations in lipid metabolism, leading to increased cholesterol and triglyceride levels and atherosclerosis

8) Other contributory and concurrent disease processes can impact on the development of CAD and lead to poorer outcomes

b. Hypertension (HTN)

1) **Sodium sensitivity:** excessive sodium intake related to increased BP, fluid retention, volume, and SVR (more common in African Americans, the elderly, diabetics, and the obese)

2) Contributory conditions that can increase the risk of HTN: elevated serum lipids, obesity (especially central abdominal upper body, also called truncal), diabetes mellitus, alcohol intake of 3 or more drinks per day, and cardiac pathology

3) Low dietary intake of potassium, calcium, and possibly magnesium can have an impact on HTN development

4) Stress responses can lead to increased risk for HTN development

3. Dietary measures used as treatment (for both CAD and HTN)

! **a.** Weight reduction is a primary treatment measure that has been proven to provide quick, effective results

b. Step therapy approach is aimed at decreasing intake of saturated fats and cholesterol and maintaining a 15% intake of protein and a 55% intake of CHO

! **c.** Cholesterol-lowering diet plans: American Heart Association—Steps I and II (see Table 6-1)

! **d.** DASH diet: dietary approaches to stop hypertension (see Table 6-2)

! **e.** Teach healthy choices, portion control, and cooking methods to lower fat in diet (see Box 6-3 for guidelines for lowering dietary fat and cholesterol, p. 166)

! **f.** Use of sodium-controlled or sodium-restricted diets (see Table 6-3, p. 166)

1) Frequently ordered diets include a 2 gram Na diet (also called low sodium diet), or a 4 gram Na diet, also called a no-added-salt (NAS) diet

2) Teach client to read labels for sodium content in foods, beverages, and over-the-counter (OTC) medications, toothpaste, mouthwashes, etc.

3) Teach client to avoid foods high in sodium (see Box 6-4, p. 167)

4) Instruct client that salt substitutes can be used because they replace sodium with potassium, but they should be used cautiously with

Table 6-1

Cholesterol-Lowering Diet Plans

Nutrient	Step I	Step II
Total fat*	25–35%	25–35%
Saturated fat*	8–10%	less than 7%
Polyunsaturated fat*	up to 10%	up to 10%
Monosaturated fat*	up to 20%	up to 20%
Carbohydrates (CHO)*	50–60%	50–60%
Protein*	15%	15%
Cholesterol	< 300 mg/day	< 200 mg/day

Saturated fat: hard or solid at room temperature (butter, red meat, coconut oil, chocolate)
Monounsaturated fat: olive and canola oils, hazelnuts, avocados
Polyunsaturated fat: corn and soybean oils, tuna, walnuts
Cholesterol: animal products and egg yolks

To calculate number of grams (g) per day:
1. Multiply total kilocalories by % of nutrient.
2. Divide by 4 kcal/g for protein and CHO; 9 kcal/g for fats.
Example: 2,000 total kilocalories × 30% = 600 kcal ÷ 9 = 66 g total fat

*Recommended % of total daily kilocalories (American Heart Association)

potassium-sparing diuretics or ACE inhibitors (if salt substitutes are allowed by prescriber)

5) Recommend use of alternative seasonings: basil, cloves, paprika, sage, pepper, oregano, chives

! **g.** Include sources of **omega–3 fatty acids** in the diet as they decrease triglyceride levels, inflammation, clotting time, and heart dysrhythmias

1) Recommend 5 ounces of coldwater fish, 1–2 times per week (mackerel, albacore tuna, salmon, sardines, lake trout, shellfish)

2) They are also found in dark green, leafy vegetables

3) The client may use supplements: 1 gram fish oil per day

! **h.** Ensure adequate intake of foods high in potassium if client is taking diuretics that decreases electrolyte levels (use cautiously with potassium-sparing diuretics or ACE inhibitors) (see Table 6-4, p. 176, for high-potassium foods)

i. Increase intake of folic acid and vitamins B_{12} and B_6 to decrease homocysteine levels

Table 6-2

DASH Diet

Grains	7–8 servings per day
Fruits	4–5 servings per day
Vegetables	4–5 servings per day
Meat, poultry, fish	2 or fewer servings per day
Low-fat or non-fat dairy	2–3 servings per day
Nuts, seeds, and legumes	4–5 servings per week
Fats and oils	2.5 servings per day

Box 6-3

Guidelines for Lowering Fat and Cholesterol in Diet

- Include up to 6 ounces of lean meat, fish, or skinless poultry per day.
- Include pasta, rice, beans, or vegetables in main dish to decrease amount of meat.
- Trim visible fat; skim fat from meat juices; drain fat after browning.
- Bake, broil, boil, roast, poach, steam, sauté, stir-fry, microwave.
- Use olive or canola oils; limit to 5–8 teaspoons per day.
- Increase use of soybean products to replace those containing animal fat.
- Increase intake of soluble fiber (legumes, oats, barley, broccoli, apples, citrus fruits) to 10–25 grams/day.
- Decrease intake of sugar.
- Use antioxidant supplements (vitamins C, E, and beta carotene).
- Choose low-fat or nonfat dairy products; avoid food products containing trans-fatty acids.
- Limit to 3–4 egg yolks per week.
- Limit intake of organ meats (liver, kidneys, gizzards).
- Include 5–6 servings of fruits and vegetables per day.
- Include 6 or more servings of breads, cereals, grains per day.
- Eat foods containing plant sterols (butter substitutes and salad dressings) in amounts of 2 grams/day to reduce LDL-C levels by 10%; these structurally resemble cholesterol and are not absorbable.

Table 6-3

Sodium-Restricted Diets

500 mg Restriction	1 gram Restriction	2 gram Restriction	4 gram Restriction
No salt in cooking	No salt in cooking	No salt in cooking	Small amount of salt in cooking
No added salt at table	No added salt at table	No added salt at table	No added salt at table
Avoid high sodium foods	Avoid high sodium foods	Avoid high sodium foods	Avoid high sodium foods
Limit milk: 1 cup/day	Limit milk: 1 cup/day	Limit milk: 2 cups/day	Limit milk: 3 cups/day
Salt-free butter, bread, vegetables, starches	Salt-free butter and vegetables		

j. Use moderation in alcohol consumption
   1) One-drink equivalents: 12 ounces beer, 4–5 ounces wine, or 1½ ounces hard liquor
   2) Limit intake to 1–2 drinks per day

k. Decrease intake of saturated fats and trans-fatty acids; increase intake of polyunsaturated fats in the diet

l. Increase soluble fiber in the diet to reduce cholesterol

m. If no response to nutritional interventions (continued hyperlipidemia or elevated BP), medication therapy can be added

4. Nutritional monitoring
   a. Fasting lipid profile and serum electrolytes

Box 6-4

Foods High in Sodium

- Mineral water
- Club soda
- Tomato juice
- Baking powder biscuits
- Commercial bakery products
- Instant cooked cereals
- Instant potatoes
- Potato chips (and other salted snack foods)
- Canned tuna
- Bacon
- Ham (and other cured meats)
- Canned soups
- Canned vegetables
- Olives
- Pickles
- Sauerkraut
- Steak sauce
- Soy sauce
- Meat tenderizer

b. Weekly weight and BP check

c. Food and activity diary

d. Set realistic target weight goal and include physical activity program to work in combination with nutritional and medical interventions

5. Disease impact

a. Heart disease continues to be a leading cause of death in United States

b. Most people have both CAD and HTN

c. Sodium sensitivity can lead to target organ damage and increased cardiovascular and renal morbidity

Table 6-4

Foods High in Calcium and Potassium

Calcium	Potassium
Milk	Avocado
Cheese	Banana
Yogurt	Orange
Spinach	Beet greens
Greens (turnip, beet)	Baked potato with skin
Broccoli	Sweet potato
Legumes	Spinach
Tofu	Chocolate

! d. Complications of poorly controlled CAD and HTN can include stroke, myocardial infarction, renal disease, and diabetic retinopathy

B. Congestive heart failure (CHF)

1. Description

   a. Characterized by decreased myocardial contractility that results in pulmonary and systemic congestion and inadequate cardiac output to meet tissue oxygen demands

   b. Primary risk factors include CAD, HTN, and advancing age

   c. Most clients exhibit some degree of biventricular heart failure in the clinical setting

   d. Fluid volume excess states and hypernatremia result in the development of edema and ascites, which further complicate the clinical course

Practice to Pass

A client is readmitted for congestive heart failure for the third time in 2 months. What admission data would be relevant in determining factors that are contributing to these frequent admissions?

2. Associated nutritional problems

   a. Body is unable to excrete enough sodium to equalize sodium intake

   b. Progressive weight gain related to fluid retention causes increasing dyspnea and fatigue

   c. Anorexia and nausea occur and are related to abdominal fullness (ascites and hepatomegaly)

   d. There is loss of muscle and fat tissue masked by edema

3. Dietary measures used as treatment

   a. Multimodal therapy: nutrition, medications, and activity

   b. Restricted sodium diet

   c. Fluid restriction for moderate to severe CHF

   ! d. Include or avoid high potassium foods (depending on type of diuretic medication) (refer back to Table 6-4 for examples)

   ! e. Coordinate diet and medications used to prevent deficiencies or excess in the clinical setting

4. Nutritional monitoring

   ! a. Measure daily weights: same time each day with same type clothing; notify primary care provider of weight gain of 2–3 pounds over 1–2 days

   b. Keep a food and activity diary

   ! c. Monitor serum electrolytes and lipid profile

   ! d. Teach client to recognize and report worsening CHF symptoms (weight gain, loss of appetite, increased shortness of breath [SOB], increased peripheral edema, and persistent cough)

! 5. Disease impact

   a. Increased mortality and morbidity is associated with the clinical diagnosis of CHF

   b. HTN and CAD have been called “silent killers” because significant damage can be done to the body before overt clinical signs and symptoms are present

   c. Heart disease impairs quality of life and restricts functional capacity

   d. Clients usually take multiple medications to treat these diseases and must be evaluated closely during treatment

IV. THE CLIENT WITH AN ENDOCRINE DISORDER

A. Diabetes mellitus (DM)

1. Description
   a. Metabolic disorder of carbohydrate (CHO) metabolism, leading to altered glucose regulation and utilization as a result of insufficient or ineffective insulin
   b. Type 1 (formerly called insulin dependent diabetes mellitus or IDDM)
      1) No insulin production, related to destruction of beta cells of pancreas
      2) Onset during childhood, usually < 20 years of age
      3) Onset usually associated with some stressor to immune system (e.g., viral infection)
      4) Genetic predisposition
   c. Type 2 (formerly called noninsulin dependent diabetes mellitus or NIDDM)
      1) Decreased cell sensitivity to insulin, increased peripheral resistance, and altered hepatic uptake
      2) Onset later in life (usually); there is increased incidence of children who are obese with type 2 diabetes mellitus
      3) Genetic predisposition
   d. Gestational diabetes mellitus
      1) Occurrence of clinical diabetes during the pregnancy state that can result in maternal effects and fetal changes (macrosomia and IDM—infants of diabetic mothers)
      2) Family history of type 2 diabetes (genetic predisposition to insulin resistance)
      3) Diet therapy needed and may require insulin injections
      4) Normal outcome of pregnancy occurs if blood glucose levels are maintained near normal throughout pregnancy
      5) Mothers are elevated to high-risk client status during their obstetrical care
      6) Mothers are more likely to develop type 2 diabetes mellitus later in life

! 2. Associated nutritional problems
   a. Obesity: especially type 2, related to insulin resistance
   b. Hyperinsulinemia occurs in response to high CHO intake
   c. Clients are at risk to develop both microvascular and macrovascular complications during the course of the disease process, which can lead to target organ (end-organ) damage
   d. There is a risk for hypoglycemia, especially if the client is taking oral hypoglycemic agents and/or insulin
   e. Rebounding blood glucose levels can further complicate dietary and treatment regimens
   f. Clients with DM have been shown to have **dyslipidemia** (abnormal lipid profile), and new research suggests that prompt treatment of this disorder will help the clinical profile and prevent the development of complications
   g. Changing insulin demands can be seen in response to individual client exercise and activity levels, illness, and stressors

3. Dietary measures used as treatment

   a. Overall goal: make changes in nutrition and exercise habits for improved metabolic control of CHO metabolism to normalize blood glucose levels (fasting: 70–140 mg/dL and 2-hour postprandial: <180 mg/dL)

   b. Three components of treatment: nutrition, exercise, and medications

   c. Daily kilocalorie (kcal) requirements: 20–30 kcal/kg of body weight; reduce by 500 kcal/day for weight loss of one pound per week

   d. Daily protein requirements: 10–20% of total daily kcals (1–1.5 grams/kg of body weight)

   e. Daily fat requirements: 25–35% of total daily kcals (follow American Heart Association Guidelines for Step I, low fat diet) (refer back to Table 6-1)

   f. Daily carbohydrate requirements: remaining 50–60% of total daily kcals

      1) Complex CHOs: fruits, vegetables, beans, dairy foods, starchy foods

      2) Table sugar (sucrose) allowed in moderation as long as counted in meal plan (1 teaspoon sugar = 4 grams CHO)

   g. Fiber: 25–35 grams/day (lowers postprandial blood glucose)

   h. Sodium: use in moderation (< 2,400 mg/day)

   i. Use alcohol in moderation and count alcohol as a CHO source

   j. Balance food intake with exercise: include nutritious snacks in meal plan monitor blood glucose levels before, during, and after exercise

   k. Sugar substitutes: free use (saccharin, aspartame)

   l. Type 1: eat at consistent times; adjust insulin dose for amount of food eaten

   m. Type 2: space meals throughout day; moderate caloric restriction (250–500 kilocalories less than average daily intake, calculated from food history)

      1) Reduced caloric intake increases sensitivity to insulin

      2) Moderate weight loss (10–20 pounds) decreases hyperglycemia, hyperlipidemia, and hypertension

   n. Gestational: frequent, small, balanced meals; slow, steady weight gain; avoid concentrated sugars

4. Nutritional monitoring

   a. Encourage compliance with meal plan

      1) American Diabetes Association Food exchange lists: foods grouped in terms of similar composition (starch, fruit, milk, CHO, vegetable, meat, fat, combination, and free foods); foods on list contain approximately equal amounts of calories, CHO, protein, and fat; one serving may be exchanged for another within the same list; emphasis on balanced diet

      2) Diabetes food pyramid: six sections or food groups; eat more servings from bottom food groups and very few from top food group (see Table 6-5); exact number of servings depends on caloric and nutrition needs, lifestyle, and diabetic goals

      3) Carbohydrate counting: diet prescribes how many CHOs per day instead of kcals; clients must learn to count CHO content of foods; clients with type 1 diabetes learn to adjust insulin dose based on number of CHOs eaten; they don't have to give up all high CHO foods as long as they are counted in meal plan

Table 6-5

Diabetes Food Pyramid

Fats, sweets, alcohol	Very few servings
Meat, fish, and poultry	2–3 servings/day
Milk	2–3 servings/day
Fruits	3–4 servings/day
Vegetables	3–5 servings/day
Grains, beans, starchy vegetables	6 or more servings/day

! **b.** Measure daily blood glucose levels (or as ordered) and have periodic monitoring of **glycosylated hemoglobin—Hemoglobin A_{1c}** (measures degree of glucose control over previous 3 months)

c. Keep diary of food intake, exercise, and daily blood glucose levels

! **d.** Teach recognition and treatment of hypoglycemia (blood glucose < 60 mg/dL, cool, clammy, diaphoresis, lethargy) by the **15-15 rule**—if blood glucose < 60, consume 15 grams CHO (2–3 glucose tablets; 6–10 Lifesavers™ candy; 4–6 ounces juice); recheck blood glucose in 15 minutes, repeat if needed

! **e.** Illness: causes increased blood glucose levels; teach to monitor blood glucose levels and adjust nutritional intake accordingly; call healthcare provider if blood glucose > 250 mg/dL; prevent dehydration and electrolyte imbalance; drink plenty of water and fluids; continue to take insulin if ordered (illness is a stressor and raises blood glucose level); eat smaller, more frequent meals

5. Disease impact

a. Type 1 DM more common in northern European races; type 2 more common in African American, Hispanic, Asian, Native American, Pacific Islander, and Mediterranean races

b. The increasing number of hospitalizations of diabetic clients leads to continued emphasis on nutritional benefits of care and close monitoring of glycemic control to minimize and prevent complications

c. Progressive nature of disease along with significant development of microvascular and macrovascular changes lead to poor outcomes

B. Thyroid disorders

1. Description

a. Thyroid gland produces three hormones: thyroxine (T_4) and triiodothyroxine (T_3), which regulate cellular metabolism; and thyrocalcitonin, which inhibits bone resorption of calcium

b. Hyperthyroidism results from a sustained increased production of thyroid hormones leading to a hypermetabolic response

c. Hypothyroidism results from insufficient levels of circulating thyroid hormones, atrophy of thyroid gland, or decreased production of thyroid stimulating hormone (TSH) by pituitary gland, leading to a hypometabolic response

2. Associated nutritional problems

a. Iodine deficiency: predisposes to both hypo- and hyperthyroidism

b. Hyperthyroidism results in increased metabolism, weight loss, increased appetite, thirst, and nausea

c. Hypothyroidism results in decreased metabolism, weight gain, and decreased GI motility

d. Altered elimination patterns occur in both clinical disease states (diarrhea in hyperthyroidism, constipation in hypothyroidism)

3. Dietary measures used as treatments

a. Hyperthyroidism

! 1) Provide high-calorie diet to satisfy hunger and prevent tissue breakdown; 6 full meals/day and snacks that are high in protein, CHOs, vitamins, and minerals

2) Replace iodine if deficient

3) Increase protein intake (1–2 grams/kg of ideal body weight)

4) Increase CHO intake (to spare protein and provide energy)

5) Avoid highly seasoned foods and caffeine (stimulant)

6) Increase milk intake (calcium and protein)

7) Drug therapy, radiation, or surgery is needed; after treatment, no diet alterations are required

b. Hypothyroidism

! 1) Medications are used to treat hypothyroidism and, when on appropriate medications, no special diet is needed; until medication is started, do the following

2) Provide low-calorie, high-protein diet (to prevent and treat weight gain)

3) Include foods rich in folic acid, iron, and vitamin C (to prevent muscle wasting and anemia) and vitamin B_{12} (usually a deficiency)

4) Replace iodine if deficient

5) Give small frequent meals due to decreased GI motility

6) Encourage 2–3 liters fluid/day (to promote bowel function)

7) Include foods high in bulk and roughage (to promote bowel function)

8) Limit salt intake

4. Nutritional monitoring

a. Food and activity diary

b. Daily weights

c. Thyroid profile, serum chemistries, CBC, transferrin, pretransferrin, and albumin levels to establish baselines, trend results, and monitor response to treatment

5. Disease impact

a. Increased incidence of hyperthyroidism is now being seen in the clinical setting

b. Greater incidence of both hypothyroidism and hyperthyroidism occurs in iodine-poor geographic locations (iodine insufficiency not prevalent in United States any longer)

c. Hyperthyroidism is more prevalent in women aged 30 to 50 years old

d. Hypothyroidism is seen typically in women > 50 years old

e. Infant hypothyroidism (cretinism) is related to maternal iodine deficiency

f. Chronic nature of disease process and acute exacerbations requires prompt management and adequate nutritional support

C. Parathyroid disorders

1. Description

a. Hyperparathyroidism: increased secretion of parathyroid hormone (PTH) that regulates calcium and phosphate levels
   1) Common cause: benign neoplasm or single adenoma in parathyroid gland (primary)
   2) Secondary hyperparathyroidism caused by: low calcium intake, GI disorders, renal insufficiency, vitamin D deficiency, and hypercalcemia of renal origin
   3) Hyperplasia of parathyroid gland and loss of negative feedback from circulating calcium (tertiary)

b. Hypoparathyroidism: inadequate levels of circulating PTH
   1) Common cause: accidental removal of parathyroid gland or damage to its vascular supply during neck surgery
   2) Also caused by congenital disorders, metastatic carcinoma, Wilson's disease, sarcoidosis, positive human immunodeficiency (HIV) status, and acquired immunodeficiency syndrome (AIDS)

2. Associated nutritional problems
   a. Hypercalcemia, loss of appetite, constipation, and osteoporosis (hyperparathyroidism) and nausea and vomiting
   b. Hypocalcemia, dysphagia, tetany, pain and altered mental status (hypoparathyroidism)

3. Dietary measures used as treatment
   a. Hyperparathyroidism: small frequent meals
      1) Include foods high in bulk and roughage and increase fluid intake (to decrease constipation)
      2) Calcium intake of 1200–1500 mg/day and phosphorus supplements
      3) Sodium replacement (8–10 grams/day)
   b. Hypoparathyroidism: vitamin D and calcium replacement with foods high in calcium (refer again to Table 6-4 for a listing of common foods high in calcium) and possibly supplements; IV calcium may be necessary in emergency situations (10% solution of calcium chloride, or calcium gluconate)

4. Nutritional monitoring
   a. Food diary, calorie counts
   b. Ionized calcium levels (both hypo- and hyperparathyroidism)
   c. Bone density measurements (both hypo- and hyperparathyroidism)

5. Disease impact
   a. Clinical course depends on underlying etiology and abnormal endocrine response
   b. Lifelong nature of disease process requires monitored treatment, medication, and diet therapy

Practice to Pass

What subjective data would be relevant when admitting a client with diabetes mellitus?

V. THE CLIENT WITH A GASTROINTESTINAL (GI) DISORDER

A. GI upset (nausea, vomiting, and diarrhea)

1. Description
   a. Vomiting center in brainstem receives various stimuli as input and initiates vomiting reflex

- **b.** Emotions, stress, unpleasant sights and odors, pain, bowel obstruction, viruses, and food poisoning can trigger vomiting reflex
- **c.** Diarrhea: increase in frequency, volume, and looseness of stools
  - **1)** Causes: decreased fluid absorption, increased fluid secretion, or motility disturbance
  - **2)** Acute: usually secondary to infection
  - **3)** Chronic: lasts longer than two weeks or reoccurs
- **d.** Nausea can be seen as a symptom of a disease and/or associated with food, smell, and activities
  - **1)** The sight and smell of food can serve as a nausea trigger
  - **2)** Activities involving balance and movement can act as triggers

2. Associated nutritional problems

- ! **a.** Dehydration and loss of essential electrolytes
- **b.** Metabolic alkalosis (loss of gastric hydrochloric acid [HCl])
- **c.** Metabolic acidosis (loss of sodium bicarbonate from small intestine)
- **d.** Malabsorption and malnutrition (chronic diarrhea)

3. Dietary measures used as treatment

- **a.** Bland diet: small frequent meals (decrease stomach acid); eliminate known GI irritants such as caffeine and alcohol
- **b.** BRAT diet: bananas, rice, applesauce, and toast: may be used for treatment of diarrhea in pediatric clients; yogurt is often included now as well
  - **1)** Allows GI tract to rest and recover while diarrhea runs its course
  - ! **2)** This is a transition diet and should not be used over an extended period of time as it may further contribute to a deficiency state
  - **3)** Clients should be monitored for response to treatment; if condition persists, notify the healthcare provider
  - **4)** Provides limited protein, food energy, and fat
  - **5)** American Academy of Pediatrics now recommends that a child's regular diet be resumed within 24 hours of the first episode of diarrhea and to avoid spicy and fried foods until diarrhea has subsided
- **c.** Nothing by mouth (NPO) until symptoms subside (vomiting)
- ! **d.** Replace fluids and electrolytes: oral solutions with glucose and electrolytes (Gatorade™, Pedialyte™); or IV fluid replacement for severe vomiting
- **e.** Begin oral diet with clear liquids at room temperature; add dry toast or crackers; progress to regular diet as tolerated

4. Nutritional monitoring

- ! **a.** Fluid intake and output (I & O) balance
- ! **b.** Serum electrolytes
- **c.** Number and consistency of stools
- **d.** Food tolerance as diet is progressed
- **e.** Daily weights

5. Disease impact

- ! **a.** Dehydration can be fatal in the elderly and very young
- **b.** Aspiration of gastric contents into lungs is more common in elderly

c. If symptoms are mild to moderate, then client is usually managed at home
d. If symptoms are severe and persistent or if contributory conditions exist, then the client is hospitalized

B. Gastroesophageal reflux disease (GERD)

1. Description
   a. Gastric or duodenal contents flow back into lower portion of esophagus
   b. Common causes: incompetent lower esophageal sphincter (LES), pyloric stenosis, intestinal malrotation, motility disorder
   c. Acidity of gastric contents causes irritation and inflammation of esophagus
   d. Intestinal secretions (trypsin and bile salts) are corrosive to esophageal mucosa
   e. Often associated with hiatal hernia
2. Associated nutritional problems
   a. Esophageal irritation can lead to problems with swallowing
   b. Increased pressure leads to reflux and possible aspiration
   c. Abdominal bloating leads to a sense of fullness and pressure (see Table 6-6 for a description of symptomatic terms)
3. Dietary measures used as treatment
   ! a. Diet: low fat (fatty foods decrease LES pressure)
   ! b. Avoid foods that decrease LES pressure: chocolate, peppermint, spearmint, coffee, tea, alcohol, nicotine, tomatoes, licorice, cola, fatty foods
   c. Small frequent meals (prevents overdistention of stomach)
   d. Avoid or limit fluids at mealtimes (reduces stomach distention)
   e. Avoid late-night eating (at least 2–3 hours before bedtime)
   f. Avoid spicy foods and acidic juices (irritate esophagus)
   g. Reduce weight if obese
   ! h. Remain upright for at least 2 hours after eating
   i. Elevate head of bed 6 to 8 inches (improves acid clearance)
   j. Chew food thoroughly
   k. Infants with reflux problems should have limited amount of formula per feeding; place in elevated prone position and avoid active play for 1 hour after feeding
   ! l. Avoid medications that irritate esophagus: nonsteroidal anti-inflammatory drugs (NSAIDs), iron, potassium, gel capsule antibiotics

Table 6-6

Common Symptoms of GERD that Affect Nutritional Status

Dyspepsia	Epigastric discomfort
Pyrosis	"Heartburn" (burning, tightness below sternum)
Regurgitation	Effortless backflow of gastric contents into esophagus or mouth
Dysphagia	Difficulty swallowing
Odynophagia	Painful swallowing
Aspiration	Movement of gastric contents into lungs
Esophagitis	Inflammation of esophagus

4. Nutritional monitoring
   a. Food and symptom diary: identify foods that irritate esophagus and increase reflux symptoms
   b. Limit foods in the diet that exacerbate clinical symptoms
   c. Institute positional methods after eating to minimize distress
   d. If symptoms persist, refer to healthcare provider for further diagnostic workup and medication therapy to manage clinical symptoms
5. Disease impact
   a. GERD is a common clinical presentation for which many people are being clinically treated with medication and diet therapy
   b. The presence of GERD symptoms can lead to the diagnosis of other contributory conditions such as hiatal hernia, gallbladder, liver and cardiac pathology
   c. Reflux is common in infants but usually disappears by 18 months of age
   d. Reflux reappears in the elderly related to poor muscle tone of LES and other contributory factors such as lifestyle/diet, alcohol, and medication use
   e. It is frequently underdiagnosed and undertreated in people > 50 years old as many clients use self-treatment methods and minimize the extent of the problem

C. Inflammatory bowel disease (Crohn's disease and ulcerative colitis)

1. Description
   a. Crohn's disease is a chronic disease of unknown etiology with clinical manifestations seen anywhere along the length of the GI tract that results in abdominal pain, diarrhea, fatigue, weight loss, fever, nausea and vomiting
   b. Ulcerative colitis is a chronic disease of unknown etiology with clinical manifestations seen throughout the colon and the appearance of symptoms outside the intestines that result in bloody diarrhea, dehydration, fever, weight loss, and anorexia
   c. Both disease states can present with acute exacerbations and may at some point require surgical management
2. ! Associated nutritional problems
   a. Depending on the exacerbation, altered elimination can be seen that can impact a client's overall nutrition/hydration status
   b. Presence of extraintestinal symptoms can lead to further changes in nutrition/hydration status and result in dehydration and electrolyte deficiencies
   c. Bowel rest may be indicated to allow the inflamed colon to rest
   d. The use of medications such as corticosteroids and immunosuppressive agents may lead to further nutritional concerns
   e. Negative nitrogen balance leads to protein catabolism and weight loss
3. Dietary measures used as treatment
   a. ! Low residue and low roughage diets should be used in clients with Crohn's disease during exacerbations
   b. ! Bowel rest along clear liquids with alternate feeding methods such as total parenteral nutrition (TPN) may be needed to provide calories during exacerbations
   c. ! Increased fiber is used during remission
   d. A consultation with a dietitian may be helpful to evaluate client's baseline status and develop a plan of care to nutritionally manage the client
   e. Supplementation with vitamins and minerals may be needed to restore levels

4. Nutritional monitoring
   - **a.** Baseline lab findings (serum chemistries and CBC) to confirm clinical status
   - ! **b.** Pertinent lab findings relative to TPN feedings (electrolytes, BUN, creatinine, blood glucose) if alternate feedings are initiated
   - **c.** Intake and output monitoring
   - **d.** If surgical intervention is necessary in order to correct complications (such as abscess, fistulas, or obstruction) or as a treatment method (colostomy, ileostomy, or resection), then greater nutritional monitoring will be indicated; refer to section on ostomy for more detail

! 5. Disease impact
   - **a.** Clients with IBD usually also have anemia and may require treatment and monitoring for this condition as well
   - **b.** Chronic nature of the disease along with acute exacerbations lead to a lifetime of nutritional problems
   - **c.** Psychological impact and component of these disease processes have a profound influence on both the client and family members
   - **d.** Frequent hospitalizations and surgical treatment interventions require lifestyle adaptations

D. Intestinal obstruction

1. Description
   - **a.** Normal peristalsis of intestinal contents is disrupted
   - **b.** Mechanical: occlusion of lumen of intestinal tract
     - **1)** Most common in small intestine: adhesions, hernias, neoplasms, or volvulus (twisting of bowel)
     - **2)** Large intestine: carcinoma, diverticulitis, inflammatory bowel disorders, or benign tumors
   - **c.** Nonmechanical: neuromuscular or vascular disorder (paralytic ileus)
2. Associated nutritional problems
   - **a.** Dehydration and electrolyte imbalance
   - **b.** Constipation with possible blockage
   - **c.** Nausea, vomiting, and abdominal pain
3. Dietary measures used as treatments
   - **a.** Nasogastric tube to low intermittent suction (empty stomach and decompress bowel) or nasoenteric tube (such as Miller-Abbott) to push past area of obstruction
   - ! **b.** NPO: maintain fluid and electrolyte balance with IV fluids
   - **c.** If feeding tube can be placed distal to obstruction, give tube feedings; otherwise TPN may be indicated
   - ! **d.** TPN to maintain nutrition and promote postoperative healing
4. Nutritional monitoring
   - ! **a.** Fluid and electrolyte balance (I & O, serum electrolytes)
   - **b.** Daily weights
   - **c.** Return of bowel function prior to oral feeding (presence of bowel sounds)
5. Disease impact
   - **a.** Severity depends on part of bowel involved

b. Surgical treatment usually required

c. Underlying etiology can be a cancerous tumor of the colon or rectum

E. Irritable bowel syndrome (irritable colon; spastic colon)

1. Description

   a. Motility disorder of small and large intestine without evidence of anatomical abnormality or organic illness

   b. Intermittent and recurrent abdominal pain, associated with alternating diarrhea and constipation

   c. Gastrocolic reflex: increased movement of intestinal contents once food enters stomach

   d. Increased colonic motility in response to emotional or environmental stress

2. Associated nutritional problems

   a. Food intolerance common

   b. Gastrocolic reflex triggers: large volume, high fat, cold temperature foods and beverages

   c. Lactose intolerance common: nausea, abdominal cramps, bloating, flatulence, diarrhea (within 30 minutes of ingestion)

   d. Alternating diarrhea and constipation

3. Dietary measures used as treatments

   ! a. Identify and remove triggers: food intolerances, eating habits, diet, emotional stressors, excessive exercise, laxative use, vitamin C

   b. Avoid lactose dairy products (if lactose intolerant)

   c. Calcium supplement (if lactose intolerant)

   ! d. Avoid carbonated beverages (increase bloating and gas)

   ! e. Avoid gas-producing foods (beans, onions, broccoli, cabbage)

   f. Avoid smoking, chewing gum, drinking rapidly (increases amount of swallowed air)

   g. Eat slowly

   h. Avoid caffeine (increases intestinal motility)

   ! i. Gradually increase fiber in diet up to 20 grams/day (to regulate bowel movements)

4. Nutritional monitoring

   a. Food and symptom diary

   b. Regular exercise (to normalize bowel function)

   ! c. Stress management and stress reduction techniques

5. Disease impact

   a. Accounts for a large proportion of all referrals to gastroenterologists

   b. Increasing incidence is seen in the United States

   c. More common in women, with onset in late adolescence or early adulthood

   d. Often triggered by emotional stress

   e. Social impact: missed workdays and social isolation

   f. Many don't seek treatment due to embarrassment, pessimism, or fear

F. Gastric surgery

1. Description
   a. Treatment methods used to remove, restore, and/or reconnect stomach cavity as a result of malignancy, infection, inflammation, obstruction, or clinical obesity
   b. Surgical procedures that can be performed include Bilroth I and II, total gastrectomy, Whipple's procedure, vagotomy, pyloroplasty, gastric banding, and gastric bypass
   c. Gastric surgical procedures can require additional nutritional support in the form of lifelong parenteral or nasal vitamin B_{12} supplementation due to the loss of intrinsic factor needed to absorb oral vitamin B_{12}
2. Associated nutritional problems
   a. High risk for malnutrition and fluid and electrolyte imbalance
   b. Higher risk for mortality and morbidity if nutritionally deficient in the preoperative period
   ! c. **Dumping syndrome** can occur when two-thirds or more of the stomach is removed; concentrated carbohydrate intake then leads to hyperperistalsis, diarrhea, abdominal pain, and vomiting 30 to 60 minutes after eating; inadequate intake and malabsorption can then lead to anemia
   d. Vitamin B_{12} deficiency can occur due to loss of intrinsic factor from surgical intervention (common for total gastrectomies; surgeons now leave small area intact to prevent this problem
   ! e. **Gastroparesis** can occur in clients undergoing surgical correction and in diabetes; this leads to decreased emptying times, abdominal pain and cramping, and multiple electrolyte deficiencies
3. Dietary measures used as treatment
   a. Preoperative period
      ! 1) Identify and correct nutritional deficiencies 2 to 3 weeks prior to surgery date
      ! 2) High protein, high CHO diet with vitamin and mineral supplements
      3) Obese: lose weight (reduces surgical risk)
      4) Stomach must be empty prior to surgery if using general anesthesia (maintain NPO status for at least 8 hours)
      ! 5) Bowel preparation: clear liquid diet 1 to 2 days before surgery, followed by bowel prep solution
   b. Postoperative period
      1) Nasogastric tube to low intermittent suction (allow for healing and return of bowel function)
      2) IV fluids: 2 liters of 5% D_5W in 24 hours will yield 100 grams of glucose (340 kcal)
      3) A client who is well-nourished prior to surgery has 5 to 7 days of nutrient reserves
      ! 4) TPN is given by 5th to 7th postop day if continued on NPO status (to provide at least 1,000 kcal/day)
      5) Progress oral feeding from clear liquid to general diet as tolerated (once bowel function has returned)

! 6) Diet should include increased: protein (to prevent infection and promote production of antibodies and WBCs), vitamin C (for collagen formation), zinc (for tissue growth, bone formation, immunity, and general host defense)

! 7) Prevent dumping syndrome: limit intake of simple sugars; eat small, frequent meals; increase protein intake; avoid drinking liquids with meals; drink low CHO beverages; avoid extremes of hot and cold foods; lie down for 30 to 60 minutes after eating

! 8) Client with gastroparesis may require antibiotic therapy (erythromycin) or metoclopramide (Reglan) to stimulate stomach emptying and/or pain management to treat clinical symptoms

! 9) Client who has undergone gastric banding should follow a **gastric bypass diet** postoperatively that will help to meet dietary goals and maintain adequate nutritional levels (see Box 6-5 for a listing of gastric bypass diet instructions)

4. Nutritional monitoring
   - ! a. Fluid balance (I & O) and daily weights
   - b. Calorie counts with progression of diet once bowel function returns
   - ! c. Monitoring for bowel sounds
   - ! d. Serum electrolytes
   - e. Inspection of surgical site
5. Disease impact
   - a. Clients with existing protein energy malnutrition (poor nutrition) are at higher risk for postop complications

Box 6-5

Gastric Bypass Diet Instructions

- Gradually progress the consistency and volume of food in the early postoperative period from liquids to solids.
- Provide a diet that is low in fat to facilitate the objective of weight loss and that is high in protein to maximize postoperative tissue healing.
- Multivitamin, mineral, and calcium supplements should be taken on a daily basis to prevent vitamin B deficiencies, nutritional anemias, and calcium deficiencies.
- Clients may experience nausea and vomiting during the initial weeks following surgery and, if this occurs, the client should go back to clear liquids to maintain hydration. If the symptoms persist, the client should contact the healthcare provider for further assessment.
- Food must be chewed completely and should be eaten slowly.
- Liquids should be taken in between meals to minimize possible nausea and to delay gastric emptying.
- Carbonated beverages can be used, but they should be sugar-free and they should be opened with the gas allowed to dissipate for at least one hour prior to drinking in order to minimize gastric distention.
- Clients may be at risk to develop lactose intolerance due to effects of surgery and may have to take lactose-free products or minimize milk consumption in order to prevent symptoms.
- Altered elimination patterns (constipation or diarrhea) may occur in response to postoperative healing but are usually self-limiting and resolved with proper hydration and fiber in the diet.

b. Lifestyle changes and adaptations are needed for clients who undergo gastric surgical procedures

G. Ostomy

1. Description
   a. Surgical opening that brings part of the intestine to the skin
   b. Done as a consequence of malignancy, for surgical correction/revision due to trauma, inflammation, or infection, and/or medical treatment for GI disease states such as IBD (Crohn's disease and ulcerative colitis)
   c. Different types of drainage will occur depending on the site of ostomy and corresponding to the degree of fluid absorption (liquid in ileostomy to varying degrees of semiformed in colostomy, depending on whether ascending, transverse, or descending)
   d. Can be permanent or temporary depending on principal indication for the procedure
   e. Clients can wear external devices or have an internal pouch or stoma cap, depending on the surgical procedure used

! 2. Associated nutritional problems
   a. Altered dietary absorption related to placement of stoma
   b. Increased fluid intake is needed to maintain hydration and prevent constipation
   c. Resumption of "normal" bowel elimination pattern occurs following surgical intervention to "take down" the ostomy and reconnect the bowel
   d. A potential for altered skin integrity exists related to stoma and type of drainage

! 3. Dietary measures
   a. Increase fluids to maintain normal hydration; increase intake of sodium and potassium to offset losses of minerals from ileostomy
   b. Avoid foods that are gas-forming such as asparagus, beer, broccoli, brussel sprouts, cabbage, and carbonated beverages, if gas production is a problem
   c. Avoid foods that can produce odors, such as eggs, fish, garlic, and onions, if odors are a problem
   d. Avoid foods that can cause possible obstruction at the ileostomy site, such as celery; foods that contain seeds; and foods with tough coatings, such as nuts
   e. Most clients with ostomies tolerate a regular diet

4. Nutritional monitoring
   ! a. An enterostomal therapy (ET) nurse should coordinate plan of care for the ostomy site
   b. A dietitian should coordinate the nutritional plan, evaluate nutritional adequacy, and help client to maintain nutritional balance
   c. Monitor pertinent lab findings (such as serum electrolytes, CBC, and albumin levels) to confirm nutritional status
   d. Monitor stoma site for normal skin integrity
   e. Monitor urine output for hydration status (especially in clients with ileostomy)

5. Disease impact
   a. Altered body image as a result of surgical intervention and stoma placement

Practice to Pass

What are nursing interventions for the client with Fluid volume deficit related to an intestinal obstruction?

b. Lifestyle changes and adaptations as a result of surgical intervention

c. Clients with stomas can have contributory disease processes unrelated to need for ostomy and therefore have a more complicated clinical course of treatment

Case Study

A 60-year-old female client came in to the office two weeks ago for an annual physical examination. The past medical history reveals a weight gain of 25 pounds over the past year since her husband died, smoking half a pack of cigarettes per day for the last 40 years, eating many canned and "fast" foods, no use of alcohol, and no regular exercise. The physical examination reveals a BP of 178/92, height of 64 inches, and weight of 170 pounds. BP has remained elevated for two weeks. The nurse practitioner has diagnosed hypertension and ordered a trial of lifestyle modifications with weekly BP checks.

1. What are the contributing physiological factors in the development of hypertension?
2. What additional risk factors does the client present with?
3. What dietary modifications will you recommend for this client?
4. What other lifestyle modifications will you recommend for this client?
5. Develop two appropriate nursing diagnoses for this client.

For suggested responses, see page 319.

POSTTEST

1 A client with anorexia nervosa has a nursing diagnosis of Disturbed body image. The nurse identifies which of the following as an appropriate outcome?

1. Verbalizes knowledge of maintenance diet.
2. Demonstrates assertiveness with family.
3. Verbalizes body size accurately.
4. Demonstrates control of obsessive behaviors.

2 The nurse encourages increased intake of which of the following foods to best assist a client who has major burns to maintain a positive nitrogen balance?

1. Meats and legumes
2. Vegetables and clear liquids
3. Fruits and nuts
4. Dairy products and shellfish

3 A client has begun therapy with captopril (Capoten) for hypertension. Which of the following foods should the nurse caution the client to avoid? Select all that apply.

1. Oranges and bananas
2. Cheese and yogurt
3. Milk and milk products
4. Potato and beans
5. Broccoli and carrots

4 As part of the teaching plan for a client with type 1 diabetes mellitus, the nurse should include that carbohydrate needs may increase under which of the following circumstances?

1. The client has an infection.
2. The client has an emotional upset.
3. The client eats a large meal.
4. The client engages vigorous exercise.

5 Which of the following dietary measures should the nurse include when planning for the nutritional needs of a client who has had a subtotal gastrectomy?

1. Low-residue, bland diet
2. Fluid intake below 1000 mL/day
3. Six small meals/day
4. Low-protein, high-carbohydrate diet

6 The mother of a 16-year-old client calls to express concern about the teen's obsession with dieting and exercising. The teen appears healthy and has not lost any weight. What might the nurse suspect?

1. Anorexia
2. Depression
3. Bulimia
4. Drug abuse

7 What would the nurse prepare to do for the client who is 6 hours post-burn and has absent bowel sounds and abdominal distention?

1. Insert a feeding tube for nutrition.
2. Insert a nasogastric tube to low intermittent suction.
3. Withhold oral intake, except for water.
4. Start a diet of clear liquids only.

8 The nurse is reviewing the results of a lipid profile, including high-density lipoproteins (HDLs), low-density lipoproteins (LDLs), and very low-density lipoproteins (VLDLs), for a client who is following a low-fat diet. The nurse concludes that the client has the desired pattern of results if the laboratory values show:

1. High HDL, low LDL, low VLDL.
2. Low HDL, high LDL, high VLDL.
3. Low HDL, low LDL, low VLDL.
4. High HDL, high LDL, high VLDL.

9 A nurse is caring for a client who has burns over 50% of the body. The client's pre-burn weight is 120 pounds. When developing the plan of care, the nurse sets a goal that client's weight will not drop below _____ pounds. Provide a numerical answer.

Answer: ______________________

10 Which of the following foods will the nurse include in the diet plan for a client with hypoparathyroidism?

1. Bananas, spinach, sweet potatoes
2. Bacon, rice, canned tuna
3. Bran cereal, lima beans, corn
4. Cheese, yogurt, legumes

See pages 185–186 for Answers and Rationales.

ANSWERS & RATIONALES

Pretest

1 **Answer: 2** It is important in the early stages of treatment that a staff member sits with the client during mealtimes to offer encouragement and help calm fears of eating. The other options are not appropriate at this time. Having the client's mother come during meals may affect the client's coping status, while leaving the client alone may cause the client to refuse to eat. Obtaining an order for a feeding tube is not warranted at this time, since there is no clinical information to support an alternate feeding approach.
Cognitive Level: Application **Client Need:** Health Promotion and Maintenance **Integrated Process:** Nursing Process: Implementation **Content Area:** Foundational Sciences: Nutrition **Strategy:** It is significant to note the client is newly diagnosed; eliminate option 4 since this would be an extreme last resort measure. Recognize the emotional and psychological nature of the disorder to direct you to option 3. **Reference:** Rolfes, S., Pinna, K., & Whitney, E. (2006). *Understanding normal and clinical nutrition* (7th ed.). Belmont, CA: Wadsworth & Thomson Learning, p. 314.

2 **Answer: 2** Total kilocalories are based on the hypermetabolism response, which is proportional to the size of the wound or total body surface area burned. Weight does figure into the formula, but not height; cause and location do not affect total kilocalorie needs.
Cognitive Level: Application **Client Need:** Physiological Integrity: Physiological Adaptation **Integrated Process:** Nursing Process: Planning **Content Area:** Foundational Sciences: Nutrition **Strategy:** The core concept is nutritional

needs and total kilocalories in a client with major burn injury. Note the connection between the types of burns, partial and full thickness, to direct you to "extent" in option 2. **Reference:** Rolfes, S., Pinna, K., & Whitney, E. (2006). *Understanding normal and clinical nutrition* (7th ed.). Belmont, CA: Wadsworth & Thomson Learning, p. 700.

3 **Answer: 3** Increased intake of salad and fresh fruits and vegetables can lead to increased flatus formation in a client with a colostomy. Eating pasta, cereal, and milk and increasing fluids are not associated with increased gas formation. It is important for both the nurse and client to recognize foods that can be gas-forming and limit their inclusion in the diet.

Cognitive Level: Application **Client Need:** Health Promotion and Maintenance **Integrated Process:** Nursing Process: Assessment **Content Area:** Foundational Sciences: Nutrition **Strategy:** The question requires you to identify which food pattern would most contribute to gas formation. Many vegetables are in this category, allowing you choose option 3. **Reference:** Rolfes, S., Pinna, K., & Whitney, E. (2006). *Understanding normal and clinical nutrition* (7th ed.). Belmont, CA: Wadsworth & Thomson Learning, p. 760.

4 **Answers: 2, 3, 5** Sodium and potassium are lost via an ileostomy, and these foods are high in potassium (oranges and potatoes) and high in sodium (tomato juice). Asparagus is not high in either and may cause an odor. Chicken breast is a healthy choice, but not to offset the electrolyte losses.

Cognitive Level: Analysis Client Need: Health Promotion and Maintenance **Integrated Process:** Nursing Process: Implementation **Content Area:** Foundational Sciences: Nutrition **Strategy:** The question requires you to determine what electrolytes are lost. Recall drainage from an ileostomy is in the ileum and the body has not had time to reabsorb all the water and electrolytes. **Reference:** Lemone, P., & Burke, K. (2004). *Medical-surgical nursing: Critical thinking in client care* (3rd ed.). Upper Saddle River, NJ: Pearson/Prentice Hall, p. 657.

5 **Answer: 1** Type 1 diabetics should monitor blood glucose levels before, during, and after routine exercise. If levels before exercise are above 100 mg/dL, no additional food is needed. Exercise will lower blood glucose, so additional insulin is not needed. Adjustment of CHO intake prior to practice is not indicated as client's blood glucose level is above 100 mg/dL.

Cognitive Level: Analysis **Client Need:** Health Promotion and Maintenance **Integrated Process:** Nursing Process: Implementation **Content Area:** Foundational Sciences: Nutrition **Strategy:** Recall knowledge of normal blood glucose levels and correlate effect of exercise on insulin utilization. Eliminate option 3 since levels are already elevated. Recall exercise will help to reduce blood glucose to choose option 1. **Reference:** Lemone, P., & Burke, K. (2004). *Medical surgical nursing: Critical thinking in client care* (3rd ed.). Upper Saddle River, NJ: Pearson/Prentice Hall, p. 495.

6 **Answer: 2** The American Diabetes Association Exchange Lists group foods according to composition (similar calories, fat, protein, carbohydrate). One serving can be exchanged for another within the same list. Milk and yogurt are on the milk list. Peanut butter is on the fat list, while ground beef is on the meat list. Carrots and eggplant are on the vegetable list, while grapefruit is on the fruit list. Bagels are on the starch/bread list.

Cognitive Level: Analysis Client Need: Health Promotion and Maintenance **Integrated Process:** Nursing Process: Evaluation **Content Area:** Foundational Sciences: Nutrition **Strategy:** Systematically review each option and eliminate options 3 and 4 since they contain foods from different groups. Eliminate option 1 since peanut butter is a fat and ground beef is a protein. **Reference:** Lemone, P., & Burke, K. (2004). *Medical surgical nursing: Critical thinking in client care* (3rd ed.). Upper Saddle River, NJ: Pearson/Prentice Hall, pp. 492–496.

7 **Answer: 4** Emotional stress, psychological factors, and food intolerances have been identified as factors that can precipitate irritable bowel syndrome. Carbonated beverages (including seltzer) increase intestinal gas; laxatives can perpetuate constipation and should be avoided; fiber and bulk help to regulate bowel movements and should be increased.

Cognitive Level: Application **Client Need:** Health Promotion and Maintenance **Integrated Process:** Nursing Process: Implementation **Content Area:** Foundational Sciences: Nutrition **Strategy:** Critical words are *irritable bowel* and *prevented.* Eliminate option 2 since daily laxative use promotes dependency and would not be recommended. Recall the emotional aspect of the disorder to direct you to option 4. **Reference:** Rolfes, S., Pinna, K., & Whitney, E. (2006). *Understanding normal and clinical nutrition* (7th ed.). Belmont, CA: Wadsworth & Thomson Learning, p. 757.

8 **Answer: 3** To minimize the risk of a client's developing dumping syndrome, the client should take several small meals throughout the day rather than large meals, which would cause increased stomach distention. Fluids should be taken either before or after meals to minimize the possibility of developing nausea. The diet should be low in simple sugars, moderate in fat, and higher in complex CHOs and protein. The addition of

milk with every meal can cause possible abdominal bloating.
Cognitive Level: Application **Client Need:** Physiological Integrity: Physiological Adaptation **Integrated Process:** Teaching and Learning **Content Area:** Foundational Sciences: Nutrition **Strategy:** Note all options are related to dietary intake. Recall the stomach size has been greatly reduced to direct you to option 3. **Reference:** Rolfes, S., Pinna, K., & Whitney, E. (2006). *Understanding normal and clinical nutrition* (7th ed.). Belmont, CA: Wadsworth & Thomson Learning, p. 757.

9 **Answer: 2, 4** Liver is an organ meat and is therefore high in cholesterol. Egg yolks are also high in cholesterol. Chicken and yogurt are low in cholesterol, while carrots are a plant product and do not contain cholesterol.
Cognitive Level: Application **Client Need:** Health Promotion and Maintenance **Integrated Process:** Teaching and Learning **Content Area:** Foundational Sciences: Nutrition **Strategy:** Critical words are *hypercholesteremia* and *limit intake*. Recall cholesterol and saturated fats contribute to the disease to choose option 2. **Reference:** Rolfes, S., Pinna, K., & Whitney, E. (2006). *Understanding normal and clinical nutrition* (7th ed.). Belmont, CA: Wadsworth & Thomson Learning, pp. 159–160.

10 **Answer: 1** The most important objective is to normalize food intake with close supervision to control purging (vomiting, laxatives, diuretics). The other options are secondary to stabilizing nutritional status.
Cognitive Level: Analysis **Client Need:** Health Promotion and Maintenance **Integrated Process:** Nursing Process: Planning **Content Area:** Foundational Sciences: Nutrition **Strategy:** Critical words are *highest priority* and *goal,* indicating one goal is more important overall. Eliminate option 4, since the focus is not on dieting at this time. Note similarities in the psychological nature of options 2 and 3 and choose option 1, since it identifies a physiological need. **Reference:** Rolfes, S., Pinna, K., & Whitney, E. (2006). *Understanding normal and clinical nutrition* (7th ed.). Belmont, CA: Wadsworth & Thomson Learning, pp. 314–317.

Posttest

1 **Answer: 3** One issue for clients with anorexia nervosa is an altered view of their body appearance (visualizing themselves as being fat even when they are emaciated). Option 1 involves a knowledge deficit; option 2 involves possible resolution of family dynamic issues; option 4 involves psychological adaptation.
Cognitive Level: Analysis **Client Need:** Psychosocial Integrity **Integrated Process:** Nursing Process: Planning **Content Area:** Psychiatric-Mental Health **Strategy:** Note similarity in option 3 of body size to body image in question to choose this option. **Reference:** Rolfes, S., Pinna, K., & Whitney, E. (2006). *Understanding normal and clinical nutrition* (7th ed.). Belmont, CA: Wadsworth & Thomson Learning, pp. 312–314.

2 **Answer: 1** Clients with burns are hypermetabolic and require increased protein levels in order to maintain a positive nitrogen balance. Vegetables (option 2 and fruits (option 3) are low in protein, although the nuts in option 3 are reasonable sources of protein. Dairy products and shellfish contain protein but are not as good sources as the foods in option 1.
Cognitive Level: Application **Client Need:** Health Promotion and Maintenance **Integrated Process:** Nursing Process: Implementation **Content Area:** Foundational Sciences: Nutrition **Strategy:** Eliminate option 2 first as the lowest protein source. Discriminate among the other three options by selecting the option that has two protein sources listed rather than one. **Reference:** Rolfes, S., Pinna, K., & Whitney, E. (2006). *Understanding normal and clinical nutrition* (7th ed.). Belmont, CA: Wadsworth & Thomson Learning, pp. 699–700.

3 **Answers: 1, 4, 5** Captopril is an ACE inhibitor that leads to an elevation of serum potassium levels. Foods high in potassium such as oranges and bananas should be avoided. Other foods to avoid are potatoes and beans, and vegetables such as broccoli and carrots.
Cognitive Level: Analysis **Client Need:** Health Promotion and Maintenance **Integrated Process:** Nursing Process: Implementation **Content Area:** Foundational Sciences: Nutrition **Strategy:** Recall that the mineral potassium is vital to cardiac function and associate it with options offered. **Reference:** Rolfes, S., Pinna, K., & Whitney, E. (2006). *Understanding normal and clinical nutrition* (7th ed.). Belmont, CA: Wadsworth & Thomson Learning, p. 841.

4 **Answer: 4** Active exercise increases insulin sensitivity, thus lowering blood glucose levels. Additional carbohydrates may be needed to balance the usual insulin dose. All of the other options will increase blood glucose levels.
Cognitive Level: Application **Client Need:** Health Promotion and Maintenance **Integrated Process:** Teaching and Learning **Content Area:** Foundational Sciences: Nutrition **Strategy:** Critical words are *Type 1 diabetes,* indicating client is insulin dependent. Systematically analyze each option for the effect on blood sugar and choose option 4 since exercise will lower blood sugar. **Reference:** Rolfes, S., Pinna, K., & Whitney, E. (2006). *Understanding normal and clinical nutrition* (7th ed.). Belmont, CA: Wadsworth & Thomson Learning, pp. 798–799.

5 **Answer: 3** Small meals prevent overdistention and rapid emptying of stomach, thus helping to prevent dumping syndrome. A low-residue diet is not necessary for this client because this diet plan is usually used as a transition diet from liquids to solid foods to allow the colon to rest. A fluid intake below 1000 mL/day is too low and could cause the client to become dehydrated. Instead, the client should drink liquids between meals. A high-carbohydrate diet is not recommended because concentrated sweets pass rapidly out of stomach and will intensify symptoms of dumping syndrome. A high-protein diet is needed for tissue repair.

Cognitive Level: Application **Client Need:** Health Promotion and Maintenance **Integrated Process:** Nursing Process: Planning **Content Area:** Foundational Sciences: Nutrition **Strategy:** Critical words in the question are *nutritional intake* and *subtotal gastrectomy.* Note correlation of small meals to reduced size of stomach to direct you to option 3. **Reference:** Lemone, P., & Burke, K. (2004). *Medical surgical nursing: Critical thinking in client care* (3rd ed.). Upper Saddle River, NJ: Pearson/Prentice Hall, pp. 567–568.

6 **Answer: 3** One form of bulimia is the "nonpurging" type. Clients with this type of bulimia use fasting and excessive exercise to compensate for food binges. Many clients with bulimia will appear in a normal weight range and perform their eating behaviors in secret. Option 1 is incorrect—anorexia presents with documented weight loss. Options 2 and 4 could be possibilities, but there is no evidence to support depression or use of drugs at the present time given the information provided.

Cognitive Level: Analysis **Client Need:** Psychosocial Integrity **Integrated Process:** Nursing Process: Analysis **Content Area:** Foundational Sciences: Nutrition **Strategy:** Note the connection between obsession with dieting but lack of weight loss to direct you to option 3. **Reference:** Rolfes, S., Pinna, K., & Whitney, E. (2006). *Understanding normal and clinical nutrition* (7th ed.). Belmont, CA: Wadsworth & Thomson Learning, p. 317.

7 **Answer: 2** The client with burns often develops paralytic ileus within a few hours, thus a nasogastric tube should be used for stomach decompression. When bowel sounds return, feeding can begin, either via feeding tube or orally.

Cognitive Level: Application **Client Need:** Physiological Integrity: Physiological Adaptation **Integrated Process:** Nursing Process: Planning **Content Area:** Adult Health: Integumentary **Strategy:** Recognize the symptoms are indicative of a paralytic ileus. Eliminate options 1, 3, and 4 since oral intake could cause complications. **Reference:** Lemone, P., & Burke, K. (2004). *Medical surgical nursing: Critical thinking in client care* (3rd ed.). Upper Saddle River, NJ: Pearson/Prentice Hall, pp. 423–427.

8 **Answer: 1** High HDL levels are associated with reduced risk for coronary artery disease (CAD) and are thought to be cardioprotective. Decreased LDL and VLDL levels are associated with reduced risk for CAD. Increased levels of LDL and VLDL are associated with increased risk for CAD as are low HDL levels.

Cognitive Level: Application **Client Need:** Health Promotion and Maintenance **Integrated Process:** Nursing Process: Evaluation **Content Area:** Foundational Sciences: Nutrition **Strategy:** Systematically review each option and eliminate all incorrect ones. If you had difficulty with this question, review lipid metabolism and coronary heart disease. **Reference:** Rolfes, S., Pinna, K., & Whitney, E. (2006). *Understanding normal and clinical nutrition* (7th ed.). Belmont, CA: Wadsworth & Thomson Learning, p. 823.

9 **Answer: 108 pounds** A nutritional goal for a client with burns is to maintain weight within 10% of the preburn weight.

Cognitive Level: Analysis **Client Need:** Health Promotion and Maintenance **Integrated Process:** Nursing Process: Planning **Content Area:** Foundational Sciences: Nutrition **Strategy:** Calculate 10% of 120 pounds by multiplying 120 by 0.10 to yield 12 pounds; subtract 12 pounds from 120 to yield a weight of 108 pounds. **Reference:** Lemone, P., & Burke, K. (2004). *Medical surgical nursing: Critical thinking in client care* (3rd ed.). Upper Saddle River, NJ: Pearson/Prentice Hall, pp. 432–434.

10 **Answer: 4** Clients with hypoparathyroidism require calcium replacement. These foods are high in calcium. Option 1 reflects foods that are high in potassium; option 2 reflects foods that are high in sodium; option 3 reflects foods that are high in starches.

Cognitive Level: Analysis **Client Need:** Health Promotion and Maintenance **Integrated Process:** Nursing Process: Planning **Content Area:** Foundational Sciences: Nutrition **Strategy:** Refer to the physiological function of the parathyroid gland and the regulation of blood calcium. **Reference:** Rolfes, S., Pinna, K., & Whitney, E. (2006). *Understanding normal and clinical nutrition* (7th ed.). Belmont, CA: Wadsworth & Thomson Learning, p. 414.

References

Cataldo, C., DeBruyne, L., & Whitney, E. (2006). *Nutrition and diet therapy* (7th ed.). Belmont, CA: Wadsworth & Thomson Learning, pp. 130–160, 413–433, 473–483, 595–618, 629–652.

Demeny, R., DeSanti, L., & Orgill, D. (2000). *The burn nutrition module* [Online]. http://www.burnsurgery.org, accessed 10/14/05.

Dudek, S. (2006). *Nutritional essentials for nursing practice* (5th ed.). Philadelphia: Lippincott, Williams & Wilkins, pp. 455–567.

Halpern, J., & Wang, N. E. (2005). *Hypoparathyroidism.* [Online]. http://www.emedicine.com/emerg/topic276.htm, accessed 10/16/05.

Kim, L., & Nwariaku, F. (2005). *Hyperparathyroidism.* [Online]. http://www.emedicine.com/MED/topic3200.htm, accessed 10/16/05.

Lutz, C., & Przytulski, K. (2006). *Nutrition and diet therapy* (4th ed.). Philadelphia: F. A. Davis, pp. 113–114, 349–395, 395–452, 409–432, 471–502.

Nix, S. (2005). *Williams' basic nutrition and diet therapy* (12th ed.). St. Louis: Elsevier Mosby, pp. 324–364.

Rolfes, S., Pinna, K. & Whitney, E. (2006). *Understanding normal and clinical nutrition* (7th ed.). Belmont, CA: Wadsworth & Thomson Learning, pp. 740–764, 791–843.

7 Nutrition Therapy for Immune, Liver, Musculoskeletal, Neurological, Renal, or Respiratory Disorders

Chapter Outline

Client with Immune Disorders
Client with Liver Disorders
Client with Musculoskeletal Disorders
Client with Neurological Disorders
Client with Renal Disorders
Client with Respiratory Disorders

Objectives

- Review basic physiological principles relevant to clients with immune, liver, musculoskeletal, neurological, renal, and respiratory disorders.
- Identify specific nutritional therapies that can be used to treat clients with immune, liver, musculoskeletal, neurological, renal, and respiratory disorders.
- Explain the importance of adequate nutritional monitoring of clients with immune, liver, musculoskeletal, neurological, renal, and respiratory disorders in order to prevent further complications.
- Review dietary measures used to treat clients with immune, liver, musculoskeletal, neurological, renal, and respiratory disorders.
- Describe the impact of acute and chronic disease states on nutritional well-being of the client.

NCLEX-RN® Test Prep

Use the CD-ROM enclosed with this book to access additional practice opportunities.

Review at a Glance

bone mineral density (BMD) examination of bone mass using radiation methods to determine integrity of bone structure

cancer cachexia starvation syndrome resulting from malabsorption and maldigestion; ultimately, there is severe depletion of lean body mass, weight loss, and wasting; end stage of cancer

carcinogenesis the process of cancer; uncontrolled growth of cells that tend to invade surrounding tissue and metastasize to distant body areas

dysgeusia an altered sense of taste; may be due to chemotherapy or radiation

dysphagia the inability to chew, swallow, digest, and absorb nutrients while passing fiber and other substances on for elimination

Harris-Benedict equation equation used to determine client's basal energy requirement

neutropenic diet diet used for clients who undergo bone marrow transplants because they are prone to develop infection due to profound immunosuppression treatment regimens; restriction of foods that are high in bacteria sources, such as fresh fruits, vegetables, raw items, and black pepper, used when client's absolute neutrophil count is < 1,000/mm^3

peak bone mass (PBM) period during which bone mineral density and calcium retention is maximum (at 20 to 30 years of age), after which bone loss begins to take place

protein-calorie malnutrition (PCM) also known as marasmus; inadequate protein and calorie intake characterized by protein catabolism and resulting in wasting despite normal serum albumin levels

purine-restricted diet restriction of foods such as organ meats, game, anchovies, herring, mackerel, sardines, scallops, and certain grains and vegetables, prescribed primarily for clients with gout

respiratory quotient (RQ) ratio measurement that looks at the volume of CO_2 produced to the volume of O_2 consumed

wasting syndrome chronic process whereby the client loses > 10% of body weight in the presence of diarrhea, weakness, or fever; leads to a cycle of malnutrition and wasting; is now classified as an AIDS-defining diagnosis in clients who are HIV-positive

PRETEST

PRETEST

1 Which one of the following actions by the nurse would be most appropriate related to diet selection for an immunosuppressed client?

1. Provide any food enjoyed by the client as long as it is thoroughly cooked (well done).
2. Limit fluids to prevent edema due to decreased protein stores.
3. Encourage fresh foods and vegetable produce, which are essential to maintain adequate nutrition.
4. Cut foods into small pieces to facilitate chewing.

2 A 47-year-old male client with renal disease doesn't understand why the nurse is instructing him to include high biologic value protein in the diet, since he has always been told to restrict protein. What explanation should the nurse give to the client?

1. High biologic value proteins help to increase urea excretion.
2. Increased protein is needed to prevent catabolism, regardless of the stage of renal disease.
3. High biologic value proteins contain essential amino acids that are necessary to maintain nutritional balance.
4. High biologic value proteins are needed during times of stress to maximize metabolic efforts only in clients on dialysis therapy.

3 When assessing a client with a history of kidney stones, the nurse notes the client is taking daily vitamin C supplements. What dietary counseling should the nurse provide to this client?

1. The client should increase daily intake of vitamin C for its antioxidant effects.
2. Fluid intake should be monitored to prevent stone formation.
3. Limit intake of supplemental vitamin C, which can exacerbate stone formation if taken in high doses.
4. Stop taking vitamin C because it is only beneficial for common cold symptoms.

PRETEST

4 What interventions should the nurse plan for in a client admitted to the oncology unit for chemotherapy who is experiencing dysgeusia?

1. Premedicate the client with an antiemetic.
2. Observe the client for signs of dehydration.
3. Use highly seasoned foods to stimulate taste buds.
4. Obtain an order for zinc and give with food or milk to treat the symptom.

5 Which dietary instruction is most appropriate for the client with chronic obstructive pulmonary disease (COPD) experiencing fatigue and shortness of breath during mealtime?

1. Include simple carbohydrates (CHO) for quick energy.
2. Eat fatty foods to increase calorie intake.
3. Eat frequent small meals to decrease energy use.
4. Eat the largest meal before bedtime.

6 A client presenting with ascites secondary to liver failure is being evaluated for fluid balance. The nurse would best assess fluid status using which of the following?

1. Intake and output measurement
2. Liver function test results
3. Caloric intake and serum protein levels
4. Dry weight calculation

7 A client who has cirrhosis of the liver is now diagnosed with hepatic encephalopathy. The dietitian has been consulted to evaluate this client for appropriate nutritional therapy. What priority information should the nurse provide to the dietician to help formulate nutritional goals for the client?

1. Client's usual weight and caloric intake pattern prior to admission
2. Client's reduced intake secondary to decreased mental status
3. Client has a preference for snack foods and sodas
4. Client has been compliant with medical treatment during this hospitalization

8 The nurse is teaching the wife of a client who has a neutrophil count of 500/mm^3 about dietary precautions that should be instituted. Which of the following instructions should the nurse include?

1. Avoid eating any raw vegetables.
2. Boil all liquids before serving them.
3. Do not let him eat any seeds or nuts.
4. Use a separate cutting board for beef and poultry.

9 The spouse of a client with Parkinson's disease asks how to best assist her husband during feeding as he is having "increasing problems with drooling and swallowing." What instruction should the nurse provide to the family member?

1. "Use thickened liquids along with upright positioning during feeding."
2. "It might be time to switch to enteral feedings if you are afraid that your husband may choke."
3. "Increase the amount of fluids he receives to decrease saliva formation and improve swallowing."
4. "Use a straw during feedings to facilitate swallowing."

10 Which of the following foods enjoyed by a client with gout would the nurse encourage the client to continue to include in the diet? Select all that apply.

1. Beets
2. Milk
3. Eggs
4. Sweetbreads
5. Sardines

See pages 226–228 for Answers and Rationales.

I. CLIENT WITH IMMUNE DISORDERS

A. Cancer and other malignancies (leukemia and lymphoma)

1. Description
   a. Cancer cells originate from preexisting cells; they demonstrate uncontrolled growth and tend to invade surrounding tissue
   b. Eventually, cancer cells detach from the tumor mass and migrate (metastasize) to a distant site where they lodge and grow in the new location; there, they form a secondary tumor mass; if left untreated, cancer ends in death

c. **Carcinogenesis,** the process of cancer production, is thought to occur in two stages

   1) Initiation—during this stage a repeated or prolonged exposure to carcinogens or radiation changes the structure of DNA, the reproductive code; this change takes place in a normal cell during reproduction; exactly why this change takes place in normal cells is unclear; a neoplasm, or abnormal growth results, which can either be benign or malignant

   2) Promotion—during this stage, neoplastic cells are activated and begin to divide (this can occur after a latency period)

d. Leukemia is a broad term used to characterize the abnormal proliferation of white blood cells that results in release of immature cells from normal bone marrow, leading to immunosuppression

e. Lymphoma is a broad term used to characterize malignancies of lymphoid tissue (Hodgkins and non-Hodgkins) that leads to immunosuppression

f. During the course of clinical treatment for cancers and malignancies, the client can experience remission, progression of disease process (metastasis), conversion of disease processes (chronic to acute leukemia), and development of secondary malignancies (such as a client with HIV/AIDS who develops lymphoma)

g. Etiology

   1) Initiators and promoters are believed to be environmental, lifestyle, and genetic in nature

   2) Diet is considered to be an important environmental/lifestyle risk factor

      a) While no one food can cause/prevent the development of cancer, there is a correlation between aspects of diet (high fat content and decreased amount of fruits and vegetables) and development of cancer

      b) Epidemiological studies suggest that some specific dietary components may increase the risk of developing some types of cancers, while others may decrease the risk

2. Associated nutritional problems

   a. **Protein-calorie malnutrition (PCM)**—a major cause of morbidity and mortality that can result from cancer but is further complicated by treatment of the disease

   b. Anorexia is multifactorial and may be caused by the disease or by treatment; it may be related to changes in taste and smell, decreased transit time and subsequent early satiety, opportunistic infection, medication side effects, or emotional or psychological factors

   c. **Cancer cachexia**—complex syndrome that results in severe wasting of lean body mass and weight loss; affects about two-thirds of all clients with cancer (refer to Table 7-1, p. 192)

3. Dietary measures used as treatment

   a. Individualize nutritional support and utilize interventions that maximize nutritional intake

   b. Nutritional adequacy in a client helps to preserve immune function (refer to Box 7-1, p. 192)

   c. Clients with an absolute neutrophil count (ANC) $< 1{,}000$ mm^3 may be placed on a **neutropenic diet** (low-bacteria diet) to attempt to prevent infection

Table 7-1

Causes of Cancer Cachexia

Factor	Effect
Vomiting, diarrhea, malabsorption, maldigestion, fistula formation	Increased nutritional losses
Altered metabolism	Increased basal metabolic rate (BMR); hyperglycemia; insulin resistance; catabolism of fat stores; decreased synthesis of fat in fat cells; hyperlipidemia; fluid and electrolyte abnormalities
Anorexia	Early satiety; severe weight loss (10% of body weight within 6 months or unintentional weight loss of 2 lbs/wk)

because the immune system is compromised (refer to Box 7-2); they can be taken off the diet when counts return to normal range

d. Managing anorexia

1) Intervene early, educate, and impart a sense of control to the client in managing his or her nutritional intake

! **2)** Refer to Box 7-3 for nutrition care related to clients who are experiencing anorexia

e. **Dysgeusia** (a change in taste)

1) Elemental zinc may correct taste abnormalities; take zinc with food or milk

! **2)** Substitute beef or pork, if unpleasant, with other high-quality protein foods such as legumes, beans, fish, dairy products, and eggs

f. Sore mouth (stomatitis) and thick saliva

1) Eat food in small pieces

! **2)** Avoid spicy, acidic, and coarse foods

3) Eat soft or blended foods; drink plenty of fluids; high-calorie, high-protein liquid supplements may be useful

4) Use straws when necessary

! **5)** Eat ice chips and sugar-free candy between meals, if necessary, to temporarily reduce mouth dryness

6) Proper oral hygiene is essential; ask physician for local anesthetic solution (lidocaine) before meals

g. Method of feeding

1) Use enteral feeding when intake is inadequate

2) Utilize parenteral feeding when GI tract is nonfunctional

Box 7-1

Benefits of Nutritional Adequacy for Clients with Cancer

- Optimizes ability to meet increased needs for protein and energy.
- Provides nutrients to enhance immune response.
- Decreases risk of complications due to surgery.
- Optimizes response to chemotherapy, radiation therapy, and other treatment modalities.
- Promotes enhanced overall stamina, which in turn improves quality of life.

Box 7-2

Neutropenic or Low-Bacteria Diet Implementation

- Wash hands before and after handling food, and eating and after using bathroom.
- Cook all meat, fish, and poultry until well-done.
- Wash fruits and vegetables thoroughly. Remove skin or peels.
- Avoid cross-contamination by using separate cutting boards for meat/poultry and after other foods.

Low-bacteria diet encourages:

- Use of proper food handling to maintain a low-bacteria count.
- Foods to be served within 1 hour at room temperature.
- No storage of leftover food for more than 24 hours.
- Cooking foods thoroughly in order to kill bacteria.

4. Nutritional monitoring
   - !a. Screen regularly for nutritional risk and initiate nutritional therapy early, when indicated; preventing malnutrition is more effective than treating existing malnutrition
   - b. Assess nutritional status to determine calorie and protein requirement
   - c. Monitor weight; not all clients develop anorexia or cachexia; clients with breast cancer may gain weight due to side effects of treatment
   - d. Assess micronutrient status; malabsorption and vomiting may put clients at risk for vitamin and/or mineral deficiencies
   - e. Consider prognosis when determining or adjusting aggressiveness of nutritional intervention
5. Disease impact
   - a. Nutritional problems may result from the disease or as a result of treatment
   - !b. The clinical diagnosis of cancer/malignancy can have physiological local and systemic effects as well as psychological effects on the individual client and family support system

Box 7-3

Nutrition Care for Clients with Cancer or HIV/AIDS Managing Anorexia

- Eat small, frequent meals every 1 to 2 hours.
- Eat nutrient-dense high-calorie/high-protein meals when appetite is best.
- Add nutrient-dense "extras" to food; for example, honey, powdered skim milk, peanut butter, butter, cheese.
- Limit liquids with meals because this can contribute to nausea.
- Use liquid supplements if too fatigued to eat or if decreased appetite is present.
- Avoid spicy, pungent foods that could reduce overall intake.
- Foods may be better tolerated cooler than warmer.
- Make the eating experience pleasurable—eat in a comfortable setting, enjoy the company of friends.
- Take anti-nausea medication prior to eating.
- Take appetite stimulants such as Megace and Marinol as ordered to promote weight gain.

c. Clients with cancer who are undergoing surgery and already experiencing PCM are at higher risks for surgical complications

d. Altered metabolic processes, including the mechanisms and actions of tumor cells, and their effects on host cells, are not fully understood; however, cancer does increase energy expenditure and affect metabolism of macronutrients

1) Carbohydrates (CHOs): impaired glucose utilization and insulin resistance

2) Proteins: decreased albumin as a result of decreased protein synthesis

3) Lipids: elevated serum lipid levels, fat wasting, and inefficient shift of metabolism from CHO to lipid

4) These areas of metabolic impact are still being explored in research

B. Human immunodeficiency virus (HIV) and acquired immunodeficiency syndrome (AIDS)

1. Description

a. An RNA retrovirus, HIV represents a chronic infection that leads to AIDS, an end-stage immune disorder caused by infection with HIV

b. HIV is spread through contact with contaminated body fluids, including blood, blood products, or semen

c. HIV can cross the placenta and thus can be spread from mother to infant during delivery; can also be transmitted during lactation (perinatal transmission)

d. The clinical course begins with mononucleosis-like symptoms—nonspecific and variable

e. AIDS-related complex (ARC) includes weight loss, diarrhea, and enlarged lymph nodes

f. AIDS is diagnosed by a blood test positive for HIV antibodies and one of three other symptoms, including an opportunistic infection, AIDS-related cancer (quite often Kaposi's sarcoma), or fewer than 200 $CD4^+$ T lymphocyte cells (T-helper lymphocyte cells) per L of blood; Centers for Disease Control (CDC) guidelines establish clinical criteria for the diagnosis of AIDS in the individual client

2. Associated nutritional problems

a. Malnutrition exists in the early stages of HIV but may be subclinical and therefore overlooked

b. Vitamin and mineral deficiencies occur in addition to a decline in body mass

c. Kaposi's sarcoma can cause lesions and obstructions in esophagus, making eating painful

! d. Wasting syndrome

1) Wasting syndrome is a separate clinical diagnosis that has been established to represent the specific weight loss that HIV and AIDS clients undergo as a consequence of the disease process

2) Weight loss through AIDS wasting is characterized by an unexplained weight loss of > 10%, leading to a cycle of malnutrition and subsequent wasting

3) Severe infections, malignancies, and therapies coupled with increased nutritional needs contribute to the wasting

4) Wasting exacerbates the illness and is associated with significant morbidity resulting in reduced quality of life

! e. Clients who are HIV positive or who have AIDS often suffer from the effects of anorexia due to disease progression, effects of medication, and/or effects of medical treatments

f. Since the HIV/AIDS client is at risk for developing opportunistic infections, there can be many nutritional consequences due to weight loss, anorexia, oral/esophageal problems, and malabsorption problems (diarrhea)

3. Dietary measures used as treatment

a. Since the HIV/AIDS client often has a very large drug treatment program (antivirals, antibiotics, and antitubercular agents), there are numerous side effects such as nausea, vomiting, diarrhea, and fluid and electrolyte imbalances that need to be monitored and treated in order to maintain a client's nutrient intake (refer again to Box 7-3 for nutrition care)

b. The HIV/AIDS client may also receive prophylactic therapy for both primary and secondary prevention of opportunistic infections such as *pneumocystis carinii* pneumonia (PCP) and tuberculosis that can result in GI side effects

c. Calorie intake should be 35–45 kcal/kg due to increased metabolic needs; protein intake should be 2.0–2.5 grams/kg to replenish losses and help maintain lean body mass

d. Limit fat intake in clients with malabsorption; supplemental medium chain triglyceride (MCT) oil may be added for additional calories

e. There may be a need to reduce intake of lactose (milk products) to control diarrhea

f. To prevent dehydration due to diarrhea, additional fluid intake may be required

g. Decrease roughage along with soluble fiber and increase insoluble fiber sources; Metamucil or other fiber supplements may also be helpful

h. Clients receiving isoniazid (INH) therapy for prophylaxis of tuberculosis are at risk for vitamin B_6 and vitamin B_{12} deficiencies and should receive additional supplementation; this drug acts as a vitamin B_6 antagonist and interferes with the absorption of vitamin B_{12}

i. Clients may receive medication therapy in the form of megesterol (Megace), an oral progesterone, or dronabinol (Marinol), a cannibus derivative that are used as appetite stimulants for clients suffering anorexia due to HIV/AIDS and other cancers

j. Enteral and parenteral feedings

1) Enteral feeding may be required if oral feeding, even with liquid supplements, is inadequate

2) May use enteral feeding in addition to oral feeding

3) Total parenteral nutrition (TPN) may be indicated when severe GI and malabsorption complications are present; risk for infection increases at the site of infusion

4. Nutritional monitoring

a. Conduct baseline and continual nutrition assessment to monitor nutritional risk

1) Measure body weight and compare to client's usual body weight and to last recording; calculate body mass index (BMI); a BMI less than 18.5 is classified as underweight and is associated with malnutrition

2) Monitor protein status; measure serum albumin, prealbumin, transferrin, and total lymphocyte count (TLC)

3) Loss of lean body mass (LBM) is characteristic of clients with AIDS; monitor shifts in LBM through bioelectric impedance analysis (BIA)

b. It is critical to prevent foodborne illness; teach food safety methods and prescribe a low-bacteria diet (refer again to Box 7-2 for details)

Practice to Pass

Describe early intervention strategies for clients with HIV/AIDS.

c. Monitor gut function, abdominal bloating, presence of diarrhea and steatorrhea, or any other symptom that may interfere with oral intake

d. Conduct dietary assessment through use of food frequency questionnaire, 24-hour dietary recall, and food diary

5. Disease impact

a. Impact on nutritional status is profound, resulting in malabsorption, malnutrition, and wasting

b. Immune function is comprised, ultimately resulting in death

c. HIV is a significant global health issue with infection rates rising throughout the world, particularly in Southern Africa and Asia

d. Socioeconomic cost of disease continues to rise both nationally and globally

C. Autoimmune disorders

1. These include rheumatoid arthritis (RA), systemic lupus erythematosus (SLE), Sjögren's syndrome, and scleroderma

2. Description

a. Rheumatoid arthritis represents an autoimmune systemic disease that affects joints in a symmetrical pattern, resulting in inflammation, pain, stiffness, deformity, and loss of function; characteristic joint deformities are present; American College of Rheumatology establishes criteria for clinical diagnosis

b. Systemic lupus erythematosus (SLE) represents an autoimmune disease that is chronic in nature, affecting multiple systems in the body as a result of the development of autoantibodies; characteristic skin lesions (butterfly malar rash or discoid rash) and sensitivity to sunlight are common presentations; American Rheumatism Association establishes criteria for clinical diagnosis

c. Sjögren's syndrome represents an autoimmune disease that affects the production of secretions in lacrimal and salivary glands, resulting in dryness of mucous membranes that can affect the entire body; primary form affects the mouth and eyes, whereas the secondary form is usually seen in conjunction with other autoimmune (RA or SLE) or disease processes

d. Scleroderma (progressive systemic sclerosis) represents an autoimmune disease of the connective tissue, which becomes thickened, hard, and fibrotic and can affect multiple systems throughout the body

3. Associated nutritional problems

a. Clients with autoimmune diseases may be receiving medical treatment such as antihypertensives, NSAIDs, steroids, or chemotherapy agents that can interfere with their efforts to maintain adequate nutrition

! b. During the acute phase or exacerbation of the disease process, clients may have other medications or therapies added to their treatment regimen that can cause nausea and/or lead to further immunosuppression

c. Clients who are affected by limitation of mobility, internal hardening, and dryness may be at risk to develop further problems as a result of inactivity, leading to protein and calcium loss and dehydration due to fluid and electrolyte imbalances

d. Since pain is a primary concern for clients with arthritic problems, the use of pain medication therapies can lead to elimination problems as a result of reduction in gut motility

e. Clients with Sjögren's syndrome suffer from xerophthalmia (dry eyes) and xerostomia (dry mouth) that can affect mucosal dryness, leading to altered taste and smell and chewing and swallowing difficulties, along with increased incidence of dental caries

4. Dietary measures used as treatment
   a. Clients with autoimmune diseases should be placed on a well-balanced diet in order to maintain ideal body weight
   b. Clients with Sjögren's syndrome should be encouraged to increase intake of fluids to maintain adequate hydration
   c. Clients with scleroderma may have problems related to the GI system such as esophageal reflux and malabsorption; treatment measures consist of:
      1) Eating small, frequent meals
      2) Sitting up for an hour after eating to prevent stomach contents from regurgitating
      3) Avoiding late-night meals, spicy or fatty foods, and alcohol and caffeine
5. Nutritional monitoring
   a. Clients with autoimmune diseases should have their baseline weight recorded; weights should then be trended during the course of therapy to establish clinical response and disease progression
   b. Refer to a dietician those clients who have autoimmune diseases due to exacerbation of chronic disease
6. Disease impact
   a. Autoimmune diseases affect millions of people in the United States
   b. SLE is the most commonly occurring autoimmune disease of childbearing women; therefore, the impact on females and pregnancy must be seriously considered in relation to maternal and perinatal outcomes
   c. Impact on mobility and quality of life is a chronic concern with autoimmune disease processes

D. Chemotherapy, radiation therapy, and their effects on nutrition

1. Description
   a. Local effects
      1) Radiation
         a) It is used to treat tumors that cannot be surgically removed and are sensitive to radiation exposure
         b) It damages rapidly replicating local normal host cells along with cancerous cells
         c) Sites primarily include head, neck, abdomen, pelvis, and central nervous system (CNS)
         d) Clients can receive external-beam radiation therapy (EBRT) or internal radiation therapy (brachytherapy) with implanted isotopes
         e) Skin irritation can occur, depending on dosage used and clinical condition of client (this ranges from mild erythema, rash, and itching to severe forms with wet desquamation—resembling second-degree burns)
      2) Chemotherapy
         a) These agents act by inhibiting steps in DNA synthesis in rapidly proliferating cells
         b) Host cells as well as malignant cells are affected

c) Chemotherapy agents can be administered by mouth, parenterally, or by intravascular catheters placed surgically in the body at specific tumor sites

b. Systemic effects

1) Clients who receive radiation therapy may develop systemic side effects following therapy or at a later date ranging from weeks to years

2) Severity and manifestations of side effects of chemotherapy depend on agents used; effects also depend on dosage, duration of treatment, rates of metabolism, accompanying drugs, and individual susceptibility

2. Associated nutritional problems

! a. Clients receiving radiation therapy are at risk to develop mucositis of the oral cavity, xerostomia, nausea and vomiting, diarrhea, dental caries, esophagitis, dysphagia, and anorexia (refer to Table 7-2)

! b. Clients receiving chemotherapy are at risk to develop anorexia, nausea and vomiting, altered elimination pattern (diarrhea or constipation), mucositis, and altered liver function (jaundice) as a consequence of impaired drug clearance (refer to Box 7-4)

! c. Associated weight loss and accompanying malnutrition correlate with impaired immunity and affect response to therapy and survival

! 3. Dietary measures used as treatment

a. If necessary, provide as much as 3,000 kcal/day and 100 grams of protein/day (depending on client's age, size, and state of disease), to meet increased demands of hypermetabolic rate to prevent tissue breakdown and weight loss

b. Give nutritionally complete liquid supplements, as necessary, to meet caloric needs

c. Provide at least minimum of RDA for micronutrients; assess individual needs based on impact of treatment on nutritional risk

d. Replace fluids lost to fever, diarrhea, and vomiting

e. Nausea and vomiting need to be managed using specific strategies

1) Symptoms may begin prior to treatment and last up to 3 days posttreatment

2) Antiemetic therapy should be aggressive; give medications 60–90 minutes before meals so that they can be most effective; anticipatory nausea and vomiting may be prevented if food-related nausea and vomiting can be controlled

3) Cool foods without odor tend to be better tolerated than warm and/or odorous foods

Table 7-2

Effects of Radiation on Nutritional Status

Area of Treatment	Effects
Head and neck	Irritation of mouth, tongue, and esophagus; dry mouth, tooth decay; gum destruction, altered taste and smell, dysphagia
Abdomen	Nausea, vomiting, diarrhea, malabsorption, gastritis
Upper spine	Irritation to stomach and esophagus
Lower spine	Diarrhea
Pelvis	Diarrhea, malabsorption

Box 7-4

Nutritional Impact of Chemotherapy

- Weight changes
- Taste changes
- Food aversions
- Dysphagia
- Irritation and inflammation of mouth, tongue, and throat
- Nausea
- Vomiting
- Dehydration
- Altered glucose tolerance
- Altered protein metabolism
- Water retention/bloating
- Electrolyte imbalance

4) Suggest high-carbohydrate, low-fat foods
5) Discourage spicy, greasy foods
6) Have client eat one to two hours prior to treatment to reduce occurrence of nausea

4. Nutritional monitoring
   a. Monitor nutritional status, particularly symptoms of cancer cachexia
   b. Monitor fluid and electrolytes
   c. Monitor client's ability to feed, chew, and consume foods
   d. Be aware of timing of client's treatment regimen relative to radiation/chemotherapy and premedicate with antiemetics as needed
   e. Assess changes in weight for trends, perform calorie counts, and keep accurate intake and output records

Practice to Pass

What strategies would you employ when working with clients who have cancer to manage anorexia resulting from chemotherapy?

II. CLIENT WITH LIVER DISORDERS

A. Cirrhosis

1. Description
   a. Cirrhosis represents a diffuse disease process characterized by fibrosis of the liver with clinical manifestations of ascites, portal hypertension, and variceal bleeding, and that can progress to hepatic encephalopathy
   b. As part of the evolution of many chronic liver diseases or metabolic disease processes, cirrhosis of the liver can progress to an irreversible stage
   ! **c.** Chronic alcoholism is a common etiology for this clinical presentation; other causative agents include medications, autoimmune diseases, and progression of viral hepatitis
   d. Initial common presenting symptoms are nonspecific and may include malaise and lethargy, dyspepsia, bloating, nausea, vomiting, and anorexia
   e. As the disease progresses, complications develop leading to jaundice, hepatomegaly, ascites, asterixis, spider angiomas, secondary infections, and hepatic encephalopathy

f. Abnormal liver function tests (resulting in elevated liver enzymes), decreased albumin, elevated ammonia levels, and alterations in coagulation are common findings

2. Associated nutritional problems

a. Nutritional status is influenced by the liver's role in the intermediate metabolism of CHOs, protein, lipids, and vitamins

b. Decline of nutritional status can further impair liver function

! c. Inadequate metabolism of CHOs results in low energy and lethargy

d. Electrolyte imbalance is common because of poor storage of minerals

! e. Vitamin deficiencies are common; nutrient intake is poor in clients with Laënnec's (alcoholic) cirrhosis prior to onset of liver disorders

f. Esophageal and gastric varices may result, requiring medical intervention, and further compromising client's ability to meet nutritional goals

! 3. Dietary measures used as treatment (refer to Table 7-3)

a. Clients need adequate calories in order to meet nutritional goals for maintaining adequate liver function

b. Protein intake should be adequate to enhance possible regeneration of liver tissue (up to 1.5 grams/kg/day) in the early stages of the disease process

c. However, clients who have hepatic encephalopathy may need to restrict protein (0.5 grams/kg/day) because of their inability to metabolize protein properly because of poor liver function (yielding increased ammonia levels)

1) Limit protein intake; high amounts of protein are believed to increase serum ammonia levels that may precipitate hepatic encephalopathy

2) Although animal proteins have higher biologic value than plant protein, clients tolerate nonanimal protein better than animal protein because ammonia is the end-product of metabolism of meat products

3) Omit foods that contain preformed ammonia—salami, bacon, ham, some cheeses, ground beef, and gelatin

4) Plant proteins contain fewer aromatic amino acids (phenylalanine, tryptophan, and tyrosine) and have more branched chain amino acids (leucine, isoleucine, lysine, and valine)

5) Branched chain amino acid (BCAA)-enriched parenteral solutions may improve significantly the complication of hepatic encephalopathy

Table 7-3

Nutritional Needs of Clients with Cirrhosis

Nutrient	Amount	Purpose
Energy	2,000–3,000 kcal/day	Minimize endogenous protein catabolism
Protein	20–40 grams/day (0.5–1.5 grams/kg/day)	Maintain nitrogen balance; provide for liver repair
Carbohydrate	300–400 grams/day	Minimize endogenous protein catabolism
Fat	Variable	Restrict if evidence of jaundice; add in moderation to make diet more palatable
Salt	Restriction 2–3 grams/day Fluid restriction	Minimize fluid retention and prevent ascites In presence of hyponatremia, restriction of fluids may be necessary.

d. Carbohydrate intake should be adequate to help minimize protein catabolism; fat intake may vary according to clinical presentation

e. Depending on presence of ascites, sodium restriction may be necessary; if hyponatremia is present, then fluid restriction may also be needed

f. Daily weights and abdominal girth measurements are critical elements in monitoring a client with cirrhosis who presents with ascites in order to determine baseline status and response to therapies

! g. Vitamins are a necessary part of diet therapy

1) Provide a multivitamin supplement daily

2) A diet containing 50 grams of protein or less may be deficient in thiamine, riboflavin, calcium, niacin, phosphorus, and iron

3) Ethanol (alcohol) intake decreases the absorption of folate, B_{12}, and thiamine

4) Give fat-soluble vitamins in water-soluble form if steatorrhea is present

h. The following recommendations may also be helpful:

! 1) Offer food in 4 to 6 small meals due to anorexia, nausea, drowsiness, or confusion

2) Provide liquid supplements in between meals to increase kcal intake

3) Reduce roughage in the diet to avoid damage to intestinal mucosa and prevent GI bleeding if esophageal varices are present

4) Use a complete formula feeding as a supplement to meals if GI varices persist

4. Nutritional monitoring

a. Monitor catabolic stress factors such as infection, trauma, surgery, or steatorrhea in order to make adjustments in protein requirement

! b. Monitor client's response to fluid restriction (ordered to prevent or decrease ascites) to maintain weight loss objective (0.5 to 1.0 kg/day)

c. Monitor renal function because potassium may need to be restricted if renal function is inadequate; correspondingly, potassium supplementation may be needed if potassium-wasting diuretics are used

5. Disease impact

a. Due to nature of disease and complications, the client is at risk to require frequent hospitalizations leading to altered nutritional intake

b. Clients receiving lactulose therapy to decrease ammonia are at risk for dehydration because of diarrhea

c. Refer client to a dietitian and recommend adherence to dietary measures to help prevent fluid and electrolyte imbalances associated with ascites (hypokalemia, hypomagnesemia, hypoglycemia, and altered calcium status)

d. As cirrhosis progresses and liver function deteriorates leading to liver failure, the client may require a liver transplant

B. Hepatitis

1. Description

a. Hepatitis A (HAV)

1) HAV is a serious and contagious liver disease that can cause fever, vomiting, stomach pain, diarrhea, and jaundice

! 2) It is usually transmitted by the fecal-oral route (contaminated food or water), but infrequently can be spread by transfusion or infected blood;

most often results from poor handwashing or inadequate stool precautions and is common in overcrowded areas with poor sanitation

3) At-risk (endemic) areas include Mexico, Central and South America, parts of the Caribbean, Africa, Asia, parts of the Middle East, and the Mediterranean basin

4) Onset is rapid, usually within 4 to 6 weeks

b. Hepatitis B (HBV)

1) Is transmitted through contaminated blood, saliva, or semen

2) Onset is usually slow, from 6 weeks to 6 months

3) It is the major form of acute and chronic hepatitis and liver cancer worldwide

c. Hepatitis C (HCV)

1) Is transmitted through contaminated blood or blood products or may present due to unknown etiology (sporadic form)

2) Like HBV, HCV onset is slow, from 6 weeks to 6 months, and can develop into chronic liver disease

3) HCV is a risk factor for liver cancer

d. Hepatitis D (HDV)

1) Hepatitis D is seen as a co-infection in conjunction with Hepatitis B infection

2) The presence of HDV increases the severity of the HBV infection

e. Clinical manifestations and risk factors

1) Nausea, fever, abdominal pain, hepatomegaly, jaundice, anorexia, dark-colored urine (cola-colored), and malaise are often seen in clients with hepatitis

2) At-risk behaviors (IV drug use, alcoholism, multiple sexual partners), occupational exposure of healthcare workers, and clients receiving hemodialysis or blood/blood products are at increased risk of contracting the infection

3) Chronic alcohol use is associated with the development of alcoholic hepatitis that can lead to chronic liver disease and cirrhosis

2. Associated nutritional problems

a. Clients require adequate caloric intake and a balanced diet in order to maintain liver function

b. Due to clinical presentation, the client may suffer from anorexia, nausea, and vomiting, which may prevent client from maintaining adequate intake

c. With the development of ascites and a need for medical intervention therapies, the client will be at risk for fluid and electrolyte disturbances

d. Vitamin/mineral deficiencies can occur because of impact on liver metabolism

3. Dietary measures used as treatment

a. HAV, HBV

1) During periods of nausea and vomiting, use hydration via intravenous (IV) fluids as necessary; otherwise, give 2,500 to 3,000 mL fluid/day to accommodate high protein intake

2) Provide a diet high in kcals (3,000 to 4,000) and high-quality protein (100–150 grams/day or 1.5–2.0 grams/kg), as tolerated

3) Provide 40% of the kcals as CHOs to promote glycogen synthesis and spare protein

4) Do not limit fat unless not well-tolerated (steatorrhea); fat imparts taste and supplies a concentrated form of calories

! 5) Supplement with multivitamin that includes vitamin B complex, especially thiamine and vitamin B_{12} because of decreased absorption and/or hepatic uptake; vitamin K to normalize bleeding tendency; vitamin C for healing; and zinc for poor appetite

b. HCV

1) Clients with chronic HCV sometimes have increased iron concentration in the liver; high iron levels may reduce response rate of clients to interferon; avoid multivitamins with iron, restrict intake of iron-rich foods such as red meats, liver, and iron-fortified cereals, and avoid cooking with iron-coated cookware

2) Provide adequate daily protein for noncirrhotic clients

3) Restrict sodium to 1,000 mg or less/day

c. Nutritional care of clients with hepatitis due to alcoholism

1) Provide a diet adequate in all nutrients

! 2) Avoid inadvertent alcohol intake in food, mouthwashes, or in over-the-counter products or medications

3) Provide parenteral support to correct fluid and electrolyte imbalance and hypoglycemia during withdrawal

4) Alcohol in the diet constitutes a source of empty calories and activates the MEOS system, leading to inefficient nutritional metabolism and multiple vitamin deficiencies that require supplementation (especially with thiamin and niacin)

4. Nutritional monitoring

a. Monitor weight

b. Monitor pertinent serum chemistries for abnormalities

c. Monitor nutritional status; define nutritional goals and measure progress toward meeting goals

5. Disease impact

a. HCV can progress to cirrhosis and its complications, and ultimately to liver failure

b. Alcoholic hepatitis can lead to cirrhosis

c. Alcohol has direct toxic effects on digestion, absorption, and metabolism of nutrients

Practice to Pass

Compare the treatment strategies and goals for clients with hepatitis A (HAV), hepatitis B (HBV), and hepatitis C (HCV).

III. CLIENT WITH MUSCULOSKELETAL DISORDERS

A. Fractures of the long bones

1. Description

a. Fractures can occur as a traumatic injury or as a consequence of metabolic disease

b. Resultant destruction of long bones requires medical/surgical intervention in order to reestablish structural integrity

! c. Clients with long bone fractures are at risk to develop complications that can range from infection, blood clots, and fat embolism to issues of nonhealing (non-union) from nature of traumatic injury and/or baseline clinical/nutritional condition

2. Associated nutritional problems
   a. Nutrient demands are increased due to healing of bone tissue
   b. Impaired mobility leads to subsequent elimination problems that can affect nutritional intake
   c. Pain management therapies can lead to altered feeding patterns and digestion in the postoperative period
   d. Contributory disease processes, if present, affect the client's nutritional status and response to medical/surgical therapies
3. Dietary measures used as treatment
   ! a. Adequate calcium and protein are needed to support bone growth
   b. Adequate calories and balanced intake are needed to meet increased protein needs
   ! c. Adequate fluid intake, fiber, and progression of exercise are needed to maintain mobility and range of motion (ROM) and prevent altered elimination patterns
4. Nutritional monitoring
   a. It is important to correct underlying medical problems in order to assist in client recovery
   b. Evaluate CBC and serum chemistries in order to determine client's baseline status and monitor response to therapies
5. Disease impact
   a. Altered mobility occurs as a consequence of surgical/medical management, which can necessitate a lengthy recovery and rehabilitation process
   b. Clients with contributory disease processes are more likely to encounter long-term problems with healing and mobility
   ! c. There are possible growth issues with pediatric/adolescent clients who have long bone fractures, because these may lead to structural deformities and altered body image

B. Osteoarthritis (OA)

1. Description
   a. Also known as degenerative joint disease, it is a painful disease that often involves hips, knees, neck, lower back, or small joints of the hands
   b. It usually develops in joints that are injured by repeated overuse in performance of a particular job or activity; repeated impact thins and frays cartilage that cushions ends of the bones in the joint; bones then rub together, causing a grating sensation
   c. Joint flexibility is reduced, bony spurs (pointy bulges of bone) develop, and the joint swells
   d. The first symptom is joint pain; pain worsens following exercise or immobility; curtailment in activity reduces joint motion, which can cause loss of joint function and may result in disability
   e. It is characterized by an increased rate of cartilage degradation and a decreased rate of cartilage production

2. Associated nutritional problems
   a. Excess body weight can put excess pressure on joints and aggravate OA
   b. Increased pain level leads to decreased activity tolerance; as a result, clients often limit their exercise/mobility, leading to further pain upon motion of joint
   c. Medication therapy used to treat clinical pain often causes GI side effects (nausea and indigestion), leading to reduced nutritional intake
3. Dietary measures used as treatment
   a. Maintain ideal body weight; if overweight, weight loss can reduce stress on weight-bearing joints and improve clinical symptoms
   b. Vitamin D is needed for effective calcium metabolism
   c. Supplements such as glucosamine and condroitin sulfate may be utilized
      1) Treatment is based on hypothesis that oral consumption may increase rate of formation of new cartilage by providing more of the necessary "building blocks"
      2) Data is inconclusive; most studies last only 1 to 2 months; however, studies have indicated that clients who received glucosamine/chondroitin experienced less pain than clients who received a placebo
4. Nutritional monitoring
   a. Monitor body weight; in obese and overweight clients, ideal body weight should be a goal
   b. Monitor calcium levels
   c. Monitor client's diet pattern for intake of calcium and vitamin D
5. Disease impact
   a. Pain reduces mobility and activity tolerance, leading to alterations of daily living activities
   b. Psychosocial aspects of dealing with pain and altered mobility can lead to depression
   c. Degenerative aspects of disease can necessitate surgical intervention, resulting in joint replacement
   d. Attempts to control pain can lead to alternative therapies for relief
   e. Financial impact of dealing with a chronic degenerative disease process can impose burdens on the client and family support system

Practice to Pass

Describe the long-term effects of osteoarthritis and their impact on nutritional needs.

C. Osteoporosis

1. Description
   a. Osteoporosis is a disease characterized by low bone mass due to loss of minerals from the skeleton
   b. Mineral loss from the skeleton results in structural deterioration of bone tissue; this increases susceptibility to fractures of the hip, spine, and wrist that often occur spontaneously; thinning of the trabecular bone and loss of structural integrity characterize osteoporosis
   c. The disease cannot be cured; it can only be prevented or minimized
   d. Over a lifetime, bone mass is continually changing; bone mineral density increases up to about age 25 to 30 years in both men and women; hence, between these years **peak bone mass (PBM)** is achieved, the most bone mass a person will ever have

e. Osteoporosis affects both females and males, but is usually associated with a dramatic decrease in bone density in females following menopause (decrease in estrogen production); male clients do not usually experience such a rapid decline in bone mass

f. After an initial rapid decline, women lose bone mass at a steady rate of about 1% per year throughout the rest of their lives; men lose bone mass at about half of the rate of women throughout their lives

g. Estrogen status, heredity and lifestyle, and diet, among other factors, influence bone health

2. Associated nutritional problems

! a. Calcium adds strength and stiffness to bones; low calcium intake is associated with low bone mass and increased fracture risk; vertebrae, hip, and wrist are sites most sensitive to fracture

b. Vitamin D (refer to Table 7-4 for daily recommended intake or DRI)

1) The elderly are at risk for vitamin D insufficiency because they do not absorb it from the diet as well as do younger people; the elderly also spend less time outdoors

2) People residing in Northern Europe and other locations at higher latitudes may be at risk for vitamin D deficiency in the winter and early spring

! 3) Vitamin D is essential for calcium absorption and normal bone mineralization; low levels of vitamin D can contribute to low bone density

c. Protein affects bone health as well

1) High protein intake may increase the calcium requirement; however, the association between protein and osteoporotic bone fractures is under investigation

2) Reduced protein intake has been linked to low femoral neck bone density in elderly hospitalized clients

d. Nutritional status can influence one's tendency to fall; thin, undernourished elderly persons who may lack sufficient muscle mass and fat mass in the hip region may be particularly prone to fracture

e. Body weight is positively correlated with bone mineral density; weight loss is associated with bone loss

1) A weight gain of 10% or more of initial body weight beginning at age 50 may decrease risk of hip fractures in older individuals

2) A weight loss of 10% or more beginning at age 50 increases the risk of hip fracture in older women and men

f. Long-term excessive intake of alcohol appears to reduce bone density

g. Caffeine consumption has been tied to increased urinary excretion of calcium; reasonable use of caffeinated beverages is acceptable

Table 7-4

Daily Recommended Intake for Vitamin D

Age	Requirement
1–18 years	200 IU
19–50 years	400 IU
51–70+ years	600 IU
70+	600 IU

3. Dietary measures used as treatment
   a. Calcium
      1) A client needs 1,200 mg of calcium/day from age 11 to 24; body is at peak capacity to absorb and retain calcium during this time
      2) RDA is 1,000 mg for individuals 25 to 50 years and 1,200 mg for those 50+ years; some recommend as high as 1,500 mg for women over age 50
      3) Foods that are good sources of calcium should be included in the diet (refer to Box 7-5)
      4) Client should receive dietary teaching regarding factors that affect calcium absorption in the body; even though a client may consume adequate calcium, there are dietary factors that may alter its absorption (refer to Table 7-5)
   b. Vitamin D
      1) Natural sources of vitamin D include cod liver oil, fatty fish, and eggs
      2) Almost all vitamin D comes from fortified foods such as milk, cereals, and margarine
4. Nutritional monitoring
   a. Monitor client's height, weight, and BMI
   b. Instruct client who takes medications such as biphosphonates to increase bone mass and density that this will require dietary adjustments (take on empty stomach upon arising with 8 ounces of water with no food or other medications in the morning in an upright position) due to side effects and potential interactions
   c. Monitor client's serum calcium and protein levels
   d. Monitor results of **bone mineral density (BMD)** tests
      1) Measure bone density at various sites of the body to be able to predict the chances of future fracture
      2) BMD testing determines presence of bone loss and correlates treatment (biphosphonates) with response (increased or stabilized bone mineral density)
5. Disease impact
   a. The effects of osteoporosis can lead to decreased stature and deformity and pathologic fractures
   b. Depending on where bone demineralization occurs, there can be a reduction in lung capacity, chronic back pain, and early satiety due to reduced abdominal volume and decreased tolerance to exercise

Box 7-5

Good Sources of Dietary Calcium

- Low-fat dairy products
- Spinach
- Kale
- Beans and legumes
- Broccoli
- Tofu
- Fortified orange juice
- Salmon
- Sardines

Table 7-5

Factors Affecting Calcium Absorption

Enhancing Factors	Impeding Factors
Vitamin D Lactose Body's requirement as in pregnancy Acidity of digestive mass Exposure to UV radiation Certain medications such as thiazide diuretics, steroids, lithium, theophylline, calcium-containing antacids, biphosphonates, and certain chemo agents	Phytic acid (phytates) and oxalic acid (oxalates) Dietary fiber Excessive phosphorus intake Laxatives Aging Sedentary lifestyle Certain medications such as antineoplastics, loop diuretics, anticonvulsants, citrate-buffered blood, gentamycin, ASA, and antacids

c. Surgery to treat fractures can lead to increased nutritional demands during the perioperative period

d. Disease can impair quality of life both physically and emotionally

e. Hip fractures as a result of osteoporosis are a real health concern, leading to lengthy rehabilitation and alterations in lifestyle

f. A woman's risk of hip fracture is equal to her combined risk of breast, uterine, and ovarian cancer

D. Gout

1. Description

a. This disorder results from deposits of needlelike crystals of uric acid in connective tissue, joint spaces, or both; results from hyperuricemia (increased levels of uric acid in the blood) as a result of overproduction or underexcretion

b. The presence of hyperuricemia can be seen in conjunction with other disease processes (tumor lysis syndrome or malignancies) or as a consequence of chemotherapy protocols

c. Medication therapy can be given PO or IV to treat clinical symptoms of gout

2. Associated nutritional problems

! **a.** Hyperuricemia may result when a person eats too many high-protein foods that are high in purines (dried beans and peas, organ meats, wheat germ, anchovies, and seafood)

b. Clients often can trigger gouty attacks with dietary intake by drinking alcohol and eating foods that are high in purine content and high in fat content

c. If client is experiencing hyperuricemia as a consequence of malignancy or chemotherapy protocols, then the client already may have underlying nutritional problems that will further affect nutritional status

3. Dietary measures used as treatment

! **a.** **Purine-restricted diet**—restrict high-protein foods such as dried beans, lentils, bran, and wheat germ; eat only 200 grams of meat, poultry, or fish twice weekly; eliminate organ meats

b. Limit high-fat diets, consumption of alcohol, and very-low-calorie diets; these tend to increase serum urate concentrations and may provoke acute gout attacks

! **c.** Increase consumption of fluids to help flush out uric acid in the renal system

4. Nutritional monitoring
   a. Monitor serum uric acid level periodically
   b. Clients with contributory disease may experience alterations in uric acid level due to medication therapy (thiazide diuretics)
   c. Monitor client's dietary intake pattern for trigger foods that may exacerbate attacks
5. Disease impact
   a. Acute pain commonly occurs due to gouty deposits, which leads to alterations in activity tolerance and tolerance for daily living activities
   b. Gout can manifest in joints in the big toe, instep, ankles, heels, knees, wrists, and fingers, thus interfering with mobility
   c. Initially, gout's characterized by recurrent acute attacks of severe inflammation in peripheral joints; gradually, episodes become more frequent and lead to chronic disability and joint destruction
   d. Adhering to a purine-restricted diet and taking medication therapy are important aspects of the client's clinical management

IV. CLIENT WITH NEUROLOGICAL DISORDERS

A. Guillain-Barré (GB)

1. Description
   a. This is also called acute inflammatory demyelinating polyneuropathy and Landry's ascending paralysis; it is an inflammatory disorder of the peripheral nerves (those outside the brain and spinal cord)
   b. It is characterized by rapid onset of weakness and, often, paralysis of the legs, arms, respiratory muscles, and face
   c. Abnormal sensations often accompany the weakness; the onset of GB is usually seen following a viral illness; exact cause is not known; however, theories suggest an autoimmune mechanism

! 2. Associated nutritional problems
   a. Nutrition becomes a priority for preserving lean body mass, especially muscles of respiration
   b. Clients tend to be hypermetabolic and catabolic because of endocrine, infectious, and inflammatory components of the disease
   c. If client requires ventilatory support or tracheostomy, then alternate forms of feeding will be required; collaboration with dietitian is essential

! 3. Dietary measures: high-energy, high-protein diet may have a favorable effect on visceral protein repletion, nitrogen balance, and resistance to pulmonary infection
4. Nutritional monitoring
   a. The preferred method of measuring caloric expenditure is indirect calorimetry
   b. Nitrogen balance studies may help to estimate protein need
   c. It is important to provide enteral and parenteral nutrition support if facial and oropharyngeal weakness occurs or if respiratory dependence jeopardizes adequate oral intake

5. Disease impact
    a. Many clients require intensive care during the course of their illness
    ! b. Recovery is long-term with significant impact on client and family system dynamics
    ! c. The nutritional management of a client experiencing this type of degenerative neurological disease is also long-term because of respiratory support measures that may be required

B. Myasthenia gravis (MG)

1. Description
    a. This disorder is caused by the antibody-mediated autoimmune attack of acetylcholine receptors at neuromuscular junctions that disrupt normal nerve impulse transmission across those junctions
    b. Symptoms include poor muscle contraction, fatigue, and weakness with paralysis of muscles of eyes, face, and throat
    c. Symptoms worsen as the disease progresses
2. Associated nutritional problems
    ! a. Occasionally, clients develop **dysphagia** (difficulty swallowing) as the disease progresses
    ! b. Enteral feeding may be necessary due to client's dysphagia and progressive muscle weakness
    c. Nutrition intervention is needed for long-term care and during respiratory crises that may arise during course of disease
    d. Clients tend to gain weight and develop hyperglycemia from medications commonly prescribed to treat this disease (steroids); because physical activity exacerbates symptoms, diet counseling is the mainstay of weight control management
3. Dietary measures used as treatment
    a. It may be helpful to use the **Harris-Benedict equation** (method of estimating calorie requirements, using appropriate stress factors) to obtain caloric requirements in consultation with dietitian
    b. Protein needs are thought to be similar to those of debilitated chronically ill clients; the protein requirement is approximately 1.0–1.5 grams protein/kg
    ! c. Some clients lose weight because of muscle fatigue and severe dysphagia; provide small, frequent calorie-dense meals modified for appropriate consistency
    ! d. Provide commercial nutritional supplements if necessary; encourage frequent "finger foods" along with resting before meals; administer medications so peak action is at mealtimes to improve abilities to chew and swallow
    e. Provide enteral support for clients too weak to meet their nutrient needs by oral means
4. Nutritional monitoring
    a. Monitor body weight to determine appropriate nutritional intervention
    b. Evaluate clients in respiratory crisis who might require ventilatory support necessitating enteral or parenteral nutrition therapy
    c. Immunosuppressive therapy used to manage this disease process may alter the client's fluid and electrolyte status; monitor serum chemistries and appropriate labs to establish nutritional baseline and response to therapies

5. Disease impact
    a. Current therapy is long-term in nature but is usually very effective and includes anticholinesterase agents, immunosuppressant treatment, and plasmapheresis for crises
    b. Removal of the thymus gland is recommended for clients between puberty and 60 years of age

C. Parkinson's disease (PD)

1. Description
    a. This is a chronic, irreversible neurodegenerative disease caused by progressive degeneration of cells in the substantial nigra, the region of the brain stem where the neurotransmitter dopamine is produced
    b. Symptoms associated with this disease are resting tremors, bradykinesia, slow movements, akenisia, cogwheel rigidity, shuffling gait, and a stooped posture
    c. Clients often show reduced facial expressions and speak in a soft voice; the disease also causes depression, personality changes, dementia, sleep disturbances, and speech impairment
    d. Symptoms are due to a deficiency of the brain chemical dopamine
2. Associated nutritional problems
    a. Gastric motility disorders may include delayed gastric emptying, constipation, anorexia, dysphagia, drooling, and aspiration
    b. Clients tend to lose body weight and body fat
3. Dietary measures used as treatment
    a. Protein
        1) Symptoms may decrease when clients taking levodopa (Sinemet) consume a diet with 7:1 CHO:protein ratio in all meals; this dietary modification is most effective for clients whose motor fluctuations are not controlled by altering the dose of levodopa
        2) Protein intake should be distributed among 4 meals so excess protein is not taken at once; high protein intake can affect binding sites for medications, thereby affecting (reducing) control of symptoms
    b. Energy
        1) The total energy needs can be based on the Harris-Benedict equation using appropriate activity factors
        2) Encourage client to alter time of consumption and type of protein; omit large neutral amino acids—valine, isoleucine, tryptophan, tyrosine, and phenylanine—so as not to interfere with medication therapy
        3) Recommend frequent small meals or liquid supplements to maintain weight
    c. Gastric motility
        1) Food is better utilized when eaten in 4 or more small meals
        2) Providing foods that are easy to chew and swallow may be helpful
    d. Using thickened liquids and proper client positioning (upright) during feedings should be done consistently to prevent aspiration if swallowing could be a problem
    e. Do not consider enteral support unless PD is advanced and weight loss is significant

f. Omit vitamin supplements containing pyridoxine, since this vitamin may increase the transformation of L-dopa to dopamine before it reaches the brain

g. It is important for clients with PD to drink water on a schedule to enhance absorption of nutrients and medications and to decrease risk of dehydration

4. Nutritional monitoring

a. Monitor BMI and lean body mass periodically

b. Monitor client's intake and output and maintain adequate hydration

c. Monitor physical impairments and assess client's level of ability to feed self independently; assist as needed

5. Disease impact

a. Clients are at risk to develop dehydration due to effects of anti-Parkinson's drugs

! b. Clients with PD may risk aspiration before, during, and after swallowing; many are unaware of this "silent aspiration" because they have a poor cough reflex or altered mental status

c. Drooling in PD clients results from an inability to swallow saliva; excessive drooling may impact on ability to swallow food and may result in difficulty in articulation speech

D. Spinal cord injury (SCI)

1. Description

a. SCI is characterized by disrupted transmission of nerve impulses from brain to peripheral nerves

b. The degree of dysfunction depends on cause, degree of transection, and level of cord injury

c. The extent of both damage and preservation of cord function may not be known until spinal shock (the initial response to SCI) subsides, which can take weeks

d. As body seeks to repair damage and preserve function, abnormal muscle activity or spastic reflexes can occur

2. Associated nutritional problems

a. Generally, the higher the level of SCI, the greater the nutritional risk as paralysis may require ventilatory support

b. Body weight

1) May appear stable during the acute phase even though tissue wasting is severe; atrophic muscle is replaced by fat, water, and connective tissue

2) Loss of weight usually is evidenced after 3 to 4 weeks following the injury; weight loss is usually attributed to loss of lean body mass

! c. Metabolic response to SCI causes markedly excessive nitrogen excretion within one week of injury, peaking at approximately 3 weeks; may result in negative nitrogen balance

! d. Metabolic response to SCI also affects micronutrients; hypercalcemia can be induced by immobilization, especially in young adolescent males; symptoms associated with hypercalcemia are anorexia, abdominal cramps, nausea, vomiting, constipation, polyuria, and dehydration

e. Excessive potassium excretion and abnormal hyponatremia may occur

f. Anemia and GI complications, including stress ulcers, pancreatitis, and decreased motility, may occur

g. Neurogenic bowel and/or bladder function may result

h. The client may experience spinal shock or autonomic dysreflexia after injury and during early recovery period, leading to increased nutrient demands

3. Dietary measures used as treatment

a. Initiate enteral feeding as soon as it is medically feasible

! b. Provide high-protein diet to counteract negative nitrogen balance during acute phase of SCI

c. Use indirect calorimetry to measure energy expenditure; in general, the higher the cord lesion the more muscle is denervated and the lower the metabolic rate; if indirect calorimetry is not available, quadriplegics require (in general) 22.7 kcal/kg/day and paraplegics 27.9 kcal/kg/day

! d. Provide a low-fat, low-cholesterol diet after rehabilitation; weight gain, especially around the abdomen due to lack of muscle, may put SCI clients at risk for heart disease

! e. Treatment for hypercalcemia may include medication, hydration, and mobilization; a calcium-restricted diet has not been shown to be advantageous, and limiting calcium-rich foods can make the diet unpalatable

! f. Provide 25–30 grams fiber and 2–3 L fluid if neurogenic bowel is present; limit foods high in fat as they may cause difficulty in regulating bowel function

! g. Fluids should be increased to 2–3 L/day in order to maintain hydration and assist with managing neurogenic bladder

4. Nutritional monitoring

a. Monitor body weight at regular intervals

b. Monitor calcium levels periodically

c. Clients with SCI are at risk for pressure ulcers; for these individuals, pressure ulcers and poor healing are closely correlated with weight loss, anemia, and hypoproteinemia; these events should be monitored and nutrition counseling, high-protein and/or high-calorie diets should be instituted

d. Collaboration with dietitian as a member of the client's healthcare team is essential to provide nutritional counseling for this long-term problem

5. Disease impact

a. Excessive weight gain can contribute to other medical conditions such as heart disease, hypertension, and diabetes

b. Hypercalciuria may last longer than one year following SCI and may contribute to the development of osteoporosis; high-protein diets may promote urinary calcium excretion and may indirectly contribute to osteoporosis

c. Clients with SCI are at high risk of developing pressure ulcers and a wound specialist (enterostomal therapist) should be included in the healthcare team to manage the client

d. Clients with SCI are at risk for developing skin lesions; low serum protein levels, poor diet, and increased or decreased body weight have been implicated in development of skin lesions and impaired healing

E. Multiple sclerosis

1. Description

a. This is a chronic degenerative disease affecting demyelination and gliosis (scarring) of the CNS, leading to varied neurological symptoms and progressive effects that can be acute and/or chronic in nature

b. Multiple theories are proposed for etiology, including autoimmune (genetics and HLA lymphocytes), viral components (geographic influence), and trigger events (stress, fatigue, pregnancy and poor health)

c. Clinical course of disease is characterized by relapses and remissions with eventual progression of CNS involvement

d. Clinical manifestations reflect extent of neurological area involved, leading to motor problems (weakness, paralysis, and muscle spasticity), sensory problems (paresthesias, visual changes, and hearing changes), emotional problems (changes in stability leading to altered emotions), and cerebellar problems (dysarthria, dysphagia, ataxia, and nystagmus)

e. Bowel and bladder function is commonly affected, leading to alterations in elimination such as due to constipation and/or development of neurogenic bladder; bladder problems can present as either spastic (urinary frequency, dribbling, or incontinence) or flaccid bladder (urinary retention)

! **2.** Associated nutritional problems

a. Symptoms of disease can lead to constipation and altered intake patterns (because of swallowing and chewing difficulties)

b. Relapsing and progressive nature of the disease leads to a decrease in client's mobility, loss of function, and nutritional problems that arise due to immobility, such as muscle wasting

c. Chronic fatigue attributed to the disease process can reduce nutritional intake, leading to poor nutritional status

! **3.** Dietary measures used as treatment

a. Adequate vitamin supplementation focusing on B vitamins and vitamin C has been suggested to be effective with the chronic relapsing nature of this disease process

b. A high-protein diet is usually recommended

c. Adequate intake of roughage and fluids helps to prevent or correct elimination problems

d. The multiple medication profile (of steroids, immunomodulators, cholinergics, anticholinergics, and muscle relaxants) can affect the client's nutritional status due to potential side effects such as edema, flu-like symptoms, constipation or diarrhea, dry mouth, and drowsiness

4. Nutritional monitoring

a. Monitor intake and output to ensure that fluid balance is achieved

b. Assess client for progressive effects of disease and evaluate whether assistance is needed with regard to nutritional management

c. Refer client and family to a dietitian for a collaborative approach to help identify and meet nutritional goals

5. Disease impact

a. This is a progressive disease process that has significant impact on the client and family members, leading to dramatic lifestyle changes and adaptations

b. Client will usually need to learn how to perform self-catherization if bladder function becomes a problem, which enhances risk of urinary infection

c. Client may require assistance with ADLs, leading to custodial living arrangement if cognitive and motor function becomes increasingly impaired

d. Disease process causes major disability in adult clients

V. CLIENT WITH RENAL DISORDERS

A. Acute renal failure (ARF)

1. Description
   a. Refers to loss of excretory functions of the kidney within a short period of time
   b. Renal failure is further divided into oliguric, diuretic, and convalescent phases whereby the kidneys try to adapt and compensate in order to maintain renal function
   c. Alterations in fluid and electrolyte status are evident, leading to profound systemic changes as renal function deteriorates
   d. Causes
      1) Prerenal: result of decreased blood pressure that may follow hemorrhage, cardiac failure, dehydration, obstruction of renal arteries, or any factor that decreases blood flow to the kidneys, resulting in a fall in glomerular filtration rate (GFR)
      2) Intrarenal failure: results when kidney is damaged directly; may be the result of nephrotoxic drugs or other chemicals, hypercalcemia, or acute glomerulonephritis
      3) Postrenal failure: results when there is obstruction to urinary excretion
2. Associated nutritional problems
   ! a. As a consequence of the low GFR, client retains sodium, water, nitrogen metabolites, and other waste products
   ! b. Potassium retention is a problem in ARF that can lead to significant cardiac manifestations
   ! c. Alterations in calcium and phosphate metabolism lead to decreased calcium levels and elevated phosphate levels
   d. Hematologic abnormalities (decreased production of erythropoetin) lead to anemia that can result in fatigue, which in turn can affect nutritional intake
   e. Risk of cardiovascular disease (usually have increased LDL and VLDL)
   f. Proteinuria leads to loss of immunoglobulins and vitamin D binding proteins
3. Dietary measures used as treatment
   a. Calculation of ideal body weight (IBW), actual body weight, and determination of protein status is warranted in order to establish nutritional goals
   b. The client may be asked to do protein counting in order to determine accurate intake of protein in the diet
   ! c. The client should follow the National Renal Diet (formulated jointly by the ADA and National Kidney Foundation) that contains food choices (exchanges) for protein, sodium, potassium, and phosphorus; in addition the diet plan should specify caloric needs and fluid requirements
   d. Early intervention in the form of dialysis may be required and is associated with an improved survival rate
   e. It is necessary to provide enteral feeding if the client is incapable of oral intake
   f. Provide conservative management if the client is capable of oral intake, if the condition is mild, or if dialysis is unavailable
      ! 1) Maintaining adequate fluid balance is critical; fluid intake should be equal to volume of urine output plus 500 to 750 mL/day for insensible losses plus drainage or vomiting; in addition, consider 400 mL/day used for metabolic

processes and fluid taken in for taking medication; anuric client would receive 1,000 mL/day

!

2) Restrict sodium to amount necessary to replenish losses, about 20–40 mEq/day (2–3grams/day); if fluid and sodium intake are appropriate, a client might lose 0.25–0.50 kg body weight/day with plasma sodium levels remaining stable

!

3) Provide calories in sufficient amounts to prevent protein catabolism, since most clients with ARF are severely catabolic

!

4) Protein: limit protein to 0.25–0.5 gram/kg body weight per day to minimize azotemia or nitrogen retention if client not being dialyzed; if client is dialyzed, liberalize protein to 1.2 grams/kg daily

!

5) Potassium: limit diet to 25–40 mEq of potassium to prevent hyperkalemia until urine volume increases during recovery

!

6) Other electrolytes: dietary phosphate may sometimes have to be restricted; since a low-phosphate diet may be poorly accepted, phosphate-binding antacids may be used; parenteral iron may be needed to enhance erythropoiesis if GI absorption is poor because of GI effects of renal disease

7) Collaboration with a dietitian is necessary in order to effectively manage the diet of a client on dialysis therapy (refer to Box 7-6)

8) The type of dialysis that a client receives can affect nutritional requirements (refer to Table 7-6)

4. Nutritional monitoring

!

a. Daily client weight is critical; weight gain indicates fluid retention and is counteracted with further sodium restriction to avoid congestive heart failure (CHF)

b. Monitor caloric intake; protein-free, low-electrolyte, high-CHO liquid supplements may be indicated

c. Provide protein of high biological value; if the client is severely catabolic, as indicated by a BUN value of 100 mg/day or more plus elevated serum potassium and acidosis state, then dialysis should be considered

Box 7-6

Dietary Measures for Treatment of Clients on Dialysis

- 1.0–1.25 grams/kg/day protein; 70% of high biological value
- 35–50 kcal/kg/day to prevent protein catabolism and maintain body weight
- Goal—15% kcals protein, 35% fat, 50% carbohydrate, primarily polysaccharides
- 2:1 ratio PUFA: saturated fat
- 0.5 kg/day sodium to limit weight gain from edema
- 500–1,500 mL/fluid/day in addition to that found in solid food
- 2,000–3,000 mg/day potassium
- 1.0 mg folate
- 10.0 mg pyridoxine
- 100.0 mg ascorbic acid
- RDA of other water-soluble vitamins
- 15 mg iron, either orally, bound to ascorbic acid, or intravenously
- Calcium supplement up to 1,200 mg/day; high calcium diet not feasible because it would increase dietary phosphorus

Table 7-6 Nutritional Requirements Relative to Type of Dialysis Therapy

Hemodialysis (HD)	Peritoneal Dialysis (PD)
Increased protein needs	Increased protein needs (> than HD)
Minimal changes in glucose	Increased glucose levels
Potential for hypokalemia	Potassium remains in relatively stable amounts
Individualized calcium requirements	Individualized calcium requirements

5. Disease impact
   a. ARF may be superimposed on chronic renal failure (CRF) by stress factors such as infection or dehydration
   b. In some cases, client may have some degree of decreased renal function for months; in contrast to CRF, it may be reversible
   c. A high mortality rate exists when ARF occurs as a consequence of multisystem failure

B. Chronic renal failure (CRF)—End stage renal disease (ESRD)

1. Description
   a. Irreversible loss of the kidneys' excretory capacity that results in increased BUN and creatinine levels, anemia, and bone disease
   b. Occurs over an extended period of time, from months to years
   c. Progression of CRF has been described as occurring in 4 stages; stages are not sharply separated but, rather, are phases of a continuing degenerative process with progressive loss of functioning nephrons; the four phases are (1) decreased renal reserve, (2) renal insufficiency, (3) renal failure, and (4) uremia or uremic syndrome

! 2. Associated nutritional problems
   a. Loss of protein occurs via the urine (proteinuria)
   b. Edema develops as result of decreased albumin levels and low colloidal osmotic pressure
   c. As the disease progresses to stages 3 and 4, the nitrogen content of the diet must be balanced to reduce accumulation of nitrogenous end products while maintaining positive nitrogen balance
   d. Dialysis as a therapeutic modality is a hypermetabolic event, which increases the client's nutrient and energy needs to maintain fluid and electrolyte balance

! 3. Dietary measures used as treatment
   a. Protein
      1) Provide foods with essential amino acids (histidine, isoleucine, leucine, lysine, methionine, phenylalanine, threonine, tryptophan, and valine)
      ! 2) Restrict protein to 60–90 grams/day when the GFR is 20–25 mL/day; lower the protein restriction to 40–60 grams/day (0.50–0.65 g/kg IBW) as the GFR falls to 10–15 mL/day
   b. Energy
      1) Provide sufficient calories to avoid metabolism of body protein stores to meet energy needs (prevent protein catabolism)

2) Use low-protein, carbohydrate/lipid-rich beverages to increase caloric content of diet

3) Collaborate with dietitian, who will calculate energy needs using the Harris-Benedict equation and calculate the UNA (urea nitrogen appearance)

c. Sodium

1) Replace moderate sodium losses with a diet containing 4 to 6 grams of salt

2) If patient becomes hyponatremic (sodium-depleted), provide additional sodium with salty foods; provide sodium chloride tablets if necessary

3) With further reduction in the number of functioning nephrons, the kidney's ability to excrete sodium is diminished and sodium retention (hypernatremia) results; restrict sodium intake depending on degree of hypertension and state of hydration

Practice to Pass

What nutrients need close monitoring in predialysis clients?

d. Potassium

! 1) If hyperkalemia results and persists, restrict daily potassium to 2,800 mg or 70 mEq or less; monitor total food intake as few foods are potassium-free

2) Distribute potassium intake evenly throughout the day as dietary potassium is rapidly absorbed

3) Provide sufficient protein and energy to prevent tissue catabolism and release of intracellular potassium

! e. Provide daily supplements of 1.0 mg folic acid, 100 mg ascorbic acid, 5.0 mg pyridoxine hydrochloride, and the RDA of the remaining water-soluble vitamins

4. Nutritional monitoring

a. Monitor sodium restriction; clinical manifestations of sodium depletion may include abdominal cramps and aching muscles, weakness and lassitude, anorexia and vomiting, and mental confusion

b. Monitor potassium restriction and serum potassium levels, as cardiac effects can be noted in the presence of altered potassium levels

c. Monitor fluid intake because client is prone to develop fluid volume excess (FVE)

d. Monitor level of renal insufficiency by trending pertinent laboratory results such as BUN, creatinine, calcium, phosphate, and RBC indices

e. Clients should not be given additional magnesium because diminished renal reserve prevents excretion, leading to possible magnesium toxicity

f. Clients in CRF are prone to develop multiple fluid and electrolyte imbalances that require therapeutic management to restore values to within normal range

! 5. Disease impact

a. Metabolic acidosis may result from renal insufficiency

b. Anemia is a common finding in uremic clients due to the decrease in erythropoesis

c. CRF causes alterations in vitamin D, calcium, and phosphorus metabolism

d. A number of disorders of CHO metabolism are associated with uremia; these include fasting hyperglycemia and a glucose tolerance curve that strongly resembles the diabetic curve; circulating insulin levels often are high and there is evidence of peripheral insensitivity to insulin

e. Wasting syndrome is observed in clients with uremia; there are aberrations in serum amino acid profiles with decreased essential amino acids and increased nonessential amino acids; plasma histadine, important in the structure of hemoglobin, is reduced

f. Hyperlipidemia and elevated triglycerides are seen; uremic clients have a high incidence of arteriosclerosis and coronary artery disease that has been related to high triglyceride levels

g. Fluid restriction leads to thirst; ulcerations of the mouth and nausea and vomiting occur; depression, anxiety, and fear accompany feelings of frustration; compliance is a challenge for the client and healthcare providers

C. Client receiving dialysis

1. Description

a. It is a treatment use for ARF and CRF; in CRF, dialysis may continue indefinitely (maintenance dialysis) or may just continue for a short period of time prior to transplantation

b. It may be used for a short period of time following a renal transplant until grafted kidney begins to function

c. Indications for beginning its use include intractable hyperkalemia (unresponsive to other treatment), severe metabolic acidosis, fluid overload, pericarditis, and uremia

d. In CRF, the client usually begins dialysis treatment when the GFR is 5 to 10 mL/min

e. Depending on the client's medical status, there are several types of dialysis procedures ranging from peritoneal dialysis to hemodialysis; clients who are acutely ill may require CRRT (continuous renal replacement therapies) in the ICU setting, as they are hemodynamically unstable

f. Appropriate access, depending on type of dialysis method, is necessary in order to administer dialysis treatment (Quinton catheter, graft, or peritoneal catheter)

2. Associated nutritional problems

! **a.** Chronic hemodialysis is a catabolic process and malnutrition is a continuing problem

! **b.** Intake of caloric nutrients must be sufficient to spare protein and to maintain body weight

c. Client may lose amino acids, peptides, and some protein during each session, along with an amount of glucose that varies with the glucose content of the dialysate; for this reason, protein restriction may be lessened slightly once dialysis begins

! **d.** Peritoneal dialysis can lead to hyperglycemia because of the glucose content of the dialysate and the length of dwell time in the abdomen; however, potassium levels do not fluctuate as quickly and protein restrictions are less severe than with hemodialysis

! **e.** Sodium and fluid may accumulate between hemodialysis treatments, leading to hypertension, edema, and CHF

3. Dietary measures used as treatment (refer again to Box 7-6)

a. Collaboration with dietitian and dialysis technician/nurse is necessary in order to ensure accurate monitoring of intake and output (I & O) and calculation of needed nutrients, fluids, and caloric intake

! **b.** Dry weights must be obtained prior to dialysis based on determination of pre- and postdialysis weights since last treatment

! c. Client must maintain accurate I & O and be aware of sodium, potassium, protein, and/or fluid restrictions during the course of therapy; dialysis does not eliminate the need to comply with prescribed diet because fluid overload electrolyte imbalances and further retention of wastes could occur

4. Nutritional monitoring
    a. Monitor for anemia; transfusion of packed red blood cells (RBCs) at intervals may be necessary; one objective of nutritional care should be provision of optimum nutrition for erythropoiesis—formation of RBCs
    b. Monitor blood pressure and body weight; use as indicators of success of sodium restriction
    c. Monitor pertinent micronutrient levels (calcium, phosphorus, and magnesium)
    d. Monitor parathyroid hormone (PTH) as ordered or indicated
5. Disease impact
    a. Hypertension, along with diabetes mellitus, is often an etiologic factor in the development of renal disease
    b. Dialysis may have an impact on various forms of bone disease
    c. It is important to monitor the client's emotional response to nutritional care; compliance may pose a concern; dialysis centers vary in the strictness of approach to "snacks" or "treats" prior to dialysis
    d. ! Clients receiving dialysis therapy can be at risk for disequilibrium syndrome (cramping, hypotension, and neurological changes) due to rapid fluid shifts during the dialysis procedure; this is more likely to occur early in the course of treatment
    e. ! Clients receiving dialysis therapy who have vascular access devices are at risk to develop infection; provide meticulous care in order to avoid infection of graft or access site
    f. Because renal failure can affect all individuals (male and female) and all age groups (pediatric to elderly), stunted growth patterns could result if protein and calorie intake are inadequate

D. Kidney stones

1. Description
    a. Also known as renal calculi, they vary from the size of a grain of sand to a large staghorn calculus that fills the entire pelvis of the kidney
    b. Reduced urine flow, increased excretion of calcium and potassium and changes in pH may increase the tendency for calculi formation
    c. In addition, calculi may form due to crystallization of organic material in the urine
    d. ! Metabolic diseases that predispose individuals to calculi formation include cystinuria, gout, hyperoxaluria, hyperparathyroidism, some bone diseases, excessive intake of vitamin D, renal tubular acidosis, and idiopathic hypercalciuria
    e. Calculi may form as a complication of GI disorders or because of immobility and mobilization of calcium from bone
    f. Genetics may play a role in the formulation of kidney stones
2. Associated nutritional problems
    a. Clients may experience GI symptoms including nausea, vomiting, abdominal distention, and constipation
    b. If the client is experiencing pain (flank pain and/or dysuria), dietary intake may be altered

3. Dietary measures used as treatment
   - **a.** Most calculi are passed spontaneously; others must eventually be removed by surgery or ultrasound; increasing water intake to 2–4 L/day is recommended
   - **b.** Mild salt restriction may be helpful
   - **c.** For most clients, calcium intake should not be restricted, since calcium restriction increases oxalate absorption from the intestine and thus increases the need for oxalate excretion
   - **d.** Limit ascorbic acid (vitamin C) to less than 4 grams/day, as it is a precursor to oxalate production; doses of greater than 4 grams/day increase oxalate excretion and the tendency to form oxalate calculi
   - **e.** For oxalate stones, reduce intake of foods high in oxalates, such as dark green leafy vegetables, nuts, chocolate, rhubarb, beets, and okra, to reduce urinary oxalate levels; this may or may not actually *prevent* stone formation
   - **f.** The client with cystine calculi usually has congenital cystinuria; low-protein or low-methione diets have been proposed; results have been inconsistent
4. Nutritional monitoring
   - **a.** Monitor client's dietary pattern for intake of foods high in oxalate, vitamin C, and calcium if prone to develop kidney stones
   - **b.** Monitor fluid intake and continue to force fluids to maintain urine output
   - **c.** Monitor pertinent diagnostic tests regarding 24-hour urine collections, urinalysis, and urine cultures to determine baseline status and/or disease process
5. Disease impact
   - **a.** Bone demineralization could occur if clients with renal calciuria are treated with reduced calcium diet
   - **b.** Some clients have oxalosis, an inborn error of metabolism in which oxalate calculi are formed
   - **c.** Oxalate calculi also form in clients with Crohn's disease and clients who have undergone jejunoileal bypass surgery for obesity

VI. CLIENT WITH RESPIRATORY DISORDERS

A. Acute airway attacks

1. Description
   - **a.** Clients experiencing asthma can be subject to mild to severe irritation of the tracheobronchial tree resulting in coughing, dyspnea, air hunger, edema, inflammation, and production of mucus
   - **b.** Bronchial spasm can lead to significant alterations in ability to ventilate and require emergency intervention to maintain adequate airway passages
   - **c.** Clients diagnosed with asthma often suffer from acute exacerbations of a chronic disease process that can be triggered by multiple factors such as exercise, stress, pollution, smoking, and allergies
   - **d.** Medical management of the asthmatic client can rely on the use of steroids, beta-agonists, methylxanthines, and anticholinergics that are administered via several routes (inhalers, PO, or parenterally) depending on nature of attack or baseline therapy
   - **e.** Clients with acute exacerbation may require respiratory assistance (nebulizer treatments) in order to manage symptoms and decrease airway inflammation

! 2. Associated nutritional problems
   a. Due to nature of asthmatic attack, food and fluid intake may be reduced due to progressive respiratory symptoms
   b. Clients receiving steroid therapy to treat acute attacks will have elevations in blood glucose in response to treatment
   c. Clients taking methylxanthine (Theophylline) can experience GI side effects such as nausea, vomiting, and diarrhea; high-protein and low-CHO diets should be avoided because they favor increased excretion of the drug, leading to ineffective serum levels

! 3. Dietary measures used as treatment
   a. Monitor protein and CHO intake in order to promote effective serum level of methylxanthine (Theophylline); low-protein and high-carbohydrate diets favor decreased excretion of the drug
   b. Remove allergic triggers in the diet that could lead to exacerbation of asthma
   c. Avoid food additives containing sulfites because this could be a possible trigger
   d. Maintain adequate fluid intake to thin mucous secretions

4. Nutritional monitoring
   ! a. Clients receiving steroid therapy should have blood glucose levels monitored in response to therapy and managed accordingly to prevent clinical effects of hyperglycemia
   ! b. Monitor weight pattern for signs of fluid retention
   c. Maintain adequate hydration by noting fluid intake and output

5. Disease impact
   a. Due to chronicity of disease pattern and likelihood of exacerbations, client must be properly managed throughout the lifespan in order to avoid complications
   b. Clients should be discouraged from smoking or being in the presence of secondhand smoke due to effects on airway tissue
   c. Acute exacerbations may require frequent hospitalizations of the client with considerable impact on client and family support systems (physically, emotionally, and financially)
   d. Long-term effects of airway disease can lead to adaptive airway changes resulting in altered acid-base imbalances and decreased activity tolerance and fatigue

B. Chronic obstructive pulmonary disease (COPD)

1. Description
   a. This disorder is characterized by persistent obstruction of bronchial airflow; affects lower airways and results in chronic long-term changes in respiratory function
   b. Diseases comprising COPD include chronic bronchitis and emphysema
   c. Long-term complications can arise including acid-base disturbances, fluid and electrolyte imbalances, adaptive and nonadaptive airway changes, and episodes where ventilatory support may be needed

2. Associated nutritional problems
   ! a. Malnutrition is usually seen in clients with COPD due to decreased serum albumin levels
   b. Respiratory muscle compromise leads to fatigue, dyspnea, wheezing, coughing, cyanosis, and pursed lip breathing, which can interfere with eating patterns

3. Dietary measures used as treatment
   a. **Respiratory quotient (RQ)** is the ratio of carbon dioxide (CO) produced to the amount of oxygen consumed
      1) Diet therapy involves giving the proper mix of nutrients to reduce CO production and maintain respiratory function and an RQ less than 1.0
      2) An RQ greater than 1.0 is evidence of CO_2 accumulation
      3) An increase in total calories contributes to increased acid production and hypercapnia
   b. Protein
      1) COPD patients are hypermetabolic; not hypercatabolic
      2) Optimally, nitrogen balance can be established; give 1.0–1.4 grams/kg/day for maintenance therapy for moderate stress and 1.5–2.0 grams/kg/day for repletion therapy and marked stress
   c. Fats
      1) Provide 35 to 50% of total calories from fat in the diet of ambulatory clients
      2) If clients require parenteral nutrition, they should receive lipid emulsions no faster than at a rate of 2 kcal/min
   d. Carbohydrates
      1) Total calorie intake should be restricted in order to maintain RQ of < 1.0
      2) Maintenance and repletion regimes for ambulatory clients with COPD can be 35 to 50% of total calories from CHOs
4. Nutritional monitoring
   a. Perform nutritional assessment frequently with particular attention to body weight
   b. Design assessment to identify clients who exhibit malnutrition and might benefit from nutritional support
   c. Indirect calorimetry can be helpful in guiding nutritional management of clients
   d. Monitor respiratory rate, vital capacity, minute ventilation, and blood gases; use information to determine caloric requirement
   e. Evaluate micronutrient status since severe hypophosphatemia results in neuromuscular dysfunction and may exacerbate pulmonary failure
5. Disease impact
   a. Malnutrition associated with COPD may have an impact on phosphorus, magnesium, and calcium status, which play a dynamic role in pulmonary structure and function
   b. Impaired immunocompetence associated with malnutrition predisposes the individual to lung infection; this is likely due to alterations in the sequence of tissue injury and repair
   c. Long-term impact of the disease process can lead to decreased activity tolerance
   d. Medication therapy aimed at decreasing inflammation, loosening secretions, and improving airway exchange is long-term in nature and requires client education and other measures to foster compliance with treatment regimens

Case Study

A 52-year-old male with a long history of hypertension and Type 1 diabetes mellitus has now been diagnosed with renal failure. The client is 6 feet, 2 inches tall and weighs 180 pounds. Vital signs are BP 138/98, pulse 72 and regular, respirations 20. Laboratory results pending are CBC with differential, chemistry profile, and urinalysis. The client has been referred to you for preliminary diet counseling to determine the client's understanding of the disease process and nutritional assessment.

1. What information do the client's height, weight, and vital signs provide with regard to the clinical diagnosis of renal failure?
2. What laboratory values might you expect to see for the CBC with differential, chemistry profile, and urinalysis?
3. What information would you obtain from the client regarding dietary intake pattern and how would this impact the clinical diagnosis of renal failure?
4. The client is concerned that dialysis will be an inevitable consequence of this diagnosis and is feeling, by his own words, "somewhat anxious." How would you help to support the client?
5. What dietary information should be conveyed to the client with a diagnosis of renal failure?

For suggested responses, see pages 319–320.

POSTTEST

POSTTEST

1 A 28-year-old client who is admitted to the unit with a relapse of multiple sclerosis (MS) is experiencing constipation. The client asks what other methods besides using laxatives can be used to prevent or treat this condition. How should the nurse respond to the client's concern?

1. Tell the client to reduce fluid intake.
2. Have the client increase roughage in the diet.
3. Have the client increase range of motion (ROM) exercises to stimulate peristalsis.
4. Call the physician regarding an order for an enema.

2 A client covering from a spinal cord injury (SCI) has been referred for nutritional counseling due to weight loss. The client states, "If I eat too much, the weight will just stay on and I will become fat." How would the nurse best respond to this statement?

1. "It is important to continue to eat a diet high in protein, carbohydrates, and fiber to maintain optimal body function."
2. "I know that you are concerned about weight gain, but you can always diet later on."
3. "Let me know what your food preferences are and I will get you additional portions of whatever you like."
4. "It is important to have extra nutrient stores in order to preserve skin integrity."

3 A client being treated for gout is being evaluated for compliance with diet therapy. Which of the following meal selections would indicate that the client has adhered to the diet plan?

1. Scrambled eggs, white toast, and coffee
2. Seafood casserole, wheat roll, and soda
3. Pizza with anchovies and soda
4. Braised liver, lentils, green peas, and tea

4 A client is to undergo bone marrow transplantation (BMT) for treatment of leukemia and is receiving pre-procedure teaching about nutrition. Which of the following postoperative nutritional support options does the nurse anticipate will be utilized?

1. Supplementation with enteral feedings to prevent catabolism
2. Oral feedings as soon as possible following BMT to prevent gastroparesis
3. Total parenteral nutrition (TPN) for a period of months to maintain nutritional balance
4. Insertion of a PEG tube following the BMT to maintain nutritional balance

5 A 42-year-old male client with acquired immunodeficiency syndrome (AIDS) is admitted with dehydration. The client states he has "difficulty eating and swallowing just about anything." The client has lost 10 pounds over a 3-week period. What does the nurse identify as the most likely etiology for the client's chief complaint?

1. The client has been too weak to go food shopping.
2. The client's medication profile is causing him to develop anorexia.
3. The client could be developing an opportunistic infection.
4. The client has not been compliant with medication regimen.

6 A 60-year-old male client who has had chronic obstructive pulmonary disease (COPD) for 15 years is experiencing weight loss despite insisting that he has been "eating a well-balanced diet." The diet history indicates the client has been consuming an adequate caloric intake of approximately 2,500 kilocalories per day composed of 15% protein, 70% carbohydrates (CHOs), and 15% fat. What recommendations would the nurse make regarding the client's weight status?

1. Maintain calories and increase percentage of fat to 35% in the diet to promote weight gain.
2. Decrease the amount of fat in the diet and increase complex CHOs.
3. Increase activity level as caloric intake and percentages of nutrients are adequate to sustain weight status.
4. Increase calories, protein, fat, vitamins, and minerals in order to prevent further weight loss.

7 When assessing a client with scleroderma, the nurse identifies that which of the following conditions associated with this disease could present a nutritional problem?

1. Diarrhea and anorexia
2. Alternating constipation and diarrhea
3. Reports of frequent heartburn
4. Increased skin turgor

8 Which of the following statements about cancer cachexia would the nurse use in response to a client with cancer who asks questions about weight loss and wasting?

1. It is no different than simple starvation because the metabolic rate declines in response to tumor growth.
2. Cancer cachexia occurs as a result of chemotherapy but not radiation therapy.
3. Cancer cachexia occurs as a result of tumor-induced changes.
4. It is usually seen in clients who have limited caloric intake.

9 A 48-year-old male client who is human immunodeficiency virus (HIV) positive is being treated prophylactically with isoniazid (INH). The nurse concludes that this client is at highest risk for which of the following nutritional problems?

1. Frequent bouts of diarrhea
2. Deficiency of B vitamins
3. Development of dental caries
4. Excessive flatus formation

10 A 52-year-old male client being treated for cancer is questioning the use of a "female hormone," megesterol acetate (Megace), as part of the treatment regimen. He is afraid that it will alter his appearance. The nurse should respond to the client's concern of altered body image by first explaining:

1. The physical changes are only temporary.
2. This medication is used for its ability to stimulate appetite.
3. His concern is realistic and that he should not take the medication if he feels that way.
4. The medication will be used for a short time and any effects will be self-limiting.

See pages 226–230 for Answers and Rationales.

POSTTEST

ANSWERS & RATIONALES

Pretest

1 **Answer: 1** Food should be cooked to reduce bacteria, which the immunosuppressed client cannot fight effectively. Option 3 is incorrect, while options 2 and 4 are not relevant to the question as stated.
Cognitive Level: Application **Client Need:** Health Promotion and Maintenance **Integrated Process:** Nursing Process: Implementation **Content Area:** Foundational Sciences: Nutrition **Strategy:** The critical word is *immunosuppressed.* Recall the client is a risk for infection to direct you to option 1. **Reference:** Rolfes, S., Pinna, K., & Whitney, E. (2006). *Understanding normal and clinical nutrition* (7th ed.). Belmont, CA: Wadsworth & Thomson Learning, p. 864.

2 **Answer: 3** Even though protein restriction is the mainstay of therapy for clients with impaired renal function, high biologic value proteins are favored due to their high content of essential amino acids. Option 1 is incorrect because high biologic value proteins help to minimize urea production by allowing synthesis of nonessential amino acids from essential amino acids. Option 2 is incorrect: Protein restriction is needed because the kidneys' ability to excrete nitrogenous end products is impaired in clients with renal disease. Option 4 is incorrect: Even though it is true the high biologic value proteins are necessary, they are not reserved only for clients on dialysis.
Cognitive Level: Application **Client Need:** Health Promotion and Maintenance **Integrated Process:** Teaching and Learning **Content Area:** Foundational Sciences: Nutrition **Strategy:** The critical words are *high biologic value.* Eliminate options 1 and 2 as incorrect information. Note the restriction of the word *only* in option 4 and eliminate it. **Reference:** Rolfes, S., Pinna, K., & Whitney, E. (2006). *Understanding normal and clinical nutrition* (7th ed.). Belmont, CA: Wadsworth & Thomson Learning, p. 863.

3 **Answer: 3** Vitamin C in megadoses can increase the risk for oxalate stone formation. It would be important to determine the amount of vitamin C that the client is taking in relation to the potential effects of stone formation. Option 1 is incorrect—even though vitamin C has antioxidant effects, the potential for stone formation outweighs the benefit of taking large doses of vitamin C. While it is important to increase fluids to prevent urinary stasis, option 2 is incorrect because the statement does not specifically address the issue of vitamin C supplements. Option 4 is incorrect: Animal protein should be decreased in order to minimize potential stone formation.
Cognitive Level: Application **Client Need:** Health Promotion and Maintenance **Integrated Process:** Teaching and Learning **Content Area:** Foundational Sciences: Nutrition **Strategy:** Identify the relationship between kidney stones and vitamin C to direct you to option 3. **Reference:** Rolfes, S., Pinna, K., & Whitney, E. (2006). *Understanding normal and clinical nutrition* (7th ed.). Belmont, CA: Wadsworth & Thomson Learning, p. 866.

4 **Answer: 4** Elemental zinc taken with food or milk will help correct alterations in taste (dysgeusia). Option 1 is incorrect because this intervention is used to treat anticipatory nausea. While it is important to assess a client for signs of dehydration (option 2), it is more important to correct altered taste sensation to enable the client to increase intake. Option 3 is incorrect because highly seasoned foods can cause nausea and irritation.
Cognitive Level: Application **Client Need:** Physiological Integrity: Physiological Adaptation **Integrated Process:** Nursing Process: Planning **Content Area:** Foundational Sciences: Nutrition **Strategy:** Recall meaning of the word *dysgeusia.* If you have difficulty with the question, recognize options 1 and 2 are applicable for many conditions and option 3 would not be recommended for a client receiving chemotherapy. **Reference:** Rolfes, S., Pinna, K., & Whitney, E. (2006). *Understanding normal and clinical nutrition* (7th ed.). Belmont, CA: Wadsworth & Thomson Learning, p. 449–450.

5 **Answer: 3** Small frequent meals provide for adequate intake with reduced fatigue and SOB. Simple carbohydrates do provide quick energy, but a mixture of nutrients reduces carbon dioxide production and maintains respiratory function. Fat consumption can lead to hyperlipidemia and should only provide approximately 30% of total calories. Most individuals have more energy in the morning than evening.
Cognitive Level: Application **Client Need:** Health Promotion and Maintenance **Integrated Process:** Nursing Process: Implementation **Content Area:** Foundational Sciences: Nutrition **Strategy:** Refer to "most appropriate" in the stem of question and option 3 that makes reference to mealtime and decrease of energy needs. **Reference:** Rolfes, S., Pinna, K., & Whitney, E. (2006). *Understanding normal and clinical nutrition* (7th ed.). Belmont, CA: Wadsworth & Thomson Learning, p. 702.

6 **Answer: 4** A client experiencing ascites due to liver failure has decreased protein levels (albumin) that lead to

third spacing of fluids. The calculation of dry weight (total weight minus the weight of ascites) is critical to determining fluid status and medical management of the client. Option 1 is incorrect because it does not address the issue of ascites specifically but rather looks at a strict volume measurement. Option 2 is incorrect because one would expect abnormal liver function tests but this information is again not specific to fluid status but rather to the status of liver function. Option 3 is incorrect—even though serum protein levels would be expected to be low, the caloric intake level would not help to define fluid status.

Cognitive Level: Application **Client Need:** Physiological Integrity: Physiological Adaptation **Integrated Process:** Nursing Process: Assessment **Content Area:** Foundational Sciences: Nutrition **Strategy:** Core concept is liver failure and ascites. Recall the fluid shifts that occur to direct you to option 4. **Reference:** Rolfes, S., Pinna, K., & Whitney, E. (2006). *Understanding normal and clinical nutrition* (7th ed.). Belmont, CA: Wadsworth & Thomson Learning, p. 775.

7 **Answer: 2** A client being treated for hepatic encephalopathy has increased ammonia levels and is likely to be experiencing mental status changes and fluid retention (ascites). It is important for the dietitian to note that the client's mental status precludes normal intake and nutrition support may be indicated. Option 1 is incorrect—although a weight and caloric baseline would be important for the dietician to review, the current nutritional goal would be to decrease factors that could lead to fluid retention and increased ammonia levels. Option 3 is less important than understanding the mental status as a basis for formulating nutritional goals. Although it is nice to know that the client has been compliant with medical treatment thus far, option 4 is incorrect because it does not specifically address the establishment of nutritional goals.

Cognitive Level: Application **Client Need:** Physiological Integrity: Physiological Adaptation **Integrated Process:** Nursing Process: Planning **Content Area:** Foundational Sciences: Nutrition **Strategy:** Core concepts are encephalopathy and nutritional support. Eliminate options 1, 3, and 4 since they do not address current eating pattern or intake. **Reference:** Rolfes, S., Pinna, K., & Whitney, E. (2006). *Understanding normal and clinical nutrition* (7th ed.). Belmont, CA: Wadsworth & Thomson Learning p. 774.

8 **Answer: 4** The neutropenic client is immunocompromised and susceptible to bacterial contamination from food. Cross contamination is avoided by using separate cutting boards. Vegetables may be eaten raw as long as they are thoroughly washed. It is not necessary to boil liquids and seeds and nuts may be eaten.

Cognitive Level: Application **Client Need:** Health Promotion and Maintenance **Integrated Process:** Nursing Process: Implementation **Content Area:** Foundational Sciences: Nutrition **Strategy:** Critical words are *neutropenic precautions.* Review new guidelines and recognize client is immunosuppressed to direct you to option 4. **Reference:** LeMone, P., & Burke, K. (2004). *Medical surgical nursing: Critical thinking in client care* (3rd ed.). Upper Saddle River, NJ: Pearson/Prentice Hall, p. 967.

9 **Answer: 1** A client with Parkinson's is at risk for aspiration. The statement by the client's wife indicates that the client is experiencing an increase in clinical symptoms—drooling and impaired swallowing. The use of thickened liquids and proper positioning can minimize the risk of aspiration and help the client's wife to feel comfortable and knowledgeable regarding feeding concerns. The spouse should also notify the physician because an adjustment in medications may be needed. Option 2 is incorrect—there is not enough information to state that the client should be switched to enteral feedings at this time. Option 3 is incorrect because merely increasing fluids in a client experiencing increased drooling and difficulty swallowing could further increase the risk of aspiration. Option 4 is incorrect—merely using a straw will not help to correct the underlying problems and could possibly increase the risk of aspiration due to inability to manage fluids.

Cognitive Level: Application **Client Need:** Physiological Integrity: Physiological Adaptation **Integrated Process:** Teaching and Learning **Content Area:** Foundational Sciences: Nutrition **Strategy:** The problem with swallowing indicates a safety concern. Eliminate options 2, 3, and 4 since they do not offer appropriate suggestions to reduce risk of aspiration. **Reference:** LeMone, P., & Burke, K. (2004). *Medical surgical nursing: Critical thinking in client care* (3rd ed.). Upper Saddle River, NJ: Pearson/Prentice Hall, p. 1422.

10 **Answers: 1, 2, 3** Organ meats, such as liver, kidney, brain, and sweet breads, are high in purines. Moderately high would be meats, seafood, and dried beans. The other choices are not high in purines.

Cognitive Level: Application **Client Need:** Health Promotion and Maintenance **Integrated Process:** Nursing Process: Implementation **Content Area:** Foundational Sciences: Nutrition **Strategy:** The core issue of the question is knowledge of foods that need to be avoided with gout because they are high in purines. With this in mind, choose the foods that are not high in purines. **Reference:** Rolfes, S., Pinna, K., & Whitney, E. (2006). *Understanding normal and* *clinical nutrition* (7th ed.). Belmont, CA: Wadsworth & Thomson Learning, pp. 867–868.

Posttest

1 **Answer: 2** A client with MS is prone to developing both bowel and bladder dysfunction as a result of this progressive degenerative neurological disease. Increasing fluids and roughage in the diet will help to facilitate evacuation by improving stool consistency. Option 1 is incorrect—the client needs increased fluids. Option 3 is incorrect because increasing ROM exercises provides for joint motion but does not necessarily exercise the abdominal muscles, which could influence peristalsis. Option 4 is incorrect because there is not enough clinical information provided to make this assessment. The nurse would have to assess further for elimination pattern and the date of the client's last BM.
Cognitive Level: Application **Client Need:** Physiological Integrity: Physiological Adaptation **Integrated Process:** Nursing Process: Implementation **Content Area:** Foundational Sciences: Nutrition **Strategy:** Note that the question addresses the need to treat constipation without laxatives to eliminate option 4. Option 3 will not have a direct effect on bowel elimination and can be eliminated. Option 1 will aggravate constipation and needs to be eliminated as well. **Reference:** Rolfes, S., Pinna, K., & Whitney, E. (2006). *Understanding normal and clinical nutrition* (7th ed.). Belmont, CA: Wadsworth & Thomson Learning, pp. 96–97.

2 **Answer: 1** Even though a client has had an SCI, the use of a diet high in protein, carbohydrates, and fiber is necessary to prevent both the catabolic process that occurs following SCI and potential problems with bowel function. Option 2 is incorrect because it reflects the belief that weight loss is an easy goal to achieve. Option 3 is incorrect because it assumes that merely getting foods that the client likes will correct the problem. Option 4 is incorrect—excess nutrient stores will not merely help to preserve skin integrity but are needed for overall support of the client's metabolism and immune response.
Cognitive Level: Application **Client Need:** Health Promotion and Maintenance **Integrated Process:** Communication and Documentation **Content Area:** Foundational Sciences: Nutrition **Strategy:** Eliminate options that do not address the client's concern (2 and 3). Choose option 1 over 4 since it provides a broader, more inclusive answer. **Reference:** Nix, S. (2005). *Williams' basic nutrition & diet therapy* (12th ed.). St. Louis, MO: Elsevier Mosby, pp. 416–417.

3 **Answer: 1** Scrambled eggs, white toast, and coffee are all foods that are low in purine content. A client who is being treated for gout should restrict dietary purine sources because they can lead to an exacerbation of the disease process. All of the other choices reflect dietary selections that range from moderate to high purine content. If dietary education is successful, then the client would avoid/limit these food selections.
Cognitive Level: Analysis **Client Need:** Health Promotion and Maintenance **Integrated Process:** Nursing Process: Evaluation **Content Area:** Foundational Sciences: Nutrition **Strategy:** Recognize that gout is affected by purine metabolism and systematically eliminate foods containing purines. **Reference:** Rolfes, S., Pinna, K., & Whitney, E. (2006). *Understanding normal and clinical nutrition* (7th ed.). Belmont, CA: Wadsworth & Thomson Learning, pp. 867–868.

4 **Answer: 3** A client undergoing a BMT will probably be fed by TPN in the post-transplant period due to potential complications affecting the mouth, esophagus, and intestines, leading to diarrhea and malabsorption. Option 1 is incorrect—supplemental enteral feedings would not help because the client's GI tract has been affected by chemotherapy and other medical treatments. In addition, merely supplementing the client will not provide sufficient calories and nutrients. Option 2 is incorrect because oral intake is usually not available due to side effects from high dose chemotherapy regimens that lead to anorexia, taste perception, nausea, vomiting, and inflammation of mucous membranes. Initiation of oral feedings will not prevent gastroparesis. Option 4 is incorrect—there is nothing to suggest that a PEG tube would be indicated. The goal with BMT clients is to return to a "normal" route-feeding regimen as soon as possible once clinical effects of immunosuppression have been resolved.
Cognitive Level: Analysis **Client Need:** Physiological Integrity: Physiological Adaptation **Integrated Process:** Nursing Process: Planning **Content Area:** Foundational Sciences: Nutrition **Strategy:** Recognize the need for prolonged nutritional therapy and to bypass the enteral system following a transplant to direct you to option 3. **Reference:** Nix, S. (2005). *Williams' basic nutrition & diet therapy* (12th ed.). St. Louis, MO: Elsevier Mosby, pp. 441–442.

5 **Answer: 3** A client complaining that he has "difficulty eating and swallowing just about anything" may have a fungal infection of the mouth and/or esophagus. A clinical diagnosis of AIDS suggests that the client is at high risk for developing an opportunistic infection. Option 1 is incorrect—even if the client may not be able to shop because of fatigue or other factors, it doesn't directly explain the client's statement. Option 2 is incorrect because the client's complaint addresses the issue of swallowing, not anorexia. Option 4 is incorrect—there is

nothing to suggest that the client has not been compliant with the medication regimen. The presence of opportunistic disease can occur even in the presence of medication therapy due to underlying immunosuppression. **Cognitive Level:** Analysis **Client Need:** Physiological Integrity: Physiological Adaptation **Integrated Process:** Nursing Process: Analysis **Content Area:** Foundational Sciences: Nutrition **Strategy:** Critical words are *difficulty eating and swallowing.* Eliminate options 1 and 4 since they do not address the problem directly. Eliminate option 2 because anorexia is not the problem. **Reference:** Nix, S. (2005). *Williams' basic nutrition & diet therapy* (12th ed.). St. Louis, MO: Elsevier Mosby, pp. 447–448.

6 **Answer: 4** A client with COPD is often hypermetabolic from the disease process and requires increased calories, proteins, vitamins, and minerals in order to maintain desired weight and meet additional energy demands. Option 1 is incorrect: Caloric intake is not adequate, and increasing fat percentage above 30% is not prudent. Option 2 is incorrect: Increasing carbohydrates in the diet can lead to increased respiratory workload due to excess acid production. Option 3 is incorrect because increasing activity level will not help to prevent weight loss. In addition, the client may not be able to increase activity level due to effects of COPD.
Cognitive Level: Application **Client Need:** Health Promotion and Maintenance **Integrated Process:** Nursing Process: Implementation **Content Area:** Foundational Sciences: Nutrition **Strategy:** Recall the need for a high-protein, high-caloric diet with COPD. Eliminate options 1 and 2 since fats and CHO should not be increased. Eliminate option 3 since this could cause further weight loss. **Reference:** Rolfes, S., Pinna, K., & Whitney, E. (2006). *Understanding normal and clinical nutrition* (7th ed.). Belmont, CA: Wadsworth & Thomson Learning, pp. 704–706.

7 **Answer: 3** A client with scleroderma often suffers from increased acid secretion and esophageal reflux. This could pose a significant nutritional problem. Option 1 is incorrect—anorexia is not commonly associated with this disease process. Option 2 is incorrect because alternating periods of constipation and diarrhea are usually seen in a client who is experiencing irritable bowel syndrome (IBS). Option 4 is incorrect—skin becomes hardened during this disease process and skin turgor is not increased.
Cognitive Level: Application **Client Need:** Physiological Integrity: Physiological Adaptation **Integrated Process:** Nursing Process: Analysis **Content Area:** Foundational Sciences: Nutrition **Strategy:** Recall that clients with scleroderma experience esophageal reflux to direct you to option 3, since clients with reflux often report heartburn. **Reference:** LeMone, P., & Burke, K. (2004). *Medical surgical nursing: Critical thinking in client care* (3rd ed.). Upper Saddle River, NJ: Pearson/Prentice Hall, pp. 1275–1276.

8 **Answer: 3** Cancer cachexia is a syndrome that occurs in clients with cancer (malignancy) that leads to a loss of muscle, fat, and body weight. It is thought to occur due to tumor-induced changes that cause profound effects on metabolism, nutrient losses, and anorexia. A cycle of wasting is established because alterations in nutrient requirements and intake lead to high cell turnover in body organs, affecting the GI tract and bone marrow. Alterations in digestion occur along with decreased immune response. Option 1 is incorrect—in simple starvation the body adapts to a lower metabolic rate. A client with cancer cachexia does not have an adaptive metabolic rate. The metabolic rate can be normal, decreased, or increased. Option 2 is incorrect because cancer cachexia occurs in the presence of both chemotherapy and radiation. Option 4 is incorrect—cancer cachexia can be seen in clients who have adequate caloric intake because it is not calorie dependent.
Cognitive Level: Application **Client Need:** Physiological Integrity: Physiological Adaptation **Integrated Process:** Nursing Process: Implementation **Content Area:** Foundational Sciences: Nutrition **Strategy:** First eliminate option 4 as too general. Recall cancer cachexia is associated with tumors to direct you to option 3. **Reference:** Rolfes, S., Pinna, K., & Whitney, E. (2006). *Understanding normal and clinical nutrition* (7th ed.). Belmont, CA: Wadsworth & Thomson Learning, p. 892.

9 **Answer: 2** A client who is receiving isoniazid (INH) as a prophylaxis for tuberculosis is at highest risk for deficiencies of vitamins, specifically vitamin B_6 (because the drug acts as a vitamin antagonist) and vitamin B_{12} (interferes with absorption). All of the other choices do not occur as a result of the action of this medication.
Cognitive Level: Application **Client Need:** Physiological Integrity: Pharmacological and Parenteral Therapies **Integrated Process:** Nursing Process: Analysis **Content Area:** Foundational Sciences: Nutrition **Strategy:** Recall significance of INH to intake of vitamin B_6 to prevent peripheral neuropathies. This will direct you to option 2. **Reference:** Rolfes, S., Pinna, K., & Whitney, E. (2006). *Understanding normal and clinical nutrition* (7th ed.). Belmont, CA: Wadsworth & Thomson Learning, p. 334.

10 **Answer: 2** Megesterol acetate (Megace) is oral progesterone that is used for both male and female clients to boost appetite and promote weight gain. It is important that all clients receive accurate information about prescribed medications and are aware of the indication for the drug, potential side effects, and expected response

to treatment. The nurse should respond to the client's concern initially with factual information because the client does not seem to understand the effect of the medication. Options 1 and 4 are incorrect because they do not address the client's concern and may further increase his anxiety about body image changes. Option 3 is incorrect—even though the client has the right to refuse any treatment, the response does not attempt to communicate pertinent factual information and may even reinforce the client's concern of body image changes.

Cognitive Level: Application **Client Need:** Physiological Integrity: Pharmacological and Parenteral Therapies **Integrated Process:** Communication and Documentation **Content Area:** Foundational Sciences: Nutrition **Strategy:** Recall the use of Megace in cancer and malnourished clients to direct you to option 2. **Reference:** Rolfes, S., Pinna, K., & Whitney, E. (2006). *Understanding normal and clinical nutrition* (7th ed.). Belmont, CA: Wadsworth & Thomson Learning, p. 886.

References

Cataldo, C., DeBruyne, L. K., & Whitney, E. (2006). *Nutrition and diet therapy* (7th ed.). Belmont CA: Wadsworth Publishing, pp. 565–583, 658–679, 705–721.

Dudek, S. (2006). *Nutrition essentials for nursing practice* (5th ed.). Philadelphia: Lippincott, pp. 603–658.

Larson, E., & Nirenberg, A., (2004). Evidence-based nursing practice to prevent infection in hospitalized neutropenic patients with cancer. *Oncology Nursing Forum, 31,* 717–725.

LeMone, P., & Burke, K. (2004). *Medical-surgical nursing: Critical thinking in client care* (3rd ed.). Upper Saddle River, NJ: Prentice-Hall, pp. 281–370, 520–541, 908–1012, 1425–1445, 1572–1665, 1787–1864.

Lutz, C., & Przytulski, K. (2006). *Nutrition and diet therapy* (4th ed.). Philadelphia: F. A. Davis Company, pp. 453–528.

National Institute of Arthritis and Musculoskeletal and Skin Diseases. (2006) *Questions and answers about gout.*[Online] *http://niams.nih.gov/hi/topics/gout/gout.htm*

National Institute of Arthritis and Musculoskeletal and Skin Diseases. (2006) *Questions and Answers about arthritis and rheumatoid disease.* [Online]. *http://niams.nih.gov/hi/topics/ arthritis/artrheu.htm.*

Nix, S. (2006). *Williams' basic nutrition and diet therapy* (12th ed). St. Louis, MO: Mosby, pp 399–418, 442–465.

Rolfes, S., Pinna, K. & Whitney, E. (2006). *Understanding normal and clinical nutrition* (7th ed.). Belmont, CA: Wadsworth & Thomson Learning, pp. 692–707, 769–785, 851–894.

Nutritional Support Methods and Therapeutic Diets

8

Chapter Outline

Objectives

- Discuss medical nutrition therapy as a first-line treatment option.
- Explain the different types of nutritional support methods and their indications for use in client treatment.
- Describe the importance of collaborative management of the client receiving nutritional therapeutics.
- Describe the different types of therapeutic diets.
- Identify short-term and long-term types of nutritional support that can be used in the clinical setting to promote nutritional balance.
- Identify specific diagnostic and monitoring tests that are utilized to assess the client's response to treatment.
- Review nursing responsibilities in the management of clients receiving nutritional support and therapeutic diets.
- Review the use of transition and test diets for clients in the clinical setting and for those who have defined health needs.

NCLEX-RN® Test Prep

Use the CD-ROM enclosed with this book to access additional practice opportunities.

Review at a Glance

altered consistency food items used in diets that have different consistency states (liquid and texture) other than solid forms

BRAT diet consists of bananas, rice, applesauce, and toast to be used on a short-term basis for pediatric (and even adult) clients who have GI symptoms resulting in increased fluid and electrolyte losses

bolus feeding delivery of a large specified amount of feeding in a small time period

cyclic feeding delivery of a specified amount of feeding over a period of several hours

enteral nutrition delivery of nutrients to a functioning GI tract in clients who have impaired ability to eat, chew, or swallow foods

medical nutrition therapy the incorporation of medical treatment based on a complete nutritional assessment that is coordinated by a dietitian and reflects nutritional principles that correlate with positive health outcomes and decreased rate of complications

peripheral parenteral nutrition (PPN) delivery of nutrients to a client via a peripheral vein

residual the amount of feeding that is left in the stomach or intestine; residuals are usually checked before each intermittent feeding, every 4–12 hours with continuous feedings, or not at all

restrictive/modified diet consists of food items that are either restricted (or limited) or modified (changed or individualized) in accordance with a physician's order based on a client's underlying clinical condition

supplemental/enhanced diet consists of food items that are added to the diet either in the form of high quality dietary sources, in the processing method or as an extra additional source in the diet

therapeutic diet a treatment diet that is prescribed to effect some clinical response for a client who has specific defined health needs

total parenteral nutrition (TPN) delivery of nutrients (hyperosmolar concentrations) via central venous access to a client who has a nonfunctioning GI tract

transition diet a diet that allows progression from one form to another (clear—full—regular) based on client's underlying clinical condition and return of GI motility (as defined by increased peristalsis, bowel movements, passage of flatus), absence of GI complaints (no nausea, vomiting, or diarrhea), or return of gag reflex (postprocedure/postanesthesia)

tube enterostomy surgical placement of a tube into the intestines to allow feedings

tube feeding delivery of feeding (enteral) via a feeding tube inserted via the nose into the stomach or small intestine

PRETEST

1 When caring for an elderly client who has difficulty chewing, the nurse identifies which of the following diets to be most appropriate to use as a long-term treatment measure?

1. A low residue diet
2. A full liquid diet
3. A high-protein diet
4. A mechanical soft diet

2 A client who receives intermittent enteral feedings has a feeding ordered during the shift. Which of the following interventions would the nurse perform prior to starting the next feeding?

1. Have the client go to the bathroom in preparation for the enteral feeding.
2. Check the residual before beginning the feeding and note the amount.
3. Place the client in a lateral recumbent position to facilitate the feeding.
4. Tally the client's intake and output for the last 24 hours.

3 Which of the following nutritional interventions would be of most assistance to a client who has recently suffered a cerebrovascular accident (CVA)?

1. Have the client eat bite-sized portions of foods to facilitate digestion.
2. Place the client on a full liquid diet.
3. Use thickening agents to minimize the risk of aspiration and monitor the client closely during all feedings.
4. Allow the client to eat alone as post-CVA clients are often self-conscious about their residual deficits.

4 The nurse would expect which of the following assigned clients to be candidates for total parenteral nutrition (TPN)? Select all that apply.

1. A client suffering from severe trauma who is in a hypermetabolic state
2. A client undergoing a cholecystectomy
3. A client with short bowel syndrome
4. A client undergoing radiation treatment for lung cancer
5. A client recovering from a cerebrovascular accident (CVA)

5 A client given a clear liquid diet tray prior to diagnostic testing states, "I'm not eating this and want some real food." Which of the following would be the best response by the nurse?

1. "I am sure that you will have a regular diet after the test, so please just try some of this for now."
2. "Would like me to get you some other type of broth of juice?"
3. "This is the diet that has been ordered for you. It is the only diet you can have right now."
4. "I understand this is not your usual diet, but it is needed to help the test establish a diagnosis."

6 The nurse determines that which of the following assigned clients has an increased need for fluid intake?

1. A client who has burn injuries
2. A client in cardiac failure
3. A client receiving blood transfusions
4. A client in the oliguric phase of renal failure

7 The nurse has conducted discharge teaching for a client diagnosed with gout. The nurse evaluates the client understood the instructions given if the client states he will refrain from eating which of the following favorite foods?

1. Steak
2. Poultry
3. Dairy products
4. Anchovies

8 A client receiving total parenteral nutrition (TPN) via central venous catheter asks the nurse why the bag isn't being changed as often as the IV bag of another client in the room, who has IV solution ordered at a rate of 150 mL/hr. The nurse responds that the TPN bag is routinely changed every _____ hours. Provide a numerical response.

Answer: ________________________

9 Which one of the following diets would the nurse recommend for a client being treated for dyslipidemia?

1. High polyunsaturated fat diet
2. Protein-controlled diet with mild sodium restriction
3. Low saturated fat diet
4. Decreased monounsaturated fat diet

10 The nurse uses which of the following best rationales in deciding to perform a dietary assessment on a client who is taking a monoamine oxidase (MAO) inhibitor?

1. It is important to determine food preferences since this may interfere with intake of nutrients.
2. Certain foods, such as cheese or chocolate, can affect drug action, leading to serious complications.
3. It is important to recognize potential food-drug allergies because this may cause serious health problems.
4. It is an expected assessment that is needed for any client.

See pages 256–258 for Answers and Rationales.

I. CONCEPT OF MEDICAL NUTRITION THERAPY

A. Definition of terms

1. **Medical nutrition therapy (MNT)** refers to a comprehensive nutritional assessment based on identified client needs upon which therapeutic treatment of disease processes can be based
2. MNT is provided by a dietitian in conjunction with collaborative management by the physician or healthcare provider
3. MNT is used to correct and replace nutrient deficiencies and provide adequate nutrition for clients with defined health problems
4. The American Dietetic Association (ADA) is recommending inclusion of MNT as a reimbursable therapy for treatment of clients in healthcare settings (both clinical and community)

B. First-line treatment

1. It is important to include nutrition as part of a sound foundation on which to base identified needs, expected outcomes, and response to treatments
2. Inclusion of MNT is now being recognized as a first-line treatment in many disease processes such as diabetes and heart, liver, and renal disorders

C. Importance of nutrition in the overall management of the client

1. Scientific research findings have provided evidence that dietary factors influence disease risk and progression
2. A stable weight pattern with body mass index (BMI) within range of 19 to 25 is associated with a decreased risk of disease progression
3. Clients feel better when they eat better and are in an acceptable weight range pattern (per BMI)

Practice to Pass

Why is medical nutrition therapy (MNT) important in the management of clients with defined healthcare needs?

II. NUTRITIONAL SUPPORT METHODS

! **A. Indications for nutritional support**

1. Client physical conditions
   a. Stress and trauma states (burns) cause increased metabolic demands on the body and require additional nutritional support
   b. Clients receiving mechanical ventilation may have increased metabolic demands and are not able to eat, so they often require additional nutritional support
2. Therapeutic bowel rest
   a. This may be indicated for clients who have GI pathology or surgical interventions that may require decreased activity of the bowel in order to regain normal integrity
   b. Bowel rest regimens can be ordered as part of the therapeutic treatment plan
3. Severe protein-calorie malnutrition (PCM) or protein-energy malnutrition (PEM)
   a. Clients with severe PCM or PEM may require additional nutritional support in the presence of significant malnutrition and loss of visceral protein stores
   b. It may be impossible to restore normal functioning and balance without the use of additional nutritional support in clients with severe PCM

B. Types of support methods

1. Oral supplements
   a. Oral supplements provide clients with calories and nutrients

Table 8-1 Types of Nutritional Formulas (all lactose-free)

Formula Type	Contents	Selection
Modular supplements (3.8–4.0 kcal/mL)	One nutrient source Not nutritionally complete by themselves Considered to be nutrient dense without increasing volume	CHO—Moducal, Nutrisource CHO, Polycosem Sumacal Lipids—MCT, Microlipid Protein—ProMod, Propac, Pro-MT, Casec, Bene protein
Polymeric (intact protein)	Essential nutrients in a specific volume based on a specified formulation	Oral supplements: Ensure, Sustacal, Resource, Meritene, Boost, Osmolite, Nutren, Isosource, Promote, Replete, Isocal, Choice DM, Glucerna
High-caloric polymeric (2 kcal/mL)	Contains intact proteins of high biologic value, complex CHOs, fats, vitamins, minerals, and trace elements	Deliver 2.0, Nutren 2.0
Elemental (predigested or hydrolyzed) (1–1.3 kcal/mL)	Provides nutrients in predigested form	Flexical, Vital, Vivonex, Criticare HN, (Nonpalatable, and hyperosmolar—best given by enteral administration)
Disease-specific	Provides formulation specific to metabolic requirements	Liver—Hepatic-Aid, Nutrihep Pulmonary—Pulmocare, Nutrivent, Respalor Renal—Travasob Renal, Nepro, Nutrirenal, Novasource Renal
Fiber-containing	Added fiber content	Jevity, Promote with fiber, Replete with fiber

b. Formulas can be found in liquid or powdered form and are usually packaged in ready-to-use formulations

! c. There are specific types of formulas available based on nutrient source, essential nutrients in specified volume, elemental formulas, and disease specific formulas (refer to Table 8-1 for a listing of specific types of formulas)

2. Tube feedings
   a. Are clinically indicated when the client has a physical condition that prevents food intake, such as swallowing and chewing problems and/or infection in the oral cavity
   b. Are clinically indicated when the client has a disease state that prevents or limits food absorption such as intestinal disease or malabsorptive states
   c. Are clinically indicated when the client has increased metabolic needs whereby oral intake cannot meet needed nutrient requirements (examples are clinical disease states such as malnutrition, burns, and trauma)
   d. Site selections for nasal tube feedings include NG—nasogastric tube from nose to stomach, ND—nasoduodenal tube from nose to duodenum, and NJ—nasojejunal tube from nose to jejunum
   e. Site selection for oral tube feedings is an orogastric tube
3. Tube enterostomy
   a. Involves placement of a tube through a surgical opening to provide nutrient/fluid intake

b. Site selections include PEG tube (percutaneous endoscopic gastrostomy), PEJ tube (percutaneous endoscopic jejunostomy), PEG/J (J-arm through PEG)

c. Is clinically indicated for clients who have specific malabsorption problems or will require long-term therapy as their primary nutrient source of intake

4. Parenteral nutrition

a. Are nutrients/fluids that are delivered through the parenteral route (intravenously) to maintain adequate metabolic balance

! b. Site selections include **peripheral parenteral nutrition (PPN)** via a peripheral vein for short-term use and **total parenteral nutrition (TPN)** (hyperalimentation) via a central vein for long-term use in clients who have increased nutrient requirements

C. Nutritional requirements for the client using support methods

1. Macronutrients

a. A Registered Dietitian (RD) or Dietetic Technician Registered (DTR) calculates requirements for macronutrients based on actual body weight and adjusted body weight

b. Calculations are further made for basal energy expenditure (BEE) and are correlated with the client's underlying physical condition

c. Pertinent baseline labs (serum chemistries, electrolytes, BUN, creatinine, albumin, prealbumin, hemoglobin/hematocrit) help to identify client's status, indicate needs, and, with subsequent testing, determine response to therapy

d. Dietary composition and recognition of fiber and residue components are included in evaluating the client's ability to handle digestion of nutrients in the clinical setting

e. Food sensitivities, food allergies, and potential food–drug interactions are evaluated for possible effects on dietary consumption and client's projected outcomes

2. Micronutrients

a. The RD also evaluates the electrolyte status of an individual client by looking at baseline serum chemistries and observing physical manifestations

b. The inclusion of trace elements is important in preventing the occurrence of clinical deficiencies that could place the client in a more compromised state during the course of clinical treatment

3. Water

a. Fluid volume may be restricted when there are concurrent or underlying disease presentations that indicate this is a need

b. It is important to calculate the required fluid volume content needed to prevent dehydration and constipation from occurring

! c. Increased fluids may be required for clients who have extensive drainage from the GI tract, endocrine abnormalities resulting in diabetes insipidus (DI), or plasma tissue losses due to burns

! d. Decreased fluids may be required for clients who have system failure (cardiac, hepatic, or renal), edema states, or who are already receiving other types of needed infusions such as blood, medication, or IV therapy

! e. Feeding tubes must be flushed with water before and after a feeding, medication administration, and periodically during a shift (every 4 hours for continuous feedings) in order to maintain patency

f. Water used as a flush or irrigation is included in the client's total I & O documentation

g. The water content of different tube feedings varies; therefore, it is likely that each client will need additional fluids during enteral feedings; however, this must be individualized according to client's tolerance and underlying medical condition

D. Collaborative management principles

1. Physician

a. The physician acts as coordinator of the healthcare team, working in conjunction with other members toward achieving client goals

b. Specific protocols may be instituted and reviewed on a daily basis

c. Trending of laboratory and diagnostic tests is ongoing to validate response to treatment protocols

d. Findings are documented in the client's medical record

e. Client education is ongoing and collaborative in nature as the client's care is reviewed in the clinical or community setting by healthcare team members

2. Dietitian

a. Performs nutritional assessment to calculate energy requirements and specific nutrient needs

b. Reviews records on an ongoing basis, looking at pertinent laboratory and diagnostic test results and daily weight monitoring

! c. The client is interviewed to determine food preferences, sensitivities, allergies, and dietary factors that may limit absorption of nutrients

d. Findings are usually documented in the client's progress notes unless there is a separate dietary section in the medical record

e. Client education is ongoing as the dietitian works closely with healthcare team members and client to meet individualized needs

3. Nurse

a. Implements physician orders and protocols in nutritional support methods

! b. Performs daily weights, measures I & O, and trends pertinent lab/diagnostic test results

c. Documentation is found on the flow sheets and client's progress notes

d. The nurse at the bedside is able to observe dietary patterns, assist the client during feedings, and monitor client tolerance and response to feeding methods

e. Client education is ongoing, as the nurse is often the mainstay of consistent therapy in the clinical/community setting

4. Client and family

a. Education related to a specific feeding regimen is necessary in order to enhance compliance and increase the likelihood of meeting desired outcomes

b. The therapeutic plan is most successful in achieving client outcomes when care is coordinated and family receives necessary support

c. It is important that both the client and family members have adequate access to resources to prevent potential complications or to obtain reinforcement of information about a selected therapy

Practice to Pass

What information is necessary in order to calculate nutritional requirements for clients receiving nutritional support therapy?

III. THERAPEUTIC DIETS

A. Altered consistency diets

1. Clear liquid diet
   - **a.** A clear liquid diet provides adequate fluid/water, 500–1,000 kcal of simple sugars, electrolytes, and is fiber free and fat free
   - **b.** It requires minimal digestion, as there is no residue, fiber, or fat
   - ! **c.** It is recommended for short-term use (3–5 days), can be used both before and after surgery or diagnostic procedures and during acute stages of illness
   - ! **d.** It consists of "see-through" foods that are liquid at body temperature—gelatin, tea, coffee, broth, or frozen ice pops
2. Full liquid diet
   - **a.** A full liquid diet provides water, calories, protein, vitamins and minerals, and dairy products (contains lactose); because milk is allowed, it contains residue
   - **b.** It may be indicated for some clients who have difficulty chewing or swallowing but may not be indicated for a client following CVA
   - **c.** It can be considered to be a **transition diet** (moving from one diet to another as the client's clinical status improves) as the client progresses postoperatively or post-procedure from liquid to solids
   - ! **d.** It consists of all foods found on a clear liquid diet, plus milk, pudding, ice cream, soups, yogurts, and all prepared liquid formulas; is contraindicated with severe lactose intolerance; may have increased cholesterol content
   - **e.** Clients who are lactose intolerant may require lactose-free supplements to prevent clinical symptoms
3. Pureed diet
   - **a.** A pureed diet provides essential nutrients in a pureed (blenderized) form for clients who are unable to chew or swallow
   - **b.** It can be used as a long-term diet—the preparation of the food items is the deciding factor
   - **c.** The use of seasoning depends on individual client preferences
   - **d.** A blender or food processor is used to change foods into pureed or blended form for use in the diet
   - ! **e.** Certain foods such as raw eggs, nuts, whole breads, raw fruits or vegetables, and foods containing seeds are not included in this type of diet
4. Dysphagia diet
   - ! **a.** A dysphagia diet consists of chopped, ground, or pureed foods and liquids that may be thickened; provided to clients who have swallowing problems and are at risk for aspiration (such as those post-CVA)
   - ! **b.** Thickening agents can be added to liquids to maximize texture and help facilitate the swallowing process
   - **c.** This diet is a modification of the soft diet with increased attention to the liquid component due to possible aspiration concerns
   - **d.** Stringy, raw, dry, and fried foods are not allowed on this type of diet due to potential aspiration
   - ! **e.** Foods that are considered to be small in size or handheld, such as popcorn, nuts, and small candies, should be avoided due to risk of aspiration

f. Positioning of the client to at least 30–45 degrees or higher and monitoring of feedings are critical during meals in order to decrease risk of aspiration and evaluate client's attempts at eating

5. Mechanical soft diet or mechanically altered diet
   a. This diet is used for clients who have problems with chewing; focuses on including all foods and seasonings in a form that is easily handled by the client
   b. Foods with soft textures, those that are tender, and chopped food items are included in the diet
   c. It can be used as either a long-term diet or a transition diet
   d. This diet is a modification of the regular diet with attention to texture
   e. Foods that are tough in nature—containing seeds, nuts, raw eggs, and fruits with pits—are not included in this diet
6. Soft diet (also called bland diet)
   a. This diet includes food items that contain small amounts of seasoning and moderate fiber content but are easy to chew, digest, and absorb
   b. Foods that are highly seasoned, fried, high in fiber, nuts, coconuts, and foods that contain seeds are not included in the diet as they could cause GI symptom upset
   c. It can be used as a progressive or transition diet and is a modification of a regular diet

B. Restrictive/modified diet

1. Carbohydrate-controlled diets
   a. The diabetic diet includes a controlled complex carbohydrate (CHO) source of 55–60%/day of total calories, protein source of 10–20%/day of total calories, a lipid source of < 30%/day of total calories, and a recommended fiber intake of 20–35 grams/day; the relationship among glucose levels, serum lipids, kilocalories, diet therapy, and insulin/medication is evaluated in response to hemoglobin A_{1c} and serum blood glucose monitoring
   b. The gestational diabetes diet provides adequate calories based on prepregnant weight status and frequent small feedings and snacks throughout the day to normalize postprandial glucose levels, maintain normal (euglycemic) levels throughout the pregnancy, and prevent ketosis
   c. A hypoglycemic diet consists of small feedings at frequent intervals to help normalize blood glucose levels; the 15-15 rule (see Chapter 6) is used to treat glucose levels < 60 mg/dL
2. Gastric bypass diet
   a. A gastric bypass diet consists of small meals eaten several times a day, drinking liquids between meals and taking multivitamin supplements with an emphasis on nutrient-dense foods
   b. The diet is low in fat and high in protein
   c. The use of carbonated beverages, simple CHOs, and foods with a high content of fiber and residue are restricted
3. Low-residue diet
   a. A low-residue diet consists of food items that minimize elimination patterns by reducing fecal volume
   b. High-fiber food sources are restricted in this diet along with milk and milk products

c. Fried foods, pepper, the use of alcohol, and heavily seasoned foods are restricted because they may cause GI upset

4. Fat-controlled diet

a. Diets where fat is restricted are used in the management of clients who have clinical conditions related to malabsorption, chronic pancreatitis, and gallbladder disease

b. Medium chain triglycerides (MCTs) are utilized in the diet because they are easily digested, along with high intakes of CHOs and protein

c. Foods that are high in fat content are omitted, and no additional fat is used in the cooking process

d. Enzyme replacements may be necessary if there is pancreatic insufficiency; fat-soluble vitamin and mineral supplements may also be needed

e. Foods that are high in oxalates (such as nuts, chocolate, green leafy vegetables, rhubarb, and beets) are limited to hinder kidney stone formation; beer and tea are also high in oxalates but may have limited bioavailability and thus may be less problematic; avoid vitamin C supplements

f. Clients who are being treated for dyslipidemia (high cholesterol and triglyceride levels) should be placed on a low saturated fat diet (increased monounsaturated ratio of fats and small amounts of PUFA) with restricted sodium and hydrogenated food products

g. Clients who have cardiovascular disease, congestive heart failure, and who have undergone transplant will have some form of fat-controlled diet for their lifelong dietary pattern (refer back to Chapter 6)

5. Protein-controlled diet

a. Clients who have renal disease (renal failure, endstage renal disease or ESRD) or liver disease (liver failure, hepatic encephalopathy, cirrhosis) require some form of protein control in dietary pattern to prevent complications from inability to handle protein solute load (refer back to Chapter 7)

b. Proteins used in the diet must be of high biologic value and protein intake is usually weight-based, starting at 0.8 grams/kg of dry weight, depending on the client's underlying clinical condition

c. Protein levels may be increased as necessary to account for metabolic response to dialysis and regeneration of liver tissue (1.5–2.0 grams/kg/day)

d. A minimum level of CHOs are needed in the diet (50–100 grams/day) in order to spare protein

e. Vitamin and mineral supplements may be indicated with clients who have liver failure

f. The dietitian is instrumental in calculating specific nutrient requirements for these clients and reviews fluid intake and output, medication profile, and daily weights to monitor client outcomes in conjunction with dialysis technicians/nurses

6. Food allergy diet

a. An egg-free diet is used for clients who have a known sensitivity to eggs; it restricts the use of eggs and egg products in the diet

b. Several common foods have allergic potential such as cow's milk, eggs, fish, shellfish, nuts (peanuts, almonds, and cashews), soybeans, and wheat; 90% of food allergy reactions are attributed to these foods; primary therapy is avoidance of the particular food item

Box 8-1

Gluten-Restricted Diet Information

- Foods that are included: cornmeal, corn flakes, popcorn, hominy, and potato chips
- Food substitutions: corn, potato, rice, soybean flour, and low-gluten wheat flour
- Foods to avoid: processed, commercially prepared foods that include wheat flour extenders, additives, or stabilizers; root beer, beer, and all products that contain identified grain sources (wheat, rye, barley, buckwheat, oats, and malt); soy sauce, or soup containing these ingredients

c. Children often present with food allergies and certain diets (Allergy I and Allergy II) are used to identify potential food allergens by eliminating intake in a controlled manner; these diets are used in a limited time frame, as they are not nutritionally complete

! **d.** A gluten-restricted diet (gluten gliaden-free diet) is used for clients who have celiac disease (malabsorption syndrome) and omits wheat, rye, barley, oats, buckwheat, and malt (gluten proteins) from the diet (refer to Box 8-1 for information about a gluten-restricted diet); allows rice and corn

1) Clinical manifestations resulting from inability to properly utilize gluten protein are steatorrhea, diarrhea, weight loss, anemia, and edema formation due to loss of nutrients

2) Clients can also have lactose intolerance and must follow dietary restrictions for that diet as well

! **e.** A lactose-restricted diet is used for clients who have lactose intolerance (due to lactase–enzyme deficiency) and may require lactase enzyme supplementation to be able to tolerate some amount of dairy products (refer to Box 8-2 for information about the lactose intolerance diet)

1) Primary lactose intolerance is seen in certain ethnic groups (African Americans, Asian, Hispanic, and Native Americans)

Box 8-2

Lactose-Restricted Diet Information

- Foods that are included: aged cheese (hard) rather than soft cheese; hard cheese is lower in lactose due to aging process
- OTC products such as Lactaid are specific formulations containing lactase are used to assist clients who have identified lactase deficiency. These products are usually available in liquid or tablet form.
- Special milk products formulated with Lactaid are available for use by lactose-intolerant clients. Products of this type are usually sweeter than regular milk products.
- Individual tolerance is variable and the client is the best judge of how little or how much "lactose" can be handled without onset of clinical symptoms.
- Many clients with lactose intolerance can tolerate ¼ to ½ cup of milk at one time
- Check food labels for milk, milk solids, casein, and whey—these can be used as additives and stabilizers in processed food products.
- Check medication ingredients because lactose can be used as a binder or filler in certain formulations.
- Lactose-restricted diets are often low in calcium, vitamin B_2 (riboflavin), and vitamin D; additional nutrient supplementation may be necessary to maintain optimal nutrient levels.
- Hidden sources are baked goods and processed foods.

2) Secondary lactose intolerance is due to another established disease process (such as infection) or medication (chemo agents that inhibit cell growth) that affect the GI tract's ability to produce lactase

3) Clinical symptoms affect the GI tract, resulting in gas, bloating, and diarrhea

f. Restriction and/or avoidance therapy is utilized to prevent or minimize food allergies

7. Purine-controlled diet

a. A purine-controlled diet is indicated for clients who have gout, tumor lysis syndrome, or multiple myeloma, and all who have elevated uric acid levels

b. Excessive purine accumulation in the body leads to an increase in uric acid, which is a normal end product of purine catabolism

! c. The diet includes the use of dairy food products and restricts foods such as organ meats, anchovies, alcohol, and seafood

8. Sodium-controlled diet

a. Various levels of restriction are available and are based on supportive evidence that high sodium diets correlate with hypertension, fluid retention, and cardiovascular disease

b. The restrictions range from mild (3,000–4,000 mg/day) to severe (500 mg/day)

c. It is important to evaluate food labels, medications, and restaurant dietary intake pattern for hidden sodium sources in the diet

! d. Sodium is often used as a preservative in many foods; thus a client may be unaware of just how much hidden sodium is being added to the total daily intake; it is imperative that clients be taught how to read food labels to detect sodium in food products

e. Clients using salt substitutes may be at risk for elevated potassium levels and should be evaluated closely for development of hyperkalemia and possibly other fluid and electrolyte imbalances

f. Referral to a dietitian may be necessary in order to accurately account for all hidden sodium sources in the diet and to plan a diet pattern that is consistent with the level of required sodium restriction

9. Tyramine- and dopamine-restricted diet

a. Tyramine is an intermediate product of amino acid metabolism formed in the conversion of tyrosine to epinephrine; it is found in many food items

b. A tyramine-restricted diet is indicated for clients who are on MAO inhibitors (monoamine oxidase inhibitors—antidepressants) because foods containing tyramine affect MAO inhibitor drug action by blocking enzyme pathways and lead to release of norepinephrine, resulting in a hypertensive crisis

c. Other amines such as dopamine are also restricted in the diet because excess accumulation can lead to similar hypertensive effects

! d. Some foods that need to be avoided on this type of diet include aged cheese, chocolate, smoked fish, bologna, bananas, liver, fava beans, and large amounts of soy sauce

! e. Foods that can be included are unfermented cheese (ricotta and cottage cheese) and small amounts of certain foods such as sour cream

f. Referral to a dietitian may be helpful to a client to obtain a more complete listing of foods to be avoided on this type of diet

g. It is critical that all members of the healthcare team be knowledgeable regarding clients who are on this type of therapy to prevent complications from drug–diet interactions

C. Supplemental/enhanced diet

1. High-fiber diet
   a. A high-fiber diet is used to stimulate peristalsis, promote regularity, and maintain normal bowel function and elimination patterns
   b. Foods included in this diet are high in complex CHOs and low in fat (legumes, whole grain products, vegetables, and fruits)
2. High-potassium diet
   a. A high-potassium (K^+) diet is used for clients who have K^+ losses due to diuretic therapy
   ! b. Examples of high K^+ sources in the diet include orange juice, apricots, cantaloupes, bananas, and most other fruits and vegetables
3. High-calcium diet
   a. A high-calcium (Ca^{++}) diet is indicated for clients who have disease states that promote Ca^{++} loss leading to bone demineralization (osteoporosis, osteopenia), endocrine abnormalities, and kidney failure
   ! b. Good sources of Ca^{++} in the diet include milk and dairy products
4. High-protein diet
   a. The use of a high-protein diet has been indicated for athletes (1.2–1.6 grams/kg/day) in order to maximize endurance, according to current research evidence; also is indicated for clients recovering from surgery or who have large wounds or pressure ulcers
   b. Amino acids and phosphocreatine have been implicated as promoting enhancement of athletic performance but there is no scientific data to confirm these reports; creatine increases intramuscular creatine and power in anaerobic activities such as weight lifting and sprinting
   c. Referral to a dietitian or physician who specializes in sports medicine/nutrition is advised before starting any type of supplement/enhanced diet program

Practice to Pass

Why is a client with a clinical history of gout placed on a purine-controlled diet?

IV. ENTERAL NUTRITION

A. Definition

1. **Enteral nutrition** refers to a method of feeding clients who have a functioning GI tract but are unable to take a diet orally or whose diet is inadequate (refer to Table 8-2 for clinical indications)
2. Feedings can be delivered either orally or via tube placement although most commonly feedings are given via tubes

B. Indications for use

1. Short-term use via nasogastric tubes or oral route
2. Long-term use via enterostomy placed surgically or percutaneously

C. Administration

1. Continuous feedings occur throughout a 24-hour period at a prescribed flow rate and a total set volume using an infusion pump
2. Intermittent infusions occur over a time frame of 30 minutes (to mimic usual eating pattern) or more with a prescribed total set volume ranging from 250–400 mL of formula using an infusion pump, gravity, or syringe

Table 8-2 Clinical Indications for Enteral and Parenteral Nutrition

Enteral	Parenteral—TPN	Parenteral—PPN
Mechanical alterations due to chewing or swallowing problems Impairment in upper GI tract leading to digestion, transport and absorption problems Alteration in intake pattern due to client's inability to eat, refusal to eat, or inability to ingest sufficient intake to meet nutritional goals Functional GI tract	Clinical disease states such as malabsorption, surgical interventions, trauma/stress, and/or related pathology of GI tract or oncologic conditions Malnourished clients who require long-term nutritional support and high nutrient requirements based on clinical deficiencies Nonfunctional GI tract Central line access or PICC line placement due to hypertonic solution	Clients with moderate nutritional deficiencies who do not have central access but still require supportive nutritional therapy to meet nutrient goals Nonfunctional GI tract Limiting dose based on amino acid and dextrose concentration Caloric and energy requirements needed are usually below 1,800 kcalories/day Peripheral site placement

3. **Cyclic feeding** occurs over a several-hour period (prescribed flow rate and a set total volume using an infusion pump) usually at night as a transitional approach to normal GI functioning
4. **Bolus feeding** occurs when there is a rapid delivery of a large amount of formula (preset volume 250–300 mL) in a short time

D. Collaborative management

1. Formula selection
   a. Characteristics of formula include protein classification, nutrient density, (see Chapter 2) and amounts of residue and fiber
   b. The dietitian and physician work together to select the best treatment option for the client
   c. It is important to be aware of client's underlying clinical condition, as this will influence the selection of formula
   ! d. Elderly clients and newborns may be unable to tolerate large volume feedings and may require modification of treatment regimen in order to meet nutritional needs
2. Monitoring response to treatment
   a. Assessment findings relevant to weight status should be documented; results should be trended and communicated to healthcare team members in order to evaluate client outcomes
   ! b. Weight gain and BUN, creatinine, and other pertinent serum chemistries should be monitored closely during the course of therapy
   c. The dietitian will evaluate a client's individual requirements for macronutrients and fluid requirements based on body weight calculations

E. Nursing responsibilities

! 1. Document baseline weight to provide basis for clinical therapy and obtain daily weights thereafter to evaluate response to therapy
2. Inspect the IV site for signs/symptoms of potential irritation and infection
! 3. Check tube placement prior to initiation of any feeding regimen or medication administration
   a. Aspirate to check for gastric contents if feeding tube tip is in stomach

b. Measure pH of gastric aspirant (preferred method)
c. Using a stethoscope, auscultate for "whoosh" due to air placement in the stomach; do not rely solely on this method because it is not always accurate

! 4. Check for **residual** on tube feedings to prevent complications and document response to therapy
a. Residuals are often checked every 4–12 hours during continuous feeds, although some clinicians do not check them
! b. When feeding is not continuous, residuals are checked before starting the next feeding

! 5. If the residual amount is greater than expected, the rate of feeding will be decreased and/or withheld in order to prevent overload complications resulting from inadequate digestion
a. For continuous feeding checked every 4 hours, if the residual is > 400 ml, then the feeding should be withheld and the residual rechecked in 1 hour to determine if the client is now able to tolerate the feeding; some policies consider 100–200 mL excessive, so check agency policy
b. For an intermittent or bolus feeding, if the residual prior to starting the next feeding > 400 mL, then the feeding should be withheld and the residual rechecked in 1 hour as with a continuous feed
c. The amount and/or method of feeding (bolus, continuous, cyclic, or intermittent) may need to be adjusted based on trends noted in residual findings

Practice to Pass

How would you interpret an obtained residual of 50 mL during a q4 hour check in an adult client who was receiving a tube feeding at an initial rate of 25 mL/hr?

6. Check pertinent labs, daily weight, and I & O to monitor response to clinical therapy
7. Communicate with other healthcare team members in order to meet individualized client goals

! 8. Refer to Box 8-3 (p. 246) for a listing of nursing interventions specific to enteral tube feedings
9. Be aware of potential complications that can arise from the use of tube feedings (refer to Box 8-4, p. 247)

V. PARENTERAL NUTRITION

A. Description

1. Parenteral nutrition refers to a method of feeding clients who do not have a functioning GI tract as a result of clinical disease (malabsorption), surgical intervention, trauma/stress, and/or malignancies; when given via a central catheter, the net dextrose content of total parenteral nutrition (TPN) is up to 25%, and it is given via central line; when given via peripheral line, the dextrose content is up to 10% and is called peripheral parenteral nutrition (PPN) (refer back to Table 8-2 for a listing of clinical indications)
2. Energy needs are calculated by determining the Basal Energy Expenditure (BEE) using the Harris-Benedict equation
a. Males—BEE (kcal/day) = 66.5 + (13.7 × weight in kg) + 5.0 × height in cm) − (6.8 × age)
b. Females—BEE (kcal/day) = 65.5 + (9.6 × weight in kg) + (1.7 × height in cm) − (4.7 × age)
c. BEE calculations are for basal metabolic conditions; activity and injury can require modification of energy calculations

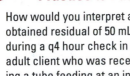

Box 8-3

Interventions Specific to Enteral Tube Feedings

- Inspect formula for particulate matter and untoward appearance that might suggest chemical breakdown.
- Do not hang more than the documented amount of formula per hospital protocol per shift—this can lead to bacterial overgrowth and chemical breakdown (usually based on manufacturer's recommendation).
- Change solution/tubing per hospital protocol to prevent risk of infection.
- Check placement of tube prior to any feeding, flush, or medication application to ensure patency.
- Flush tube with water per hospital protocol in order to prevent dehydration that can occur if only formula feedings are used as the sole fluid replacement.
- Include the amounts of flush or irrigation used in the client's I & O.
- Position the client to ensure patency and raise head of bed at least 30 degrees prior to and after feeding.
- Monitor pertinent labs per hospital protocol and document daily weights.
- Work with healthcare team members (dietitian and enterostomal therapist) in order to maintain nutritional balance and skin integrity.
- Incorporate the concepts of altered nutritional status and body image in developing plan of care.
- Be aware that the placement of feeding tubes may be long term in nature given the client's underlying medical condition.
- Hang new feeding container and tubing every 24–48 hours according to agency policy.

3. Nutrient needs are calculated by a dietitian
    a. Macronutrient needs include CHO, protein, and lipids
    b. Micronutrient needs include vitamins and minerals
    c. Fluid needs are determined and correlated with above nutrient needs (refer to Table 8-3 for a listing of TPN calculation requirements and Table 8-4 (pp. 248–249) for a listing of nutrient composition of TPN)
4. TPN solutions can be viewed as prescriptions based on the individualized requirements of the client
    a. There are standard solutions that have specific dextrose, amino acid, and electrolyte content; these solutions can be further specified to meet individual needs in the clinical setting
    b. The additive content of a solution is clearly labeled with instructions that nothing should be added to any TPN solution on the nursing unit
    c. ! Be sure to use the specified necessary filters (change every 24 hrs) and follow hospital policy/procedure while infusing this type of therapy
5. Feedings are delivered via a central vein access or peripheral site depending on the concentration of solution

B. Indications for use

1. Short-term use is via a peripheral vein site
2. Long-term use is via a central vein access or a peripherally inserted central catheter

C. Administration

1. ! Continuous feedings are done throughout a 24-hour period at a prescribed flow rate and a set total volume using an infusion pump

Box 8-4

Complications Related to Tube Feedings

- Mechanical complications include clogged tube, tube dislodgment, or use of an infusion pump that is not functioning correctly.
- Metabolic complications include dehydration, electrolyte imbalances, and altered blood glucose levels (usually hyperglycemia).
- Complications related to formula selection and client tolerance include diarrhea, cramps, abdominal distention, constipation, or nausea and vomiting.
- If the client is experiencing diarrhea from enteral feedings, then a decrease in rate and volume of the solution may be indicated. The interval of feeding may have to be altered to allow the client to absorb and process the feedings. Check medications for those with laxative effects, such as stool softeners, lactulose, magnesium, or sorbitol-containing elixirs. Check for *clostridium difficile* in stool.
- The formula may have to be switched to an isotonic or less hypertonic formula in order to minimize the possibility of the client's experiencing the clinical manifestations of dumping syndrome.
- Dermatologic complications include irritation at the site of the feeding tube (enterostomy) due to possible leakage of formula feeding or in response to skin applications/dressings at the site.
- Potential complications can arise from the use of medications via the feeding tube that are either not in correct form, leading to clogging of tube or causing potential side effects due to formula–drug interactions.
- It is important to monitor the ordered amount of feeding and fluid replacement (water) each shift; note both the shift and 24-hour totals to minimize the risk of dehydration and maintain fluid balance.
- Clients who have nasogastric tube feedings may be at risk for potential aspiration due to positioning or decreased gastric emptying. Maintain adequate client position by elevating the head of the bed during feedings and checking residuals as ordered to prevent this potential complication.

Table 8-3

TPN Calculation Requirements

Nutrients	Calculations
Carbohydrates (dextrose)	3.4 kcal/gram Provides at least 50% of total calories Primary TPN constituent
Protein (amino acids)	4.0 kcal/gram 1 gram of nitrogen = 6.25 grams of protein 0.8 gram/kg for client under no stress Stress states increase metabolic requirements up to 2.0 grams/kg
Lipids 10% Lipids 20% Lipids	9.0 kcal/gm 10% provide 1.1 kcal/day 20% provide 2.0 kcal/day Comprise 10 to 40% of daily calorie needs <1 gram/kg for adults 4 grams/kg for children
Fluids	Young adults 30–40 mL/kg/day Elderly clients 30 mL/kg/day Changes in fluid requirements occur in response to losses, increased drainage, and metabolic demands. Client can experience both FVD and FVE if fluid requirements are not calculated correctly in connection with the overall TPN formulation.

Table 8-4

Listing of Nutrients and Additives for TPN Solutions

Nutrients	Functions/Effects
Dextrose (carbohydrate source)	Primary fuel energy source. Has the greatest total concentration of nutrients in solution. Should not exceed oxidative limit of the body (> 5 mg of glucose/ kg/minute), because this will cause metabolic stress leading to fatty liver changes and increased CO_2 production. Clients who have significant respiratory history may be at risk to develop CO_2 production with high dextrose solutions requiring adjustment of TPN concentration (decrease CHO and increase lipid content) to minimize CO_2 production. TPN solution > 10% dextrose is infused via a central line access. Increased CHO source leads to increased blood glucose and increased insulin requirements.
Amino Acids (protein source)	Used to maintain nitrogen balance and are used for protein synthesis and support of immune function. Available in crystalline form with solutions that vary in concentration (3 to 15%). In addition, the solutions are available with or without electrolytes. Specialized amino acid preparations such as BCAA (branched chain amino acids) are available for clients who are in high stress states with liver or renal problems.
Lipids (fat source)	Secondary energy source of TPN solutions that is needed to prevent essential fatty acid deficiency (EFAD). Exist in different concentrations ranging from 10 to 30%, but all are considered to be isotonic and therefore can be infused via a peripheral line. Fat emulsions can increase calories of the solution but do not affect the osmolality. Lipid solutions contain egg yolk phospholipids; clients who have allergies to eggs should NOT be given these solutions. Diabetic clients may require a greater percentage of their TPN concentration in lipid form, especially if they have persistent hyperglycemia due to dextrose load. Clients who have abnormal lipid metabolism (hyperlipidemia or pancreatitis) should have serum triglyceride levels checked during IV lipid infusion to see if they have adequate lipid clearance; lipids should be withheld if serum triglycerides are > 350 mg/dL. Lipid emulsions contain both LCT and MCT (medium chain triglycerides). MCT do not contain essential fatty acids but are more easily used by the body in times of severe metabolic stress. Excessive levels of lipids and increased rate of administration are associated with clinical problems ranging from inadequate lipid clearance, impaired immune response, and altered functioning of the RES (reticuloendothelial system).
Electrolytes	Calcium is needed to support muscles, bones, nerve integrity, and coagulation. In response to low albumin levels, calcium level will have to be adjusted to reflect status of protein bound calcium in the body (adjusted Ca level = [4.0 × serum albumin] × 0.8 + serum calcium). Phosphorus is needed to support metabolism of macronutrients (15 to 30 mM/day). Magnesium is needed to support enzyme function in multiple metabolic body processes (8–24 mEq/day). Potassium is needed to maintain cardiac function and acid-base balance. Sodium is needed to maintain plasma osmolality and acid-base balance. Sodium and potassium are added to TPN solutions in the form of salts and thus accompany other electrolytes. In response to the client's underlying clinical condition, electrolyte values may be further depleted at time of therapy or in response to medications used during therapy such as diuretics and antibiotics. The majority of malnourished clients will present with multiple electrolyte imbalances.

Table 8-4 (*cont.*)

Nutrients	Functions/Effects
Micronutrients	Several trace elements have been identified as being essential in TPN formulations. They include zinc, copper, chromium, manganese, selenium, iodine, and iron. There are specific formulations such as MTE-4 (contains Zn, Ch, Cu, and Mn) and MTE-5 (same as for MTE-4 plus selenium) that can be used to supply these needed trace elements. MTE-5 is preferable. Zinc is needed for participation as a co-enzyme in multiple enzyme systems. Chromium affects glucose metabolism. Manganese participates as a co-enzyme in protein and energy metabolism. Iodine aids in the synthesis of thyroid hormones and supports endocrine function. Iron functions as a participant in enzyme systems and is an essential constituent of several proteins, especially hemoglobin and myoglobin. There may be problems with bioavailability and compatibility related to iron, so check with the pharmacist for clarification. Note iron is not a part of most TPN solutions. The presence of selenium is indicated in TPN solutions as clinical deficiencies causing cardiomyopathy (Keeshan disease) have occurred. Selenium participates in enzyme systems.
Vitamins	Most TPN solutions use MVI formulations to meet vitamin needs, including vitamin K.
Additives	Common additives to TPN solutions include regular insulin, heparin, histamine H_2 receptor antagonists. It is important to check for stability and potential incompatibility of additives. To prevent potential complications from arising, pharmacists who are well versed in these areas should always mix TPN solutions.

2. Cyclic feeding occurs over a several hour period (8–12 hours a day) at a prescribed flow rate and a set total volume using an infusion pump; this method normalizes insulin levels and allows for fat sources to be used for energy and/or essential fatty acid formation
3. Peripheral parenteral nutrition (PPN) is the delivery of nutrients through a peripheral vein
   a. PPN solutions contain amino acids, dextrose, and lipids and have a decreased osmolality
   b. Lipid emulsions can be administered through PPN as they are considered to be isotonic solutions

! 4. A total nutrient admixture (TNA) represents a specific type of TPN formulation that contains all 3 macronutrients in a 24-hour supply
   a. It is also referred to as a 3-in-1 bag because it contains all of the macronutrients in one system
   b. TNA reduces nursing and pharmacy time and pump use
5. Specific TPN formulations are used for clients with significant metabolic disease and/or stress

! a. Branched chain amino acid (BCAA) enriched solutions—valine, leucine, and isoleucine may be used as part of special amino acid products for the clinical treatment of clients with liver disease because they are subject to large losses of these three amino acids; this formulation is contraindicated if the client is anuric
   b. Clients with liver disease also have high levels of aromatic amino acids and therefore can have problems with handling standard amino acid preparations

! **c.** Clients who have renal disease also have problems handling protein; therefore, it is critical that the amino acid formulations used contain essential amino acids in order to prevent excess renal solute load; the renal client must be evaluated for acid-base and electrolyte balance and sufficient blood volume to maintain excretion of solute load

d. Clients who are suffering severe metabolic stress respond by going into a hypermetabolic pattern of metabolism that requires more protein and replacement of lost BCAA due to stress states; the client under severe stress must be evaluated for acid-base and electrolyte imbalance and this formulation is contraindicated if anuria is present

e. There are no good clinical outcome studies to date that show benefit to the use of BCAA solutions

D. Collaborative management

1. A dietitian calculates nutrients and recommends an individualized formula of macronutrients, micronutrients, and fluid based on individual energy requirements (see Box 8-5 for nutrient calculation)
2. This solution is prepared by the pharmacist

a. Solution is mixed in a laminar flow hood under sterile conditions

b. Nurses should not mix solutions

! **c.** Solutions should be refrigerated prior to administration unless the mixture is prepared immediately for use

! 3. The nurse monitors response to treatment (see Box 8-6 for assessment parameters for TPN therapy)

a. Document assessment findings per hospital protocol

b. Trend pertinent labs and diagnostic tests and measure weight daily to confirm response to treatment

Box 8-5

Nutrient Calculation for Parenteral Feeding

- The percentage of dextrose in a solution will provide the amount of grams of dextrose that are present in 100 mL of the solution. For example, in a 10% dextrose solution there are 10 grams of dextrose per 100 mL. Multiply the number of grams of dextrose by 3.4 kcalories per gram to get the total kcalories present in the solution.
- Similarly, the percentage of amino acids in a solution will provide the amount of grams of amino acids that are present in 100 mL of the solution. For example, in a 4.25% amino acid solution there are 4.25 grams of amino acids per 100 mL. Multiply the number of grams of amino acid by 4.0 kcalories per gram to get the total kcalories in the solution.
- Lipid solutions are usually available in 10–20% solutions with 1.1 kcal/mL and 2 kcal/mL provided.
- A specific volume, rate, and prescription are found in central base (TPN) and peripheral base (PPN) solutions focusing on amino acids, dextrose, and lipids.
- PPN solutions have a maximum final concentration of 4.25% amino acids and 10% dextrose.
- Additives are calculated and added to solution based on usual daily doses of electrolytes, multivitamins, and trace elements.
- Medications such as regular insulin or H_2 antagonists are added to solution based on client's clinical response to therapy.

Box 8-6

Assessment Parameters for TPN Therapy

Baseline Assessment Parameters

- Weight, height, BMI, actual body weight vs. usual body weight
- Serum chemistry profile (chem. 24), CBC, coagulation profile, iron, total iron-binding capacity (TIBC), and Mg
- Lipid profile (triglycerides and cholesterol)
- Liver function tests
- Individualized energy, nutrient, and fluid needs

Ongoing Assessments

- Q shift—vital signs and I & O
- Daily weights and 24-hour I & O
- Pertinent labs on daily and weekly basis that reflect client's response to therapy (electrolytes and serum chemistry panels)
- 24-hour urine to evaluate urine urea nitrogen level
- Evaluation of client's progress towards resumption of "normal" feeding route and consideration of client's body image and other psychological support issues
- Monitoring of client's underlying condition and response to treatment

E. Nursing responsibilities (see Box 8-7 (p. 252) for interventions specific to TPN therapy)

1. Document baseline weight to provide basis for clinical therapy and ongoing daily weights to confirm response to treatment
2. Inspect IV site looking for signs/symptoms of potential irritation and infection
3. Check pertinent labs, daily weight, and I & O to monitor clinical response
4. Use a dedicated line for infusion and proper equipment (infusion pump with filter) during course of therapy
5. Change solution bag every 24 hours per agency protocol to decrease risk of infection; hypertonic solutions have high glucose levels that can lead to bacterial overgrowth
6. Two RNs must verify solution prior to hanging
   a. Verify prescription of treatment
   b. Validate contents of bag with original order
7. Communicate with other healthcare team members
   a. Confirm TBA at the end of shift to validate ordered treatment
   b. Document shift and 24-hour I & O totals to determine clinical progress
   c. Verify that dressing changes to IV site have been done per protocol and that IV access is patent
8. Be aware of potential complications that can result from the use of parenteral nutrition therapy (refer to Box 8-8 (p. 253) for potential complications)

Practice to Pass

Why are TPN solutions changed every 24 hours as part of the treatment protocol?

VI. TEST DIETS

A. Glucose tolerance test (GTT) diet

1. This diet is used to monitor, evaluate, and assess clients for potential imbalances in glucose metabolism

Box 8-7

Interventions Specific to TPN Therapy

- Verify TPN prescription with two RNs using 5 Rights of Medication administration.
- Run TPN through a dedicated line.
- Change TPN solutions and tubing per protocol every 24 hours.
- Ensure that a pharmacist mixes all TPN solutions.
- Inspect TNA product prior to hanging for "cracking" (lipid separation). Do not hang TNA solutions that have "cracking." Return them to pharmacy.
- Infuse TPN using an infusion pump per protocol.
- Follow TPN protocols regarding client assessments, diagnostic testing, and evaluation of response to treatment.
- Assess client for complications specific to this type of therapy.
- When client is progressing and TPN therapy is to be stopped, follow protocol for discontinuing therapy. Do not stop TPN therapy abruptly—this can cause rebound hypoglycemia to develop.
- As TPN is stopped, enteral feeding routes (oral or tube) are increased to a greater percentage of the total intake.
- Collaborate with dietitian and physician in the assessment and evaluation of client response.
- Be aware of client and family member concerns regarding TPN therapy. Answer questions and provide support to client and family members.
- Document pertinent findings relative to TPN therapy.
- Clients with significant nutritional and medical problems may require permanent TPN administration.

2. The diet consists of a specified glucose content (150 grams CHO daily) for at least 3 days prior to testing
3. ! The client should then remain NPO on the day of testing when a prescribed glucose load will be administered and then serial blood draws will be done to evaluate the client's response to the imposed glucose load
4. This diet can be used prior to glucose testing because clients who are either not eating well or are using weight reduction methods may have altered results of the GTT if they do not have an adequate level of CHOs in the diet

B. Intravenous pyelogram (IVP) test diet

1. This diet is indicated for clients who are undergoing IVP testing
2. The diet consists of clear liquids the evening preprocedure; fluids are allowed until midnight, and then the client is NPO

Practice to Pass

Why is it necessary to follow a test diet in the clinical setting?

C. 100-gram "fecal fat" test diet

1. This diet is used to establish a clinical diagnosis of malabsorption and steatorrhea in the clinical setting
2. The diet consists of 100 grams of fat/day for a period of 3 to 6 days during which time stool specimens are collected for fecal fat excretion

D. Vanillylmandelic acid (VMA) test diet

1. This diet is used to establish a clinical diagnosis of pheochromocytoma
2. VMA is an end-product of catecholamine metabolism and is found in the urine

Box 8-8

Complications Related to Parenteral Nutrition

- Catheter-related complications include occlusion due to thrombosis, development of air embolism due to air or obstruction, incorrect placement of catheter or migration of catheter leading to changes in chest wall pressures (pneumothorax), infection or phlebitis, or sepsis.
- Metabolic-related complications include potential acid-base imbalances, electrolyte imbalances, deficiencies in vitamins and minerals and fatty acids, and volume disturbances leading to dehydration or fluid retention depending on client's underlying clinical condition and/or response to clinical treatment.
- A gain of > 1 kg/day indicates fluid overload.
- Alteration of rate (infusing too fast or too slow) can lead to significant complications ranging from fluid overload to neurological impairment (seizures and coma) and death. Infuse solution at prescribed rate and monitor closely for client tolerance.
- Allergic reaction to potential components and sepsis can occur.
- Clients suffering from profound malnutrition/starvation are at risk to develop refeeding syndrome (decreases in phosphorus, potassium, and/or magnesium) upon initiation of TPN therapy due to increased cellular uptake. To prevent this, monitor electrolytes closely and give half of the identified energy requirements based on client's dry body weight.
- Dramatic glycemic responses can occur because TPN solutions are hypertonic, hyperosmolar, and place an increased metabolic demand on the body. The client's blood glucose is often monitored with a sliding scale of regular insulin given in response to TPN protocols; regular insulin may be used as an additive in the solution.
- Hypoglycemia can occur if the TPN solution has run out before the next solution is due to be hung. It is imperative to follow established hospital protocol to maintain the client's blood sugar (either using $D_{10}W$ or D_5W at the prescribed rate) until the next solution is available.
- In order to prevent possible complications related to incorrect TPN solution being hung, it is imperative to follow protocol and have two RNs verify the prescription, validate ingredients with the original order, and check the client's identification prior to hanging the TPN solution.

! **3.** Certain foods such as bananas, caffeine, chocolate, and vanilla can cause increased VMA levels and should be restricted in the diet prior to this test

E. Serotonin (5-HIAA) test diet

1. This diet is used in conjunction with urine testing to determine the amount of 5-hydroxyindoleacetic because an excess of this substance is associated with carcinoid tumor and malignancies

! **2.** The test diet restricts the use of foods that can increase urinary excretion of this substance such as avocados, bananas, butternuts, eggplant, hickory nuts, kiwi, pecans, pineapple, and plantains

3. The use of aspirin can also affect urinary excretion of this substance and must not be used in the 24-hour period prior to testing

VII. TRANSITION DIETS

A. Postsurgical procedures

! **1.** Progressive diet (clear, full, soft, to regular)

! **a.** Clients are started on a progressive diet once gag reflex returns and after gastric suction tube is removed (if in place)

b. Clients are then progressed in their diet depending on return of bowel sounds, evidence of GI motility (passing gas and bowel movements), and tolerance of fluids and food without nausea or vomiting

c. "Diet as tolerated" orders allow for collaborative practice among nurses, physicians, and dietitians in meeting nutritional goals for a client

1) This order can be used postprocedure and postoperatively

2) This order incorporates client's preferences and may facilitate compliance in meeting nutritional goals

2. Postcardiac catheterization diet

! a. This diet is indicated for clients postcardiac cath procedure; it is eaten with the head raised only 30 degrees and has food items that can be picked up by the client

b. It consists of a turkey sandwich, pickup fruit (such as grapes on stem), and vegetable slices

3. Post oral surgery (modified consistency) diet

a. This diet consists of soft foods and liquids to minimize chewing and ease swallowing

b. Depending on client's condition and tolerance of food, the diet may be followed for several days

! c. The client may need rinses with warm water and/or peroxide solution mixes to cleanse the mouth area and to promote comfort

d. The client may be unable to tolerate extreme temperature differences and certain textures of foods

B. Post gastrointestinal upset diet

1. BRAT diet

a. The BRAT diet is indicated for short-term use in pediatric (sometimes adult) clients when GI symptoms (nausea, vomiting, and diarrhea) prevent normal dietary intake

! b. The diet consists of bananas, rice, applesauce, and toast and is progressive in nature

c. Fluid support is progressed as the client's GI symptoms subside

2. Progressive diet (clear, full, soft, to regular)

a. Clients who have GI symptoms may utilize a progressive diet plan based on urgency of symptoms and abdominal discomfort

b. Clients often select their own version of a progressive diet based on what has worked for them in the past and in response to family rituals and customs

c. It is important to obtain pertinent history regarding food habits and customs used by clients in response to GI upset so that proper hydration can be maintained and treatment expectations can be met

Practice to Pass

Explain the rationale for the use of progressive diets used in the postoperative period.

Case Study

A 60-year-old male client is receiving total parenteral nutrition (TPN) in the postoperative period to meet nutritional support needs. The TPN protocol has been in place for several days and the client is experiencing no observable clinical symptoms related to complications of TPN therapy. VS are stable with BP of 100/70, pulse 72, respiration 20, and temperature of 98°F.

1. What assessment parameters were most likely measured as the initial baseline for this client?
2. How often should this client be weighed?
3. During your shift, the client has a blood glucose level of 175 mg/dL. What nursing actions would you take and why?
4. The client's wife is upset and confused over "all this tubing" and wants to know why her husband "can't just eat." How would you respond to this statement?
5. How would you evaluate the client's response to treatment?

For suggested responses, see page 320.

POSTTEST

1 A client with an acute exacerbation of Crohn's disease is having oral intake resumed after having been NPO and receiving total parenteral nutrition (TPN) for 3 weeks. The nurse plans to do which of the following in order to ease transition of feeding methods?

1. Allow client to have only ice chips for the first 2 days.
2. Gradually begin oral feedings as parenteral solution is decreased.
3. Infuse the TPN solution during the nighttime only when client is sleeping.
4. Begin oral feedings of soft foods and stop TPN infusion.

2 Which of the following should the nurse include in a plan of care for a client receiving total parenteral nutrition (TPN)?

1. Withhold oral medications while the TPN is infusing.
2. Change TPN solution every 24 hours.
3. Flush the TPN line with water prior to initiating nutritional support.
4. Keep client on complete bedrest during TPN therapy.

3 Which of the following should the nurse plan to do in order to maintain normal glucose levels in a client receiving total parenteral nutrition (TPN) therapy?

1. Monitor blood glucose every 4–6 hours depending on the client's acuity and follow regular insulin sliding scale.
2. Decrease rate of TPN solution to maintain euglycemic levels.
3. Increase the rate of TPN solution to maintain euglycemic levels.
4. Use NPH insulin as an additive in TPN solutions to help maintain euglycemic levels.

4 The nurse anticipates which type of enteral feeding formula will be selected for a client who has problems with severe digestion or absorption of nutrients?

1. Modular
2. Polymeric
3. Elemental
4. Ensure

5 A client with a history of food allergies asks how to decrease the likelihood of allergic potential. What response by the nurse would be best?

1. "Eat only small amounts of a food if it has allergic potential."
2. "Increase the fluid content of the diet to minimize risk of food allergies."
3. "Avoid food items identified as potential allergens."
4. "Take antihistamines to prevent allergic reactions and eat what you like."

6 A client is placed on a low residue diet. The nurse evaluates that the client understood dietary instructions given if the client states that she will refrain from eating which of the following favorite food items?

1. Orange juice
2. Baked potatoes
3. Toasted white bread
4. Milk

7 The nurse considers which of the following factors to be necessary in order to allow progression of the diet in a postoperative client?

1. Passage of a bowel movement
2. Increased flatus production and slight abdominal distention
3. Presence of bowel sounds and passage of flatus
4. Client reports feelings of hunger

8 The nurse suggests which of the following diet selections for a client placed on a full liquid diet?

1. Beef bouillon, cranberry juice, and tea
2. Decaffeinated tea, gelatin, and Popsicles
3. Poached egg, coffee, and orange juice
4. Plain yogurt and apple juice

9 Which of the following should the nurse include as a primary focus in the teaching plan for a client placed on a transition diet?

1. The diet will be used on a long-term basis.
2. The focus of the diet is on meal planning and diet selection technique.
3. The client should understand the types of food items that are restricted on this diet.
4. This diet plan will be a temporary dietary measure.

10 The nurse should include which of the following in a plan of care for a client who is mildly lactose intolerant?

1. Remove all dairy products from the diet.
2. Consume only ½ cup of dairy products at one time.
3. Drink small amounts of milk on an empty stomach.
4. Spread out selection of dairy products throughout the day.

See pages 258–260 for Answers and Rationales.

POSTTEST

ANSWERS & RATIONALES

Pretest

1 **Answer: 4** A mechanical soft diet can be used as part of a long-term treatment plan because it includes most foods found on a regular diet, except the texture is modified to assist clients who have chewing problems. All of the other options reflect diets that should not be used on a long-term basis. Clear and full liquid diets are not nutritionally complete and are missing calories, protein, vitamins, and electrolytes. In order to meet nutritional goals, a full liquid diet would require additional source supplementation. Option 3 is incorrect because a long-term high-protein diet can place additional renal demands on the individual client because of imposed solute loads.

Cognitive Level: Application **Client Need:** Health Promotion and Maintenance **Integrated Process:** Nursing Process: Planning **Content Area:** Foundational Sciences: Nutrition **Strategy:** Critical words in the question are *long-term* and *difficulty chewing.* Recognize option 2 would not provide sufficient nutrients for long term and eliminate it. A low-residue diet (option 1) helps reduce diarrhea but is not appropriate for the client who has difficulty with chewing. Long term high protein intake could also be

ANSWERS & RATIONALES

harmful so eliminate option 3 as well. **Reference:** Cataldo, C., DeBruyne, L., & Whitney, E. (2003). *Nutrition and diet therapy* (6th ed.). Belmont, CA: Wadsworth & Thomson Learning, pp. 417–418, 452–453.

2 **Answer: 2** It is important to check residuals prior to intermittent feedings (and every 4 hours for continuous feedings) in order to evaluate if the client is able to process the feeding. Option 1 is incorrect—going to the bathroom prior to a feeding will not affect the feeding status, and the client may also not be able to physically comply with this request. Option 3 is incorrect—placing the client in this position is not warranted and can cause potential problems relative to impaired feeding or potential aspiration. Although monitoring of the client's intake and output for the last 24 hours is important, it is not as critical as checking for a residual at this point in time.

Cognitive Level: Analysis **Client Need:** Health Promotion and Maintenance **Integrated Process:** Nursing Process: Planning **Content Area:** Foundational Sciences: Nutrition **Strategy:** A critical word is *prior.* Eliminate option 1 since it does not pertain to the feeding. Recognize option 3 would be dangerous to eliminate it. Note the similarity in the word *prior* in the question with the word *before* in option 2 to direct you to the correct answer. **Reference:** Cataldo, C., DeBruyne, L., & Whitney, E. (2003). *Nutrition and diet therapy* (6th ed.). Belmont, CA: Wadsworth & Thomson Learning, pp. 425, 506–507.

3 **Answer: 3** The use of thickening agents is recommended for clients who have had CVA and have residual deficits that affect swallowing. The thickening agents are added to maximize texture, facilitate the swallowing process, and minimize potential aspiration risks. Option 1 is incorrect—bite-sized portions of foods may increase the risk of aspiration if they are swallowed and occlude the airway. The diet should be soft. Option 2 is incorrect—merely placing the client on a full liquid diet gives no indication that the client is being assessed for potential aspiration or neurological deficits. Option 4 is incorrect because clients who are post-CVA often encounter this type of problem; therefore, they should be properly monitored and assessed.

Cognitive Level: Application **Client Need:** Safe Effective Care Environment: Safety and Infection Control **Integrated Process:** Nursing Process: Implementation **Content Area:** Foundational Sciences: Nutrition **Strategy:** Focus on the critical words *assistance,* suggesting client should not be left alone, and *CVA* to consider a risk for aspiration. **Reference:** Cataldo, C., DeBruyne, L., & Whitney, E. (2003). *Nutrition and diet therapy* (6th ed.). Belmont, CA: Wadsworth & Thomson Learning, pp. 457–458.

4 **Answer: 1, 3** TPN is indicated for disease states such as trauma/stress, surgical interventions, and/or related pathology of GI tract or oncological conditions. TPN is more appropriate for long-term nutritional support. All other options are clinical indications for enteral nutrition.

Cognitive Level: Analysis **Client Need:** Health Promotion and Maintenance **Integrated Process:** Nursing Process: Analysis **Content Area:** Foundational Sciences: Nutrition **Strategy:** Focus on knowledge of indications for TPN, especially the long-term indicator. **Reference:** Cataldo, C., DeBruyne, L., & Whitney, E. (2003). *Nutrition and diet therapy* (6th ed.). Belmont, CA: Wadsworth & Thomson Learning, p. 525.

5 **Answer: 4** It is important to follow test diet instructions prior to diagnostic testing to ensure reliability and consistency of test results. Conveying the indication for the use of a clear liquid tray will help the client to understand the treatment plan and foster compliance. Although option 1 may represent an accurate statement, it will not help the client to deal with the present situation. Option 2 does not provide an adequate explanation to the client. Although option 3 is technically true, this response may serve to alienate the client as the nurse is not being sensitive to the client's needs.

Cognitive Level: Analysis **Client Need:** Physiological Integrity: Reduction of Risk Potential **Integrated Process:** Communication and Documentation **Content Area:** Foundational Sciences: Nutrition **Strategy:** The critical word is *best,* indicating some options are correct, but one answers the question more thoroughly. Eliminate option 1 since it may offer false reassurance. Eliminate options 2 and 3 since they do not offer the best explanation or adequately answer the client's question. **Reference:** Cataldo, C., DeBruyne, L., & Whitney, E. (2003). *Nutrition and diet therapy* (6th ed.). Belmont, CA: Wadsworth & Thomson Learning, p. 452.

6 **Answer: 1** Increased fluid needs are indicated for a client who has burn injuries due to release of plasma fluids through tissue destruction. All of the other options reflect clinical conditions that require a decrease in fluid needs.

Cognitive Level: Application **Client Need:** Physiological Integrity: Physiological Adaptation **Integrated Process:** Nursing Process: Analysis **Content Area:** Adult Health: Integumentary **Strategy:** Systematically evaluate each condition, recognizing fluid is retained in the conditions in options 2 and 4 and eliminate them. Recall the extensive fluid losses and shifts that occur in burn injuries to direct you to option 1. **Reference:** Cataldo, C., DeBruyne, L., & Whitney, E. (2003). *Nutrition and diet therapy* (6th ed.). Belmont, CA: Wadsworth & Thomson Learning, p. 690.

7 **Answer: 4** A clinical diagnosis of gout is associated with high uric acid levels in the body. Uric acid represents the end product of purine catabolism in the body; therefore, foods that are high in purines should be avoided. Anchovies are high in purine. All of the other options represent diet selections that are low in purine.
Cognitive Level: Application **Client Need:** Health Promotion and Maintenance **Integrated Process:** Nursing Process: Evaluation **Content Area:** Foundational Sciences: Nutrition **Strategy:** The critical word is *gout.* Recall physiology of this metabolic disorder and need to restrict foods high in purines to choose option 4. **Reference:** LeMone, P., & Burke, K. (2004). *Medical surgical nursing: Critical thinking in client care* (3rd ed.). Upper Saddle River, NJ: Pearson/Prentice Hall, p. 1235.

8 **Answer: 24** The bag of TPN solution is changed every 24 hours. By reducing the number of times the TPN tubing needs to be connected and disconnected from the central venous catheter, the risk of infection is reduced, especially since high glucose levels in TPN can lead to bacterial growth.
Cognitive Level: Application **Client Need:** Health Promotion and Maintenance **Integrated Process:** Nursing Process: Implementation **Content Area:** Foundational Sciences: Nutrition **Strategy:** This question requires knowledge of factual information. Consider the common procedure for TPN bag changes to formulate a response. **Reference:** Nix, S. (2005). *Williams' basic nutrition & diet therapy* (12th ed.). St. Louis, MO: Elsevier Mosby, pp. 417–422.

9 **Answer: 3** A client being treated for dyslipidemia has an abnormal lipid profile that is high in cholesterol and triglycerides. The client needs a diet low in saturated fats with an increase in monounsaturated fats, small amounts of PUFA, and restricted sodium and hydrogenated food products. Option 1 is incorrect because high intake of PUFAs will cause a further increase in lipid levels. Option 2 is incorrect because protein-controlled diets are usually indicated for clients who have renal disease. Option 4 is incorrect because monounsaturated fats should be increased, not decreased.
Cognitive Level: Application **Client Need:** Health Promotion and Maintenance **Integrated Process:** Nursing Process: Implementation **Content Area:** Foundational Sciences: Nutrition **Strategy:** A critical word is *dyslipidemia.* Recall saturated fats contribute to lipid formation to eliminate options 1, 2, and 4. **Reference:** LeMone, P., & Burke, K. (2004). *Medical surgical nursing: Critical thinking in client care* (3rd ed.). Upper Saddle River, NJ: Pearson/Prentice Hall, pp. 812, 814.

10 **Answer: 2** MAO inhibitor drug therapy can be complicated by excess intake of foods are high in tyramine (an intermediate product of amino acid metabolism), such as chocolate and cheese. These can alter drug action, resulting in hypertensive crisis. Although all of the other options are also important, they are not the priority consideration when assessing a client on MAO therapy.
Cognitive Level: Analysis **Client Need:** Health Promotion and Maintenance **Integrated Process:** Nursing Process: Assessment **Content Area:** Foundational Sciences: Nutrition **Strategy:** Critical words are *rationales* and *MAO inhibitors.* Note option 1 does not address the medication to eliminate it. Eliminate option 3 since allergies are not the problem, and eliminate option 4 because it is too general. **Reference:** Cataldo, C., DeBruyne, L., & Whitney, E. (2003). *Nutrition and diet therapy* (6th ed.). Belmont, CA: Wadsworth & Thomson Learning, p. 403.

Posttest

1 **Answer: 2** Clients should have a transition period from TPN to oral feedings. The GI tract will need time to adjust, and the client may experience some GI upset, so TPN is not stopped abruptly. Restriction to ice chips would not be necessary; diet can be resumed starting with fluids or as tolerated. The client may not eat sufficient calories during the day, so rate of TPN is usually tapered, rather than only infusing it at nighttime.
Cognitive Level: Application **Client Need:** Health Promotion and Maintenance **Integrated Process:** Nursing Process: Planning **Content Area:** Foundational Sciences: Nutrition **Strategy:** The core concept of the question is transitioning from TPN to oral intake. Recall the bowel has not been metabolizing food for 3 weeks while client was NPO. Recognize the need to ease the transition and associate the word *gradually* in option 2 to this process. **Reference:** Lutz, C., & Przytulski, K. (2006). *Nutrition and diet therapy: Evidence-based applications* (4th ed.). Philadelphia: F.A. Davis, pp. 318–319.

2 **Answer: 2** TPN solutions should be changed every 24 hours in order to prevent bacterial overgrowth due to hypertonicity of the solution. Option 1 is incorrect—medication therapy can continue during TPN therapy. Option 3 is incorrect—flushing is not required for TPN administration. Option 4 is incorrect because the initiation of TPN does not require a client to remain on bed rest during therapy. However, other clinical conditions of the client may affect mobility issues and warrant the client's being on bed rest.
Cognitive Level: Application **Client Need:** Physiological Integrity: Physiological Adaptation **Integrated Process:** Nursing Process: Planning **Content Area:** Foundational Sciences: Nutrition **Strategy:** Review principles related to administration of TPN and recognize the actions in options 1, 3, and 4 are not necessary. Recall any intravenous solution should be changed after 24 hours to choose option 2. **Reference:** Rolfes, S., Pinna, K., & Whitney, E. (2006). *Understanding normal and clinical nutri-*

tion (7th ed.). Belmont, CA: Wadsworth & Thomson Learning, pp. 676–680.

3 **Answer: 1** TPN solutions are hypertonic, hyperosmolar solutions that lead to an increased glycemic load. In response to this hyperglycemia, often a sliding scale insulin (with regular insulin) is used to restore, prevent, or control the effects of the hyperglycemia. Options 2 and 3 are incorrect because the TPN rate is individualized to the client and should not be adjusted unless directed by the physician because of changes in the client's clinical conditions. Option 4 is incorrect—only regular insulin is used as an additive in TPN solutions.
Cognitive Level: Application **Client Need:** Physiological Integrity: Physiological Adaptation **Integrated Process:** Nursing Process: Implementation **Content Area:** Foundational Sciences: Nutrition **Strategy:** Note options 2 and 3 are opposite and require a physician's order to eliminate them. Recognize regular insulin is the only insulin that can be given intravenously and eliminate option 4. Recall the high glucose content of TPN to direct you to option 1. **Reference:** Rolfes, S., Pinna, K., & Whitney, E. (2006). *Understanding normal and clinical nutrition* (7th ed.). Belmont, CA: Wadsworth & Thomson Learning, p. 683.

4 **Answer: 3** Elemental formulas represent predigested formulations of macronutrients that are beneficial to clients with severe digestive or absorption problems. Option 1 is incorrect—modular formulas are not nutritionally complete because they provide only one nutrient source. Options 2 and 4 represent intact protein sources that are not suitable for a client with digestive or absorptive problems.
Cognitive Level: Application **Client Need:** Physiological Integrity: Physiological Adaptation **Integrated Process:** Nursing Process: Planning **Content Area:** Foundational Sciences: Nutrition **Strategy:** Critical words are *severe digestive problems* and *absorption.* Recall content of the various formulas in the options, noting the client has severe problems and option 1 contains only 1 nutrient source. If you had difficulty with this question, review content of the various nutritional formulas. **Reference:** Rolfes, S., Pinna, K., & Whitney, E. (2006). *Understanding normal and clinical nutrition* (7th ed.). Belmont, CA: Wadsworth & Thomson Learning, p. 754.

5 **Answer: 3** Avoidance and restriction of food items known to cause allergies is the most effective way to prevent the development of potential food allergies. Option 1 is incorrect—even small amounts of "allergic" food items can trigger a response (sensitizing—challenging dose). Option 2 is incorrect—increasing fluids does not affect allergy development. Option 4 is incorrect because the use of antihistamine medication may alleviate symptoms of allergic responses but should not be used as a prophylactic measure in assisting dietary selection.
Cognitive Level: Application **Client Need:** Health Promotion and Maintenance **Integrated Process:** Nursing Process: Implementation **Content Area:** Foundational Sciences: Nutrition **Strategy:** The core concept is avoidance of food allergens. Eliminate options 1 and 4 since they are unsafe advice. Recognize option 2 is not true so eliminate it. **Reference:** Rolfes, S., Pinna, K., & Whitney, E. (2006). *Understanding normal and clinical nutrition* (7th ed.). Belmont, CA: Wadsworth & Thomson Learning, p. 527–528.

6 **Answer: 4** Milk and milk products are limited in low-residue diets. All of the other diet selections can be used for this type of diet and indicate client understanding.
Cognitive Level: Application **Client Need:** Health Promotion and Maintenance **Integrated Process:** Nursing Process: Evaluation **Content Area:** Foundational Sciences: Nutrition **Strategy:** A critical term is *low-residue.* Recall knowledge of residue and systematically eliminate options 1, 2, and 3. **Reference:** Rolfes, S., Pinna, K., & Whitney, E. (2006). *Understanding normal and clinical nutrition* (7th ed.). Belmont, CA: Wadsworth & Thomson Learning, p. 612.

7 **Answer: 3** Presence of bowel sounds accompanied by passage of flatus indicates gastric motility and return of "normal" GI functioning. Option 1 is incorrect—postoperative clients are progressed in diet to assist in the restoration of "normal" bowel activity. A bowel movement is not the initiating factor for diet progression. Option 2 is incorrect—abdominal distention may indicate a potential problem affecting GI motility. Option 4 is incorrect—even though client hunger may be present, it is not the deciding factor in diet progression.
Cognitive Level: Application **Client Need:** Physiological Integrity: Reduction of Risk Potential **Integrated Process:** Nursing Process: Evaluation **Content Area:** Foundational Sciences: Nutrition **Strategy:** Critical words are *progression of diet* and *postoperative.* Recall peristalsis is temporarily stopped secondary to anesthesia. Determine safety to begin feeding is present with return of peristalsis, indicated by passage of flatus and bowel sounds to direct you to option 3. **Reference:** LeMone, P., & Burke, K. (2004). *Medical surgical nursing: Critical thinking in client care* (3rd ed.). Upper Saddle River, NJ: Pearson/Prentice Hall, p. 187.

8 **Answer: 4** A full liquid diet contains all food items found on a clear liquid diet plus dairy products and prepared liquid formulas. Options 1 and 2 represent selections that are only found on a clear liquid diet. Option 3 represents a selection found on a low-residue diet.
Cognitive Level: Application **Client Need:** Physiological Integrity: Physiological Adaptation **Integrated Process:**

Nursing Process: Implementation **Content Area:** Foundational Sciences: Nutrition **Strategy:** The core concept in the question is a full liquid diet. Eliminate options 1 and 2 since they reflect clear liquids. Eliminate option 3 since it contains a solid food. **Reference:** LeMone, P., & Burke, K. (2004). *Medical surgical nursing: Critical thinking in client care* (3rd ed.). Upper Saddle River, NJ: Pearson/Prentice Hall, p. 417.

9 **Answer: 4** Transition (or progressive) diets are used on a short-term basis to help the client move toward resumption of a regular diet pattern. A transition diet can progress rapidly from one meal to the next if the client tolerates the feedings. Option 1 is incorrect because a transition diet is not given on a long-term basis. Even though option 2 includes meal planning and diet selection techniques, this is not the primary focus in establishing a plan of care for this client in this short-term therapy. Option 3 is important, but again, it is not the primary focus for this short-term therapy.
Cognitive Level: Analysis **Client Need:** Health Promotion and Maintenance **Integrated Process:** Nursing Process: Planning **Content Area:** Foundational Sciences: Nutrition **Strategy:** The critical words are *primary focus* and *transitional diet.* Note the similarity in the word *transition* in the question with the word *temporary* in option 4. **Reference:** Cataldo, C., DeBruyne, L., & Whitney, E. (2003). *Nutrition and diet therapy* (6th ed.). Belmont, CA: Wadsworth & Thomson Learning, p. 452.

10 **Answer: 2** Most clients with lactose intolerance can tolerate ½ cup milk at one time, and it provides a calcium source. Option 1 is incorrect—elimination of all dairy products can lead to significant clinical deficiencies of other nutrients and may not be necessary. Option 3 is incorrect because drinking milk on an empty stomach can exacerbate clinical symptoms. Drinking milk with a meal may benefit the client because other foods (especially fat) may decrease transit time and allow for increased lactase activity. Option 4 is incorrect because although individual tolerance should be acknowledged, spreading out the use of known dairy products will usually exacerbate clinical symptoms.
Cognitive Level: Analysis **Client Need:** Physiological Integrity: Physiological Adaptation **Integrated Process:** Nursing Process: Planning **Content Area:** Foundational Sciences: Nutrition **Strategy:** The critical words are *mildly intolerant.* Recognize the information in options 3 and 4 would not be recommended to eliminate them. Recall small amounts may be tolerated to choose option 2. **Reference:** LeMone, P., & Burke, K. (2004). *Medical surgical nursing: Critical thinking in client care* (3rd ed.). Upper Saddle River, NJ: Pearson/Prentice Hall, p.666.

References

Cataldo, C., DeBruyne, L. K., & Whitney, E. (2006). *Nutrition and diet therapy* (7th ed.). Belmont, CA: Wadsworth, pp. 495–529.

Dudek, S. G. (2006). *Nutrition essentials for nursing practice* (5th ed.). Philadelphia: Lippincott, pp. 415–451.

Grodner, M., Anderson, S. L., & DeYoung, S. (2005). *Foundations and clinical applications of nutrition: A nursing approach* (3rd ed.). St. Louis, MO: Mosby, pp. 399–440, 499–524.

Kozier, B., Erb, G., Berman, A. J., & Burke, K. (2004). *Fundamentals of nursing: Concepts, process, and practice* (7th ed.). Upper Saddle River, NJ: Prentice Hall, pp. 1116–1120, 1139–1164.

LeMone, P., & Burke, K. (2004). *Medical-surgical nursing: Critical thinking in client care* (3rd ed.). Upper Saddle River, NJ: Prentice Hall, pp. 655–657.

Lutz, C., & Przytulski, K. (2006). *Nutrition and diet therapy* (4th ed.). Philadelphia: F. A. Davis, pp. 172–175, 273–291, 318–322, 477–479.

McClere, S. A., Lukan, J. K., Stefzker, J. A. (2005). Poor validity of residual volumes as a marker of risk for aspiration in critically ill patients. *Critical Care Medicine, 33,* 449–450.

Nix, S. (2005). *Williams' basic nutrition and diet therapy* (12th ed.). St. Louis: Elsevier Mosby, pp. 411–430.

Rolfes, S., Pinna, K. F. Whitney, E. (2006). (1998). *Understanding normal and clinical nutrition* (7th ed.). Belmont, CA: Wadsworth, pp. 611–620, 650–690.

Nutritional Supplements and Weight Control Issues

9

Chapter Outline

Phytochemicals
Herbal Therapies
Nutritional Supplements
Nursing Responsibilities
Weight Control Issues

Objectives

- Explore the concept of phytochemicals and their use in the body to promote nutritional balance and disease-altering capabilities.
- Explain the concept of herbal therapies as a form of alternative medicine (integrative/complementary therapy).
- Review the importance of performing a thorough nutritional assessment, including use of herbal supplements and over-the-counter preparations, as they may substantially impact the client's health status.
- Describe the use of nutritional supplements to boost an individual client's nutrient levels.
- Identify specific treatments that can promote weight control in a client.

NCLEX-RN® Test Prep

Use the CD-ROM enclosed with this book to access additional practice opportunities.

Review at a Glance

adjunctive therapy treatment or medication that is used to exert a different effect than the primary indication but can be equally effective in reaching treatment goals

alternative therapy medical treatment that is not based on standards of osteopathy or allopathic medicine and as such may not have demonstrated efficacy supported by clinical research

complementary therapy term used to note the combination of alternative and traditional medical treatments in a holistic approach; the new term being used to describe this therapy is integrative therapy

ergonomic aids supplements that are used to enhance work performance, muscle growth, and endurance

functional foods food items that correlate with health benefits

herbal therapies therapies that consist of plants to promote health and prevent disease

integrative therapy newer term used to note the combination of alternative and traditional medical treatments in a holistic approach

leptin a protein hormone identified with obesity that influences energy requirements and satiety

malnutrition a state of under- or over-nutrition whereby there are adverse metabolic consequences to the body

nutraceuticals a term used to note natural products (botanicals and phytomedicine) that provide nutrient/health benefits

nutritional supplements additional products that are included in the diet to provide sources of nutrients, they can be available in several packaged forms ranging from capsules to separate food product items

obesity a BMI index of > 30 without co-morbid conditions and a BMI index of ≥ 27 with co-morbid conditions, increased weight and fat stores in excess of normal expected body mass index

phytochemicals nonnutrient chemical substances found in plants that provide health benefits

underweight a BMI index of < 18.5 that presents with health consequences; a weight that is less than expected based on body frame, height, age, and activity

very low kcalorie diet (VLCD) a clinical treatment diet used under close supervision to effect weight loss that consists of specified calorie and nutrient intake

visceral protein stores stores of protein in the body that reflect the amount of protein in the internal organs

PRETEST

1 A 53-year-old male comes to the clinic for a routine physical examination. During the intake screening, the nurse notes the client's weight is 216 pounds and height is 66 inches. The body mass index (BMI) is calculated at 35. The nurse interprets that the client's weight:

1. Is within normal limits, so a weight reduction diet is unnecessary.
2. Is lower than normal, so education about nutrient dense foods is needed.
3. Indicates obesity so weight reduction and exercise are needed.
4. Indicates an overweight status, so dietary modification and exercise are needed.

2 When evaluating a client for malnutrition, the nurse utilizes which of the following to provide information about the client's nutritional status?

1. Triceps skin fold measurement
2. Fasting blood glucose level
3. Hemoglobin A1c level
4. Serum lipid profile results

3 A client states that he has been told ketchup is a beneficial food and asks how can this be true. What would be the nurse's best response to answer the client's concern?

1. "Ketchup is considered to be a food enhancer and intensifies taste perception."
2. "Ketchup contains lycopene, which has been shown to be effective against heart disease and prostate cancer."
3. "Ketchup contains sodium, which provides health benefits."
4. "Ketchup provides a fiber source in the diet that protects against cancer."

4 The nurse interprets that which of the following clients is at increased risk to develop obesity?

1. A client with decreased visceral fat stores in the abdomen
2. A waist-to-hip ratio of greater than 1.0 in a male client
3. A BMI of 19 in a female client
4. A male client who is 6 feet tall and weighs 162 pounds

5 A client has heard information about functional foods and asks how he can include them in his diet. Which of the following suggestions should the nurse provide?

1. Increase milk in the diet.
2. Limit refined food products in the diet.
3. Use vegetables as main dish ingredients.
4. Season food to taste with salt.

6 The nurse would make which of the following responses when questioned by a client about the role of leptin in the body?

1. "It increases food intake in clients of normal weight, thereby promoting obesity."
2. "It assists in the regulation of steroid hormones."
3. "It increases the total fat mass of people who are obese."
4. "It decreases the total fat mass in the body of those who are obese."

7 The nurse is assessing a client who is taking orlistat (Xenical) for weight reduction. The nurse suspects incorrect use of the drug when the client reports which of the following?

1. Increasing fluid intake to 8–10 glasses /day
2. Having urgent bowel movements since starting the medication
3. Taking fat-soluble vitamin supplements 2 hours after the medication
4. Taking the medication with meals and following a low-fat diet

8 When performing a nutritional assessment on a female client, which of the following data would indicate to the nurse the client is underweight?

1. A body mass index (BMI) of 22
2. Being 0.5% above ideal body weight (IBW)
3. A waist/hip ratio of less than 0.8
4. A BMI of 18

9 The nurse determines which one of the following clients should consider pharmacotherapy for the treatment of obesity?

1. A 20-year-old college student who wants to lose weight quickly
2. A 32-year-old male with a history of dieting for the past 6 months who has lost 20 pounds
3. A 28-year-old female who has been trying unsuccessfully to lose weight for 6 months following lifestyle and exercise changes
4. A 12-year-old adolescent female who is tired of being overweight and does not have a social network of supportive friends.

10 A client with renal insufficiency expresses interest in starting a low-carbohydrate (CHO) diet. The nurse discourages the client from doing so, recognizing it could have which of the following implications?

1. As long as the client eats a minimum of 30 grams of CHO/day, there should be no problem.
2. The client's clinical condition is a contraindication to starting a low CHO diet.
3. Calcium supplements should be utilized to prevent the development of osteoporosis while on a low CHO diet.
4. As long as the client eats foods that are high biologic protein sources, there will be no problems with following a low CHO diet.

See pages 281–283 for Answers and Rationales.

I. PHYTOCHEMICALS

A. Definitions and descriptions

1. **Phytochemicals** are the nonnutrient chemical substances found in plants that correlate with health benefits in disease treatment and prevention
2. The term **functional foods** refers to food items (nutrients) that correlate with health benefits; this is a newer term being used to assess the therapeutic effects of foods that contain phytochemicals
3. **Nutraceuticals** refers to naturally made products consisting of botanicals and phytomedicine; this is a newer term that is being used to bridge the gap between nutrient, nonnutrient, and chemical (it is not recognized by the FDA at this time)

! B. Indications for use and availability

1. Some phytochemicals function as antioxidants and may be effective in cancer prevention (breast, lung, prostate, and stomach), decreasing risk of cardiac disease, osteoporosis, macular degeneration, and alleviation of menopausal symptoms
2. Phytochemicals are found in plant sources (fruits and vegetables), whole grains, tea, and soy products
3. Many foods contain several phytochemicals and therefore can exert multiple effects on many body systems
4. A good way to increase fruits and vegetables in the diet (as they contain phytochemicals) is by using them as main ingredients, snack items, and alternate food selections (to try new choices in the diet)

C. Types of phytochemicals

1. Carotenoids
   a. Found in colorful fruits and vegetables that are green, orange, red, and yellow in color
   b. Chemical classification includes beta-carotene and lycopene (found in tomatoes and tomato products, such as sauces and ketchup); they function as both a prooxidant and antioxidant
   c. Health benefits include retinal protection, decreased risk of coronary artery disease (CAD), lung, prostate and breast cancers, with enhanced immune effects in elderly clients
2. Indoles
   a. Found in vegetables such as broccoli, cauliflower, cabbage, and kale
   b. Chemical classification includes organosulphur compounds; they are members of the cruciferous vegetable family
   c. Health benefits include hormone stimulation to make estrogen less effective, therefore decreasing the risk of nonhormone-dependent breast cancer and protection against carcinogen development by influencing DNA enzyme activity
3. Isoflavones
   a. Found in soy foods (tofu, soy milk, and soybean products), and black and green tea
   b. Chemical composition includes phenylpropanoids that include the flavonoid group (also found in nuts, wine, and oregano)
   c. Health benefits include inhibition of cancer cell growth (breast, prostate, and endometrial), alleviation of menopausal symptoms, and prevention of osteoporosis by increasing bone density

Practice to Pass

Compare and contrast phytochemicals, functional foods, and nutraceuticals in the treatment of health problems.

4. Phenolic acids
   a. Found in coffee beans, fruits and vegetables, green tea, wine, and soybeans
   b. Chemical structure includes phenylpropanoids, which act as antioxidants and bind metals to promote excretion of carcinogenic substances
   c. Health benefits include decreased risk of certain cancers (skin, lung, and stomach) and beneficial effect on glycemic control
5. Terpones
   a. Found in the oil of citrus fruits, lemon peel, and menthol
   b. Chemical structure includes isoprenoid
   c. Health benefits include protection against carcinogens
6. Phytoestrogens
   a. Found in vegetables, plants, soybeans, and whole grain fruits and berries
   b. Chemical structure falls under the phenylpropanoids and specifically includes isoflavones and lignans
   c. Health benefits include protection against cardiac disease, cancer prevention (breast and prostate), and prevention of osteoporosis
7. Catechins
   a. Found in teas
   b. Chemical structure includes phenylpropanoids; they are rich in phenolic acid
   c. Health benefits include possible antioxidant activity, prevention of cancer, and anti-hypertensive effects

! **D. Health applications**

1. Antioxidant function and cancer prevention ability have led to great interest and continued research in the area of phytochemicals as a "natural" approach to therapeutic treatment
2. The recommendation is to increase fruits and vegetables in the diet to at least 5 servings daily
3. The "natural" approach of including functional foods that provide phyto-chemicals to the body can be incorporated into one's lifestyle
4. Phytochemicals are being used as part of therapeutic treatment in clients with cancer, CAD, and hypercholesterolemia
5. Dietitians can assist in selection of food products that contain phytochemicals
6. **Alternative therapies** or **complementary/integrative therapy** are terms used to denote therapeutic treatment that is not based on a conventional medical model
   a. Many recognized forms of alternative therapies are utilized by clients, such as acupuncture, chiropractic, herbal supplement use, homeopathy, and naturopathy
   b. In the realm of nutritional therapeutics herbal, botanical, and nutritional supplements are considered to be forms of alternative therapies (see section to follow)
   c. Since many clients are now utilizing alternative therapies, it is critical for the nurse as a member of the healthcare team to be aware of these possible therapies

II. HERBAL THERAPIES

A. Definitions and descriptions

1. The term refers to the inclusion of plant products packaged as dietary supplements to treat medical health problems
2. An alternate term such as botanical therapies may be more inclusive because it includes herbs, stems, roots, and shrubs
3. Some herbals/botanicals have provided the basic structure for recognized drug products (e.g., morphine comes from the opium poppy)
4. Regulation of herbal therapies when packaged as dietary supplements is under the jurisdiction of the FDA
5. Alternative/complementary/integrative therapy
   a. Is the inclusion of alternate healing methods that are not based on conventional medical models to treat health problems
   b. Integrative therapies are receiving attention in public, medical, and nursing schools because many reflect the diversity of cultural beliefs
   c. Herbal therapy can be included as a form of alternative therapy

! B. Indications for use and availability

1. They are used to treat many common health complaints and disease states ranging from headaches to clinical depression
2. Their availability in natural food products, packaged supplements, and OTC preparations can lead to confusion about reliable sources and bioavailability
3. Since this is a developing field, additional interest and research is being generated to obtain a more standardized approach to labeling and stricter regulation of products; it is important for consumers to be educated on the research, best brands, and contraindications
4. See Box 9-1 for general considerations for use of herbal therapies

Practice to Pass

What teaching would be warranted for a client who wants to start taking an herbal product for health benefit?

C. Types of herbals (see Table 9-1 (p. 268) for a selected listing of herbals and dosages)

1. St. John's wort (*Hypericum perforatum*)
   a. Used for emotional and mood support in the treatment of anxiety and depression (mild and moderate depression) along with other therapy and nerve and wound healing
   b. This should not be used for severe clinical depression or bipolar disorder; it is not considered to be a monotherapy treatment
   c. Photosensitivity can be seen with the use of this herbal
   d. It is available in several different types of preparations, including capsules, tea, tinctures, and topicals
2. Gingko (*Ginkgo biloba*)
   a. Health claims include increased cerebral circulation (vasodilation), decreased blood viscosity and dementia, improved peripheral vascular status, reduced asthma symptoms, and relief of vertigo
   ! b. Drug interactions can occur with anticoagulants, aspirin, and nonsteroidal anti-inflammatory drugs (NSAIDs) when used in combination; also increases bleeding
   c. It is available in several different preparations ranging from capsules and tinctures to extracts with varying recommended dosages for desired effect

Box 9-1

General Considerations for Herbal Therapies

- It is important that all members of the healthcare team be knowledgeable about the use of herbal products.
- It is important to read labels regarding product information, dosages, indications for use, side effects, and contraindications.
- This type of therapy is often self-initiated by the client; it is important that any kind of herbal therapy be included in the client's health history.
- Herbal products are available in several different forms (capsules, tinctures, teas, and topicals), each with defined dosages and applications.
- Many herbal products require several weeks before their health benefits are recognized.
- Both the client and healthcare practitioners must keep current with information related to herbal therapy use.
- If a client is scheduled for surgical procedures, it is important that all herbal therapies be stopped for at least 2 to 3 weeks prior to minimize potential complications from anesthesia induction and blood pressure changes. The Board of Anesthesiologists has made this recommendation.
- It is important to note that the client may have health problems and/or potential drug interactions that may preclude the usage of certain herbal therapies.
- The client should be encouraged to contact his or her healthcare provider before starting any herbal therapy.
- Regulation and standardization of herbal therapies is not firmly established in the United States; however, in Germany, the German Commission E regulates botanical therapies in that country. In the United States, specific labeling laws (DSHEA—Dietary Supplement Health Education Act of 1994) address specific regulations concerning the labeling requirements for dietary supplements.

3. Garlic (*Allium sativum*)
   - a. Health claims include lower cholesterol and triglyceride levels, inhibition of platelet function, antimicrobial activity, and lowering of blood pressure
   - ! b. Drug interactions can be seen when taken with anticoagulants (increased risk of bleeding) and antiplatelet agents (potentiated activity)
   - c. It is available in several different forms, ranging from capsules to individual food source (cloves)
4. Echinacea (*Echinacea angustifolia, Echinacea purpurea, Echinacea pallida*)
   - a. Health claims include treating of infections, enhanced immune system function, and managing common cold symptoms
   - b. They are available in several different forms, including capsules, tincture, freeze-dried plants, fluid extract, and powdered extracts
5. Feverfew (*Ranacetum parthenium*)
   - a. Health claims include treatment of migraine headaches and anti-inflammatory activity
   - ! b. Drug interactions are seen with anticoagulants (increased bleeding) and may potentiate activity of antiplatelet agents
   - c. It is available in several different forms including capsules, fresh herbs, and tinctures
6. Valerian (*Valeriana officinalis*)
   - a. Health claims include treatment of sleep disorders (insomnia), decreased menstrual cramping, and minimizing GI symptom complaints

Table 9-1

Selected Herbals and Dosages

Herbal	Dosages*
St. John's wort	Capsule: 300 mg TID (0.3% standard hypericin) Tea: 1 tsp in 8 ounces water (15–20 minutes) Tincture: available; check concentration; normally TID application
Gingko	Capsule: 3 capsules TID (40 mg standard) Tincture: available; check concentration; normally TID application Specific dosages identified for dementia and PVD, vertigo, and tinnitus**
Garlic	Capsule: 500–600 mg TID Food: 1 clove of garlic every day Specific dose identified for lipid-lowering effect**
Echinacea	Capsule: 300–400 mg up to 9 a day Tincture: available; check concentration, 4–6 times a day Available in different forms: freeze-dried, juice, fluid extract, and solid extract
Feverfew	Capsule: 25 mg freeze-dried leaves Fresh herb: 2 servings a day Tincture: available; check concentration; normally TID
Valerian	Capsule: 300–400 mg every day (0.5% standard) Tea: 1 tsp in 8 ounces water (20–30 minutes), 1–3 cups daily Tincture: available; check concentration; normally TID Fluid extract: Check concentration

* Standard Dose Regulations: Based on clinical findings and manufacturer's suggestion. It is important to recognize that all herbal products are not universally standardized, and this may lead to problems with dosage strength and overall clinical effects.

** Check formulary book for specific dosages related to defined health problems.

Herbal forms:

(1) Available in foods.

(2) Teas (infusions) that increase absorption of herbs may have "bad" taste and/or require increased volume for administration that will affect compliance.

(3) Tinctures (composed of ETOH and H_2O)—mixture increases activity of herb, but ETOH ingredient may be a concern.

(4) Fluid extracts (very concentrated) require a smaller dose, yet are usually more potent due to concentration.

(5) Dried extracts (powdered forms) have no taste, can be put in capsules, can have altered bioavailability.

!

b. Drug interactions are seen with other sedatives because it can potentiate drug action

c. It is available in several different forms, including dried root, capsules, fresh tincture, tea, and fluid extract

III. NUTRITIONAL SUPPLEMENTS

A. Definition and descriptions

1. FDA guidelines maintain specific requirements for products to be called nutritional supplements
2. A nutritional supplement is an additional product that is added to the daily diet; it can contain vitamins, minerals, herbs, botanicals, amino acids, and/or enzymes and extracts
3. Also included in this category are **ergonomic aids,** which include a variety of items that are used to enhance body performance and promote muscle growth; (refer to Table 9-2 for a selected listing of ergonomic aids)

Table 9-2

Selected Ergonomic Aids and Indications

Ergonomic Aids	Indications
Anabolic steroids	Body building effects—HARMFUL
Carnitine	Fat burning effect; spares glycogen
Creatinine	Promotes muscle strength and energy
Metabolite	Promote growth and increase muscle mass

- A wide variety of products are being marketed as ergonomic aids. Some of them can cause dramatic side effects.
- Consider the product, the claim, and scientific evidence that supports the use of any product that claims to be an ergonomic aid.
- It is important to read labels and verify accuracy of statements with regard to ergonomic aid products. Certain products can be associated with steroid hormones, such as DHEA (dehydroepiandrosterone), and therefore may pose health concerns for the client.

a. Amino acids are often used to promote anabolism and maintain strength in the form of glutamine and branch chain amino acids (BCAA); protein is increased, often to the level of 1.3–2 grams/day

b. Carbohydrate loading (glycogen loading) consists of high glucose ingestion in relation to intense exercise in order to increase glycogen stores and delay the onset of fatigue

c. Metabolic end products are often used as ergonomic aids (creatine and steroids) in the body

! **4.** Although many products claim to be ergonomic aids, clinical research does not support all of the claims; it is important to evaluate each product prior to using it in order to prevent potential harm and/or determine available benefit

5. Several of the herbals, botanicals, and vitamins already mentioned may fall under these categories, such as arginine

! **B. Indications for use and availability**

1. Nutritional supplements are used to decrease risk of disease, to support the body's increased needs during growth and stress periods, and improve overall body functioning

2. Selected clients who fall into at-risk categories due to life cycle concerns (pregnant or lactating women, children), underlying disease states (illness, stress, or malabsorption), or inadequate intake of nutrients (strict vegans or constant dieters) may need nutritional supplements

3. Supplements are available in several different forms ranging from oral formulations (pills, liquids) and powders to incorporated food substances (such as power bars)

C. Types of supplements

1. Glucosamine–chondroitin

a. Used to treat osteoarthritis

! **b.** Interaction can be seen with sodium warfarin (Coumadin), and it also may affect glucose metabolism

c. This supplement is used with hyaluronic acid and is recognized as an FDA-approved therapy for osteoarthritis in the clinical setting

d. Clinical progress is usually seen following several weeks of therapy

e. Several clinical studies show improvement in pain control with this product

2. Shark cartilage
   a. Used for its "cancer protective" effect, because misleading claims previously stated that sharks do not get cancer—this has been shown to be untrue—but this supplement is still being advocated for its potential anti-cancer action
   b. Available in capsule powders and tablets; has a fishy odor that may be accompanied by a fishy taste
   c. There is no scientific evidence for the use of shark cartilage
3. Metabolite™
   a. Used as an ergonomic aid to boost growth and muscle mass
   b. Is a newer product being advertised and marketed in this field
4. MSM (Methylsulfonylmethane)
   a. Used to treat arthritic pain and for possible autoimmune regulation
   b. Available in powder or tablets; represents a natural organic sulfur compound found in fruits and vegetables
5. Creatine
   a. Used as an ergonomic aid to increase energy balance and exercise endurance
   b. Is reported to be useful in decreasing fatigue, increasing muscle strength and size, and increasing body mass (anabolic effect)
   c. Is effective when used as an accompaniment to short-term exercise (repetitive patterns) because it prevents the build-up of lactic acid
   d. Supported use is related to stimulation of creatine phosphate found in muscle cells that, when increased, can lead to greater performance levels
6. Chromium (chromium picolinate)
   a. Used as an ergonomic aid to increase lean body mass and decrease total body fat
   b. ! Chromium can affect glucose metabolism and, because of this, clients should be advised of potential glycemic reactions
   c. ! There is speculation based on emerging clinical research that chromium in the form of chromium picolinate may be associated with metabolic problems such as renal failure due to greater absorption; clinical research is ongoing in this area related to picolinate portion, long-term usage, and dosing limit
   d. Chromium bound to niacin has a greater bioavailability
   e. Studies show no reduction in weight or fat with use of chromium
7. Arginine
   a. Is a conditional essential amino acid in the body
   b. Is reported to have positive benefits in wound healing and improving immune function and response
   c. ! Evidence promoting arginine as an ergonomic aid is not conclusive but it has been reported that it promotes lean muscle mass

Practice to Pass

What information would you give to a diabetic client who states that he is going to start taking chromium as a nutritional supplement?

IV. NURSING RESPONSIBILITIES

A. Knowledge about new products

1. It is important to read labels and understand information to make sound decisions about whether to incorporate supplements into a diet pattern
2. It is also important to obtain information about the use of nutritional supplements during the hospital admission assessment conducted by a nurse and the comprehensive nutritional assessment conducted by a dietetic professional

Box 9-2

Nutritional Supplement Data That Should Be Assessed in the Health History

- Have you altered your dietary pattern recently?
- Do you include supplements as part of your normal dietary pattern?
- Do you use OTC preparations to help in meeting dietary goals?
- Do you use foods (or supplements) for their health benefits?
- Have you experienced any reactions from any of the supplements that you have been taking?
- How long have you been using supplements?
- Have you realized any health benefits since you started taking the supplements?
- Is your physician aware that you are taking nutritional supplements?

B. Awareness of impact on client's health history and current health status

1. Correlate specific information regarding the use of nutritional supplements (type, dosage, and length of treatment) with client's past medical history (PMH) and current health status
2. Observe/assess for possible effects of supplements and potential drug interactions that may compromise a client's health status
3. Many nutritional supplements are contraindicated for use during pregnancy and lactation; teach clients that even though the supplement may enjoy current popularity with the public, it might not be appropriate for all individuals

C. Communication with healthcare team members

1. Document findings in admission history and nurse's notes about the use of nutritional supplements (this is often found in a newly added section to many hospital admission forms throughout the country—refer to Box 9-2 above for specific questions to ask when obtaining a health history)
2. Initiate discussion and referrals to appropriate members of the healthcare team; coordinate information-sharing about therapies used
3. It is important that all healthcare team members be aware of the medications, treatments, and therapies that their clients are participating in for their potential impact on their overall health status

Practice to Pass

Why is it so important for the nurse to obtain information about the use of nutritional supplements for any client receiving healthcare?

D. Monitoring of client during course of therapy

1. Accurately note trends in results of pertinent laboratory findings when potential drug interactions or side effects are noted
2. Assess client's level of consciousness (LOC), vital signs (VS), and elimination pattern for potential impact
3. Educate clients to report changes in their nutritional supplement practices during the course of medical treatment for its potential impact on health outcomes

V. WEIGHT CONTROL ISSUES

A. Obesity

1. Fat cell development
   a. Fat cell development as a result of hyperplasia (an increase in number of cells) and hypertrophy (an increase in size of cells) leads to increases in fat cell deposition

b. Genetic factors include leptin, uncoupling proteins, and amount of brown/white fat in the body
   1) **Leptin** (ob/ob recessive obesity gene–protein hormone) is expressed in fat cells' coding for the protein that reacts to the percentage of fat cells in the body; leptin works to increase energy expenditure and decrease food intake via hypothalamic control; obese clients have insensitivity or resistance to the effects of leptin; leptin can affect other body hormones such as insulin
   2) Uncoupling proteins refer to specific proteins involved in energy metabolism and fat storage
   3) The amount of brown/white fat in the body correlates with energy production in the form of heat and fat storage in the form of adipose tissue; residents of cold climates and newborns have a higher proportion of brown fat to aid heat retention and body insulation

c. Presence of central obesity (intra-abdominal fat) leads to an increase in the development of obesity because excess fat is converted to LDL in the liver

d. There is an increased risk of obesity associated with smoking, use of alcohol, body frame profile (apple versus pear), and gender issues (postmenopausal females)

e. There is a high correlation between fat intake/composition of diet and increased incidence of obesity; in addition, activity status can impact dietary patterns and weight control

2. Metabolism of obesity

a. Lipoprotein enzyme (LPL) promotes fat storage in both fat and muscle cells by increasing fat cell size and responds to an individual's predetermined set point in helping to maintain body weight; weight loss can trigger LPL activity in an attempt to maintain the body's set point

b. The set point theory proposes that each individual has a specific weight range that the body seeks to maintain; it is based on individual characteristics that are not gender-based and that do not change in response to metabolic or life cycle events

c. An interplay of genetic and environmental factors is most likely responsible for individual patterns of fat development
   1) Social, economic, psychological, and nutritional factors contribute to the presence and development of obesity
   2) Obesity is therefore considered to be a multifactorial phenotypic expression

! 3. Impact of obesity

a. Alterations in glucose metabolism result in decreased insulin sensitivity, high insulin secretion, and impaired glucose tolerance

b. Development of cardiovascular disease occurs, including CAD, HTN, and stroke; overall risk of cardiac events also increases

c. Increasing weight can lead to osteoarthritis and degenerative joint disease

d. An increased incidence of other disease processes occurs, including type 2 diabetes mellitus, cancer, and gallstones

e. An altered body image and psychological profile affect the client both physically and emotionally

4. Diagnosis of obesity
   a. A BMI of 30 or above indicates obesity; 25.0 to 29.9 indicates overweight status; 18.5 to 24.9 is normal; less than 18.5 is underweight
   b. Anthropometric measurements such as triceps skin fold (TSF) measurements and mid-arm circumference (MAC) provide information about skeletal muscle mass and fat stores
   c. Determining the fat distribution profile, looking at the differences between "apple" (intra-abdominal/truncal obesity) and "pear" shape (hips and thighs), and waist-to-hip ratio (> 1.0 in males and > 0.8 in females) can help establish a diagnosis of obesity
   d. Examination of body type aids is diagnosis: endomorph (stocky), ectomorph (tall), and mesomorph (middle range), along with upper body (android) and lower body (gynecoid) categories
   e. Calculation of body weight as ideal body weight (IBW), % usual weight, and determination of recent weight changes also assist in clinical diagnosis
5. Goals of diet therapy
   a. The FDA maintains that goals of dietary therapy are effective when weight loss has been maintained for a period of at least two years
   b. A key goal is to maintain a realistic livable weight based on body mass index
   c. Weight control requires a lifestyle commitment with education, activity, and family support to reach desired goals
   d. Clients who are obese are at risk to develop adverse health consequences; those clients who already have existing co-morbid conditions are at a greater risk than clients who are healthy
6. Types of diets
   a. **Very low kcalorie diet (VLCD)** consists of 800 kcalories, 1 gram high-quality protein/kg of body weight, 50 gram minimum CHO, little or no fat, vitamin and mineral supplements; indicated for short-term use (4 months) under medical supervision
      1) There are limited foods found on this type of diet, focusing on lean meats, fish, poultry, and powdered formulas
      2) Frequent feeding schedule is used in this diet plan
      3) Indicated for clients who have critical weight issues; not recommended for clients who are < 30–40% above IBW
   b. Low-carbohydrate diets may pose a problem for clients because they deplete glycogen stores, promote water loss, use fat as the primary energy source (promote ketosis), promote dehydration, and lead to a decrease in energy
   c. Liquid weight loss diets are often used to effect weight loss and provide 800–1,200 kcalories per day (OTC preparations)
   d. The use of fad diets (not based on sound nutritional principles) can often lead to further health consequences because the client can suffer nutritional deficiencies and be prone to develop weight cycling (yo-yo dieting), which often leads to further weight gain
   e. Lifestyle and behavioral changes are needed in regard to portion-controlled meals and helping the client to distinguish between hunger and food cravings
   f. Goals of diet therapy are aimed at decreasing weight to a healthy level based on client's BMI, activity status, and energy requirements (basal energy expenditure or BEE)

Box 9-3

Clinical Implications for Clients Taking Meridia

- Medication works by inhibiting the uptake of norepinephrine, serotonin, and dopamine.
- Dosage ranges from 10–15 mg PO daily and can be taken with or without food.
- Side effects include dry mouth, anorexia, insomnia, constipation, and increased diastolic blood pressure.
- Medication is contraindicated for clients with cardiac history, renal or liver dysfunction, hypertension, pregnancy, or who are lactating or taking centrally acting appetite suppressant drugs.
- This medication has been approved for use up to 1 year in a monitored weight loss program.

7. Treatment options

a. Medications

1) Sibutramine hydrochloride monohydrate (Meridia) is an FDA-approved centrally acting drug used for long-term treatment of obesity (refer to Box 9-3 for pertinent information about this medication)

2) Orlistat (Xenical) is an FDA-approved peripheral-acting drug used for long-term treatment of obesity (refer to Box 9-4 for pertinent information about this medication)

3) Diuretics, amphetamines, and laxatives are not indicated as effective weight loss regimens due to their potential side effects and interactions that affect fluid and electrolyte balance and elimination patterns

! **b.** Medications used to treat obesity are indicated for clients who are not able to lose 1 pound per week after 6 months of lifestyle changes

c. Nonprescription weight-loss medications (numerous herbal/botanical preparations including St. John's wort and Chitosan) have been used as OTC methods to maintain weight loss; Chitosan has been shown to be ineffective

d. Surgical interventions for obese clients can include gastric bypass, gastric banding, and gastroplasty; clients who undergo these types of procedures must follow specific postprocedure diets (refer to Box 9-5 for surgical procedures for the obese client and Box 9-6 for postoperative concerns for the client who has had gastric surgery)

Box 9-4

Clinical Implications for Clients Taking Xenical

- Medication works by its action as a pancreatic lipase inhibitor and therefore can also inhibit the absorption of fat-soluble vitamins.
- Dosage is 120 mg PO 3 times a day with meals, during meals, or up to 1 hour following meals that contain fat.
- Side effects include rectal incontinence and oily stools that manifest with a sense of urgency.
- If a client is eating high-fat meals, urgent elimination will occur. This can be an indication that the client is not being compliant with the proposed therapy.
- Medication serves as a negative reinforcement as excessive ingestion of fat in the diet can cause a greater incidence of side effects.
- Medication is contraindicated for clients who have chronic food absorption or gallbladder problems or who are pregnant or breastfeeding.
- This medication should not be taken together with cyclosporine or vitamin D and beta-carotene but rather after a 2-hour wait period.

Box 9-5

Surgical Interventions for the Obese Client

- Gastric bypass refers to a surgical procedure that reroutes the path that food normally travels in the body and results in a smaller stomach capacity (direct outlet to the jejunum).
- Gastric banding refers to a surgical procedure that alters the size of the stomach and results in a smaller stomach capacity. This is a form of gastric partitioning whereby the stomach is sectioned into a smaller compartment. Gastric stapling is a surgical procedure that staples sections of the stomach together, thereby decreasing stomach size. These procedures decrease the outlet and delay food passage.
- Gastroplasty refers to any surgical procedure whereby the shape of the stomach is altered.

!

e. Lifestyle/behavioral adaptations are necessary for the obese client and include eating plans that are both realistic and adequate (refer to Box 9-7 on p. 276 for a discussion of realistic eating plans for the obese client)

B. Underweight Client

1. Etiologies

a. Genetic influences can predetermine body structure/frame and, as a result, some individuals can have trouble maintaining weight within "healthy" range

b. An **underweight** client has a BMI < 18.5 and may or may not suffer poor health

c. Physical conditions related to disease processes or as a consequence of medical treatment can lead to development of underweight status

d. FTT (Failure to thrive) infants are defined as failing to meet expected growth curves and developmental milestones and are clinically malnourished; weight and height are below the expected percentile; these infants start out underweight and can proceed to have further weight loss or weight imbalance

e. Psychological conditions (anorexia, bulimia, and depression) can lead to decreased intake and poor nutrition beginning with being underweight and leading to severe health consequences

Box 9-6

Postoperative Concerns for the Obese Client Who Has Undergone Gastric Surgery

- Weight loss is the expectation for all gastric surgeries of this type.
- Complications specific to gastric surgeries include: GI complaints related to eating too much food, possible obstruction, and potential to develop dumping syndrome.
- A specific diet pattern (focusing on food selection and intake pattern) must be followed postoperatively to prevent GI symptoms.
- Consistency of food is altered during the immediate postoperative period and clients should be encouraged to chew all foods adequately, eat small volume meals, and drink the majority of fluids between meals.
- Vitamin supplementation is usually required and the client is closely monitored during the postoperative period to assess for compliance with diet therapy, pattern of weight loss, and potential risk of complications.
- Clients who have had gastric surgery often report a change in taste perception with foods (may taste sweeter) and develop aversions to selected foods (such as red meat).
- Clients who have had gastric surgery may be at risk to develop calcium deficiencies leading to osteoporosis because the absorption of calcium is affected. This can present as a long-term risk and the client should be evaluated for adequate calcium intake.

Box 9-7

Realistic Eating Plans for the Obese Client

- Include client and support members at the beginning of the treatment plan to yield the best results.
- Promote nutritional knowledge by educating client and support members as to what constitutes a healthy eating plan.
- Be aware of portion size—most individuals usually eat amounts greater than a recommended portion size.
- Use visualization of portion sizes to educate client as to what constitutes an average serving (e.g., a deck of cards = 1 serving of meat).
- Pay attention to what you are eating, focusing on good healthy foods that are high in complex CHOs and low in fat. Be aware of hidden food sources that may contain added nutrients (fats, proteins, and CHO), which contribute to weight gain.
- Drink fluids and keep hydrated but be aware of empty calories that can arise from alcohol ingestion.
- Combine physical activity as part of the eating plan, paying attention to not eating the heaviest meal at a time when most sedentary.
- Become restaurant wise by decreasing overall portion intake by sharing foods or bringing half of the portion home. Most restaurant portions are more than one serving.
- Create a reasonable weight loss time frame. It took a long time to gain weight, so it makes sense that it may take time to take the weight off. A key goal is maintaining muscle mass and adequate body stores to achieve a healthy body frame.
- Guidelines to remember: 1 pound of fat = 3,500 kcalories. It is recommended that a loss of ½ to 1 pound a week is a reasonable weight loss pattern.
- Be *realistic!* Set target goals and timeframes that are realistic and attainable.

! **2.** Metabolic concerns for the underweight client
   - **a.** A loss of **visceral protein stores** (body storage) results in negative nitrogen balance
   - **b.** Underweight clients may experience adverse health effects if further compromised because of stress, injury, or infection

! **3.** Goals of diet therapy
   - **a.** Restore weight to a reasonable level based on BMI, height, frame, and energy requirements
   - **b.** Calculate nutrient energy needs to help client reach normal weight range
   - **c.** As weight nears normal range and body stores are replaced, client will have better health outcomes and increased stamina to meet metabolic needs and encountered stresses

! **4.** Nutritional methods to promote weight gain
   - **a.** Increase the intake of calories by establishing a regular meal pattern to promote weight gain
   - **b.** Increase the intake of foods that have high nutrient density (highest kcal/food) in order to meet outcomes
   - **c.** Calculate estimated nutrient needs based on basal energy expenditure
   - **d.** Refer to Box 9-8 for a discussion of a realistic eating plan to promote weight gain

5. Medication therapy
   - **a.** Megestrol acetate (Megace) is an oral progesterone that is used as **adjunctive therapy** to boost appetite

Box 9-8

Realistic Eating Plans for the Underweight Client

- Make sure not to skip meals. It is important to start an eating pattern that is based on eating all scheduled meals.
- Increase portion sizes and add nutrient-dense foods to the eating plan. Now is the time to add on, taste new foods, and sample old foods.
- Drink fluids and make sure to include them as sources of energy by using fruit juices and milkshakes to add to dietary intake.
- Incorporate physical activity in order to maintain muscle tone, gain strength, and promote endurance.
- Supplemental feedings may be required via the enteral route to realize dietary goals.
- Reasonable weight gain expectations should be noted and weight gain over time is more likely to stay on than if one tries to force feed on a daily basis.
- Medications may be prescribed to boost appetite and stimulate weight gain. If experiencing any nausea or other GI symptoms, additional medications may be prescribed to minimize these symptoms so as to allow for an adequate eating pattern.

b. Drobabinol (Marinol) is an antinausea agent that is used as adjunctive therapy to boost appetite

c. These prescribed medications can be used both in the clinical and home setting on a long-term basis

d. Clients who have altered intake and anorexia due to effects of systemic disease such as cancer, HIV, and AIDS use these medications to boost appetite and improve nutritional status

C. Malnutrition

1. Description and etiologies

a. State of poor nutrition whereby either a clinical deficiency or clinical excess exists, leading to compromised nutritional health and metabolic consequences

b. Undernutrition (inadequate dietary intake, increased metabolic demands, or increased nutrient losses) and overnutrition (excess calories or nutrients) can be included in this broad category because they both place metabolic stress on the body

c. Protein-calorie malnutrition (PCM) or protein-energy malnutrition (PEM) is included in this category reflecting specific energy, calorie, and protein deficiency states

d. Hospitalization and contributory disease processes can further exacerbate malnutrition as it affects all systems in the body

! **2.** Metabolic concerns for the malnourished client

a. Loss of visceral protein stores leads to poor growth response

b. Decreased physiological integrity occurs because the body is lacking essential and nonessential nutrients that function as coenzymes in metabolic processes in the body

c. Loss of immune function occurs due to lack of essential/nonessential nutrient function

d. Client may develop fluid shifting due to low protein levels resulting in third spacing (ascites as seen in kwashiorkor) and edema states (dependent and/or periorbital) due to electrolyte imbalances

e. Clients may present with dermatologic changes resulting in brittle hair (that can fall out), nail changes (brittle with ridges), pruritus, impaired healing status, dermatitis, cheilosis, and mucositis

f. The client is prone to develop hormonal imbalances that will affect all body systems including neurologic (irritability, paresthesias, and decreased reflex response), musculoskeletal (decreased muscle tone, cramping, and deformities), and cardiac (altered blood pressure, development of murmurs, cardiac enlargement)

g. A thorough physical examination may reveal clinical evidence of malnutrition (sores, oral cavity changes, and decreased hydration status) and these findings should be established as baseline and used thereafter to trend results of therapy and client's response to treatment

! 3. Goals of diet therapy

a. Restore weight based on BMI, activity, and energy requirements

b. Restore protein levels to replace visceral body stores

c. Maintain appropriate weight to reduce stress on body and prevent further depletion of body stores

! 4. Nutritional methods to improve nutritional status

a. Nutrient calculation is usually done by the dietitian using BEE, BMI, activity level, and pertinent laboratory test results

b. A significant increase in caloric intake is required to effect weight gain; an extra 3,500 kcalories per week is needed for a 1-pound weight gain (results in an extra 500 kcalorie per day)

c. A supervised program is useful to work toward achieving individual client goals

d. Supplemental feedings may be required, using the enteral or parenteral routes in order to achieve client goals

e. A frequent feeding regimen is utilized to prevent hypoglycemia and hypothermia from occurring; these can cause further tissue catabolism to occur

f. A controlled regimen is used for children (not < 80 kcalories/kg/day up to > 100) and for adults (usually 30–40 kcal/kg/day) in order to meet nutritional goals

g. Documentation and trending of pertinent laboratory results and weight status needs to be done and correlated with client's underlying medical condition

D. Health concerns for clients with weight control issues

! 1. Impact of nutritional problems on client's ability to maintain homeostasis

a. Decreased specific nutrient intake can lead to development of nutritional anemias

b. Poor nutrient patterns can contribute to possible disease processes both in short-term and long-term applications

c. Clients with existing co-morbid conditions have an increased risk while trying to obtain nutritional balance as their body system is already compromised due to underlying disease process

d. Malnutrition can result in decreased cardiac output, renal failure, endocrine imbalance (thyroid, glucose), and depressed immune system function

2. Increased stress levels

a. If nutritional stores are inadequate, then the client's body is not able to withstand additional life stressors

b. Release of hormones (catecholamines and epinephrine) can lead to increased metabolic response and energy needs for which the client may be unprepared

3. Baseline nutritional status as a predictor of outcomes
   a. Assess for presence of dietary risk factors that may contribute to cardiovascular disease (high saturated fat and sodium intake)
   b. Assess clients for potential altered glucose metabolism by looking at blood glucose levels, hemoglobin A_{1c} levels, and lipid profiles to establish level of glycemic control
   c. Assess lipid profile to evaluate for potential dyslipidemia, cholesterol, and triglyceride imbalance
   d. Assess dietary intake pattern for evidence of pica that is associated with iron deficiency anemia

Practice to Pass

How can the nurse assist the client in meeting defined weight goals?

4. Weight cycling
   a. "Yo-yo" effect describes a weight loss/weight gain situation in which the client may end up at an even higher weight than when diet therapy was started
   b. This is usually seen in response to unrealistic goals and/or altered dietary patterns without the benefit of activity/lifestyle changes
   c. ! In order for weight control to be effective, there should be a combination of dietary, lifestyle, behavioral, and activity changes to result in changes in overall dietary lifestyle, not merely changes in food intake
5. ! Client teaching aspects
   a. Promote nutritional knowledge for both the client and family support systems
   b. Offer emotional support to client and support system because weight control issues are often of an ongoing nature and client may experience weight cycling
   c. This can be a lifelong problem for the client and family members—weight control issues influence not only the physical demeanor but also the underlying emotional structure
   d. A collaborative healthcare team effort is needed with the client at the center of the multidisciplinary approach; the physician, nurse, dietitian, and family support members provide guidance and encouragement throughout the weight control cycle
   e. Weight control is a multifactorial process; therefore, its evaluation requires a comprehensive therapeutic treatment plan that looks at all factors (refer to Box 9-9 for a listing of weight control factors)

Box 9-9

Weight Control Factors

- Demographics—age, race, gender, culture/geography, religion, genetic influence, and body frame structure
- Dietary—diet composition, intake and output, preferences, dietary habits, and pattern of eating
- Health and disease profile—contributory disease processes and medications (prescriptions and OTC)
- Life cycle issues—recognizing growth periods
- Behavioral and social issues—adaptation and environment
- Recognition of body image factors and use of figure rating scales to allow client to indicate body image perception
- Metabolic rate—activity, stress, and illness
- There usually is an interplay of several factors occurring at any one given time. Even though each factor can be assessed individually, all factors should be evaluated together for their potential impact on the client as a whole.

Case Study

A 28-year-old female client with a significant history of obesity for several years comes to the clinic to get some medication to help her lose weight. Physical exam reveals a BMI of 30 and a review of systems reveals no history of contributory disease.

1. What medications might be indicated for this client?
2. What other information would be relevant before starting medication therapy?
3. What follow-up would be advised for this client?
4. What other factors would be helpful in setting realistic goals for this client with regard to weight loss?
5. The client states that she is "depressed" over her weight status and asks, "Will I always be like this?" How would you respond to this concern?

For suggested responses, see page 320.

POSTTEST

1 The nurse evaluates that an obese client understands the need for a healthy weight loss pattern by indicating an intention to lose:

1. 10 pounds in one month.
2. 5 pounds in one week.
3. 1 pound in one week.
4. 3 pounds in one week.

2 Which of the following statements would the nurse use to best describe a very-low-kilocalorie diet (VLCD) to a client?

1. "This diet is low in calories and high in protein and must be used under close medical supervision."
2. "This is a long-term treatment measure that will assist obese people who can't lose weight."
3. "The VLCD consists of solid food items that are pureed to facilitate digestion and absorption."
4. "A VLCD diet contains very little protein."

3 A 40-year-old female client with a family history of coronary heart disease (CAD) expresses interest in modifying her diet to include foods to reduce associated risk factors. The nurse suggests she increase intake of foods high in carotenoids by including which of the following? Select all that apply.

1. Cauliflower and cabbage
2. Strawberries and oranges
3. Black and green tea
4. Soy products
5. Green peppers and squash

4 When explaining to a group of adolescents why creatine is being suggested as beneficial for athletic performance, the nurse would explain that creatine:

1. Is an efficient fuel source in the body that promotes catabolic effects.
2. Is effective for long-term endurance performance.
3. Decreases lean body mass and increases muscle strength.
4. Assists the body in repetitive short-term activity that requires energy bursts.

5 A client states that he is considering using herbal therapy as a natural source to aid in dietary health. What suggestion should the nurse give to the client to assist with this decision?

1. "Herbal therapy treatments reflect standard doses so all similar products will provide the same biologic effect."
2. "Herbal therapy requires a prescription and may be an expensive treatment modality."
3. "It is important to inform your healthcare practitioner about your choice to start herbal therapy."
4. "Herbal therapy is a natural form of treatment with very few side effects."

6 The diet history of a client receiving anticoagulants indicates the client eats a lot of garlic. The nurse plans to include which of the following information when teaching the client about possible drug–food interactions?

1. Garlic can enhance the coagulation process and accelerate clot formation.
2. Garlic has no effect on blood coagulation.
3. Garlic helps to support immune function but does not affect coagulation.
4. Bleeding can occur because garlic inhibits platelet aggregation.

7 The nurse encourages eating foods high in which of the following phytochemicals as a possible preventive measure for a female client concerned about developing osteoporosis? Select all that apply.

1. Phenolic acids
2. Isoflavones
3. Indoles
4. Carotenoids
5. Phytoestrogens

8 Which of the following does the nurse discuss with the client as a realistic goal for a client who is 5' 6" tall and weighs 250 pounds and is starting a weight loss program?

1. Maintain present physical activity level and decrease caloric intake.
2. Eat only when hungry.
3. Demonstrate understanding of caloric intake, weight control, and physical activity.
4. Maintain an intake of 1,000 calories or less with 30% of calories from fat.

9 Which of the following instructions should the nurse give to a client who takes numerous herbal supplements and is being scheduled for an outpatient surgical procedure?

1. "Take your supplements as usual until the morning of the surgical procedure."
2. "Stop herbal and botanical products at least 2 to 3 weeks prior to the day of surgery."
3. "Maintain usual doses of herbal products and stop 1 day prior to surgery."
4. "Consult with the dietician prior to surgery about effects of herbal therapies."

10 The nurse instructs the underweight client to consume an extra _____ kilocalories per day for a 1 pound weight gain per week? Provide a numerical response.

Answer: ______________________

See pages 283–285 for Answers and Rationales

POSTTEST

ANSWERS & RATIONALES

ANSWERS & RATIONALES

Pretest

1 **Answer: 3** Obesity is defined by BMI of 30 or above with no co-morbid conditions. It is calculated by utilizing a chart-nomogram that plots height and weight. This client's BMI is 35, indicating obesity. The other responses represent inaccurate interpretations of the client's BMI.

Cognitive Level: Analysis **Client Need:** Health Promotion and Maintenance **Integrated Process:** Nursing Process: Assessment **Content Area:** Foundational Sciences: Nutrition

Strategy: Note the question indicates that client has a high weight and is not very tall. This is a clue that options 1 and 3 are incorrect. Recall the categories for BMI to choose between options 3 and 4. **Reference:** Nix, S. (2005). *Williams' basic nutrition and diet therapy* (12th ed.). St. Louis, MO: Elsevier Mosby, p. 268.

2 **Answer: 1** Objective anthropometric measurements such as triceps skin fold and mid-arm circumference (MAC), along with weight, are usually used to diagnose malnutrition. While all of the other choices represent tests that may provide useful information, they also may be affected by variables other than malnutrition.
Cognitive Level: Application **Client Need:** Health Promotion and Maintenance **Integrated Process:** Nursing Process: Assessment **Content Area:** Foundational Sciences: Nutrition **Strategy:** Critical words are *malnutrition, evaluation,* and *nutritional status.* Note options 2 and 3 measure glucose levels only to eliminate them. Recognize option 4 is used to measure coronary artery disease risk and eliminate it. **Reference:** Rolfes, S., Pinna, K., & Whitney, E. (2006). *Understanding normal and clinical nutrition* (7th ed.). Belmont, CA: Wadsworth & Thomson Learning, p. 266.

3 **Answer: 2** Ketchup contains lycopene—a phytochemical that has health benefits. Option 1 is incorrect—it does provide flavor to food products, but does not address the concern about health benefits. Option 3 is incorrect because even though ketchup contains a large amount of sodium, this is not a health benefit and even can be viewed as a "hidden" source of sodium in the diet if used in excess. Option 4 is incorrect—ketchup is not a source of fiber in the diet.
Cognitive Level: Application **Client Need:** Health Promotion and Maintenance **Integrated Process:** Communication and Documentation **Content Area:** Foundational Sciences: Nutrition **Strategy:** The critical word is *beneficial.* Recognize what health and nutritional benefits are provided by lycopene in ketchup to direct you to option 2. **Reference:** Rolfes, S., Pinna, K., & Whitney, E. (2006). *Understanding normal and clinical nutrition* (7th ed.). Belmont, CA: Wadsworth & Thomson Learning, p. 392.

4 **Answer: 2** A waist-to-hip ratio of greater than 1.0 in a male client indicates an increased risk to develop obesity. This indicates a larger amount of abdominal fat and correlates with an apple body shape. Option 1 is incorrect because a decrease in visceral fat stores in the abdomen would improve a client's health status. Option 3 is incorrect—a BMI of 19 is associated with being underweight. Option 4 is incorrect because a male client who is 6 feet tall and 162 pounds has a BMI of 22, which is considered within normal range.
Cognitive Level: Analysis **Client Need:** Health Promotion and Maintenance **Integrated Process:** Nursing Process: Analysis **Content Area:** Foundational Sciences: Nutrition **Strategy:** The critical words are *increased risk* and *obesity.* Recall norms of BMI and waist-to-hip ratio to choose option 2. **Reference:** Rolfes, S., Pinna, K., & Whitney, E. (2006). *Understanding normal and clinical nutrition* (7th ed.). Belmont, CA: Wadsworth & Thomson Learning, p. 265.

5 **Answer: 3** Using vegetables as a main dish ingredient will help to increase the amount of functional foods that have phytochemical activity. Option 1 is incorrect—even though milk is a good source of vitamin D and calcium, it will not by itself increase the amount of functional foods in the diet. While limiting the amount of refined food products is beneficial (option 2), this does not increase the amount of functional foods in the diet. Option 3 is incorrect—seasoning to taste may be important with regard to sodium level; however, it does not specifically relate to functional foods.
Cognitive Level: Application **Client Need:** Health Promotion and Maintenance **Integrated Process:** Nursing Process: Implementation **Content Area:** Foundational Sciences: Nutrition **Strategy:** Specific knowledge of functional foods is required to answer this question. If you cannot recall this material, note the question addresses what food should be included. Eliminate option 2, since the food is eliminated and option 4, since salt is not a food, but a seasoning and electrolyte. **Reference:** Rolfes, S., Pinna, K., & Whitney, E. (2006). *Understanding normal and clinical nutrition* (7th ed.). Belmont, CA: Wadsworth & Thomson Learning, p. 467.

6 **Answer: 3** Leptin is a protein hormone that is secreted by adipose tissue; it is called the obesity gene. Leptin increases the total fat mass in obese clients. Option 1 is incorrect—the presence of leptin usually decreases food intake in normal weight individuals. Option 2 is incorrect because it does not affect the regulation of steroid hormones but does have some effect on insulin release.
Cognitive Level: Application **Client Need:** Health Promotion and Maintenance **Integrated Process:** Teaching and Learning **Content Area:** Foundational Sciences: Nutrition **Strategy:** Specific knowledge of leptin is necessary. If you had difficulty with this question, review content on leptin. **Reference:** Rolfes, S., Pinna, K., & Whitney, E. (2006). *Understanding normal and clinical nutrition* (7th ed.). Belmont, CA: Wadsworth & Thomson Learning, p. 282.

7 **Answer: 2** A side effect of orlistat, a lipase inhibitor that aids in weight loss, is rectal incontinence, and/or oily stools that are associated with urgency. The fact that the client is presenting with complaints of this symptom suggests he or she is not following the treatment regi-

men and is eating high-fat meals. Options 3 and 4 reflect compliance with the treatment regimen. Increasing fluid intake does not affect compliance. Systematically eliminate options 1, 3, and 4 since behaviors are correct.
Cognitive Level: Analysis **Client Need:** Physiological Integrity: Pharmacological and Parenteral Therapies **Integrated Process:** Nursing Process: Evaluation **Content Area:** Foundational Sciences: Nutrition **Strategy:** Note the question asks for an indication that the drug is taken incorrectly, indicating three of the options will have correct information regarding use of orlistat. **Reference:** Adams, M., Josephson, D., & Holland, L. (2005). *Pharmacology for nurses: A pathophysiologic approach.* Upper Saddle River, NJ: Pearson/Prentice Hall, p. 543.

8 **Answer: 4** A BMI of less than 18.5 is considered to represent a client who is underweight and possibly at risk for malnutrition. Option 1 is incorrect because a BMI of 22 is considered within normal range. Option 2 is incorrect—being above IBW is not consistent with being underweight. Option 3 is incorrect because a waist/hip ratio of less than 0.8 in a female client represents a normal finding. It is important for the nurse to be aware of objective anthropometric measurements (both normal and abnormal values) so that the data can be interpreted adequately.
Cognitive Level: Application **Client Need:** Health Promotion and Maintenance **Integrated Process:** Nursing Process: Assessment **Content Area:** Foundational Sciences: Nutrition **Strategy:** The critical word is *underweight.* Eliminate option 2 since it reflects an overweight status. Recall knowledge of BMI to choose option 4. **Reference:** Rolfes, S., Pinna, K., & Whitney, E. (2006). *Understanding normal and clinical nutrition* (7th ed.). Belmont, CA: Wadsworth & Thomson Learning, p. 301.

9 **Answer: 3** Pharmacotherapy for obesity is indicated when a client has been unable to achieve weight loss of 1 pound/week after 6 months of therapy while following lifestyle changes. Option 1 is incorrect—this is not a quick process decision. Option 2 is incorrect because the client has already demonstrated a reasonable weight loss pattern. Option 4 is incorrect—pharmacotherapy is not indicated for an adolescent client.
Cognitive Level: Analysis **Client Need:** Health Promotion and Maintenance **Integrated Process:** Nursing Process: Planning **Content Area:** Foundational Sciences: Nutrition **Strategy:** Critical words are *pharmacotherapy* and *obesity.* Read each stem and determine history of weight loss attempts and risk factors. Eliminate option 1 since this reflects an unhealthy choice. Eliminate option 2 since the client has already lost weight. Choose option 3 since the client has had unsuccessful attempts with other modalities. **Reference:** Rolfes, S., Pinna, K., & Whitney, E. (2006). *Understanding normal and clinical nutrition* (7th ed.). Belmont, CA: Wadsworth & Thomson Learning, p. 300.

10 **Answer: 2** A client with renal insufficiency should not start a low CHO diet—this implies that protein and fat levels will be increased, resulting in an increased renal solute load. Option 1 is incorrect—30 grams of CHO is not enough to spare protein, thereby making fat the primary energy source and leading to the development of ketosis, which will further compromise the client's clinical status. Option 3 is incorrect—osteoporosis is not associated with being on a low CHO diet but rather is due to multifactorial losses involved with calcium. Option 4 is incorrect because a client with renal insufficiency is unable to handle protein. While high biological value sources are warranted, the protein intake must be monitored cautiously to prevent further metabolic imbalances.
Cognitive Level: Analysis **Client Need:** Physiological Integrity: Physiological Adaptation **Integrated Process:** Nursing Process: Evaluation **Content Area:** Foundational Sciences: Nutrition **Strategy:** The critical words are *renal insufficiency* and *low CHO diet.* Recall nutritional needs related to decreased renal function in regards to restriction of protein and need for CHO as a caloric source. **Reference:** Rolfes, S., Pinna, K., & Whitney, E. (2006). *Understanding normal and clinical nutrition* (7th ed.). Belmont, CA: Wadsworth & Thomson Learning, p. 861–864.

Posttest

1 **Answer: 3** A recommended weight loss pattern for the obese client is 0.5 to 1 pound per week. Option 3 offers the best possibility of maintaining weight loss. All of the other options are incorrect because too great a loss may predispose the client to weight cycling or loss of lean body mass.
Cognitive Level: Application **Client Need:** Health Promotion and Maintenance **Integrated Process:** Nursing Process: Evaluation **Content Area:** Foundational Sciences: Nutrition **Strategy:** Critical words are *healthy weight loss.* Recognize that only 0.5 to 1 pound per week is the recommended healthy guideline to direct you to option 3. **Reference:** Rolfes, S., Pinna, K., & Whitney, E. (2006). *Understanding normal and clinical nutrition* (7th ed.). Belmont, CA: Wadsworth & Thomson Learning, p. 292.

2 **Answer: 1** VLCD diets are used in the clinical treatment of obesity under close medical supervision. The diet is low in calories, high in quality protein, and has a minimum of carbohydrates in order to spare protein and prevent ketosis.

Cognitive Level: Application **Client Need:** Health Promotion and Maintenance **Integrated Process:** Teaching and Learning **Content Area:** Foundational Sciences: Nutrition **Strategy:** The critical word is *best,* indicating all or some options may be correct, but one answers the question more thoroughly, as is the case in option 1. **Reference:** Lemone, P., & Burke, K. (2005). *Medical surgical nursing: Critical thinking in client care* (3rd ed.). Upper Saddle River, NJ: Pearson/Prentice Hall, p.525.

3 **Answers: 2, 5** Carotenoids are phytochemicals that have been found to decrease risk of CAD and are found in green, orange, red, and yellow fruits and vegetables. Option 1 is high in indoles. Options 3 and 4 are high in isoflavones.

Cognitive Level: Application **Client Need:** Health Promotion and Maintenance **Integrated Process:** Nursing Process: Implementation **Content Area:** Foundational Sciences: Nutrition **Strategy:** This question requires identification of foods high in carotenoids. If you have difficulty remembering this specific information, the word *carotenoid* is similar to carrots, which are orange in color and would help direct you to options 2 and 5. **Reference:** Lutz, C., & Przytulski, K. (2006). *Nutrition and diet therapy: Evidence-based applications* (4th ed.). Philadelphia: F.A. Davis, p. 98.

4 **Answer: 4** Creatine has been demonstrated to improve the body's response in an exercise pattern consisting of repetitive short-term activities. Option 1 is incorrect—creatine is supposed to promote anabolism, not catabolism. Option 2 is incorrect because creatine has not been proven effective for long-term exercise patterns. Option 3 is incorrect because creatine does not decrease lean body mass.

Cognitive Level: Application **Client Need:** Health Promotion and Maintenance **Integrated Process:** Teaching and Learning **Content Area:** Foundational Sciences: Nutrition **Strategy:** The critical phrase is *beneficial for athletic performance.* Eliminate option 1 since a catabolic effect would be a negative consequence. Recall use of creatine to muscle physiology to choose option 4. **Reference:** Nix, S. (2005). *Williams' basic nutrition and diet therapy* (12th ed.). St. Louis, MO: Mosby, Inc., pp. 301–303.

5 **Answer: 3** It is important to inform the healthcare provider at the start of herbal therapy, because this can prevent problems from potential drug interactions, verify indication for therapy, and acknowledge client's concerns over common complaints. Option 1 is incorrect—it is critical for the client to read all labels in order to be an informed consumer. Even though there are standard products, herbal therapy ingredients can vary in different types of formulations. Option 2 is incorrect—no prescription is required, but herbal therapy can cause a financial burden to the client. Option 4 is incorrect—herbal therapy can cause side effects.

Cognitive Level: Application **Client Need:** Health Promotion and Maintenance **Integrated Process:** Teaching and Learning **Content Area:** Foundational Sciences: Nutrition **Strategy:** Read each option, systematically eliminating those with incorrect information regarding herbal supplements. Recall importance of potential for interactions with herbal and OTC products to direct you to option 3. **Reference:** Rolfes, S., Pinna, K., & Whitney, E. (2006). *Understanding normal and clinical nutrition* (7th ed.). Belmont, CA: Wadsworth & Thomson Learning, p. 633.

6 **Answer: 4** Garlic is a food/herbal product that has long been recognized for its health benefits (lowers cholesterol/triglycerides, improves immune function, and decreases BP). Garlic can inhibit platelet aggregation and therefore prevents blood clot formation. A client who is taking anticoagulation therapy should be advised of potential interactions with excessive amounts of garlic in the diet. Option 1 is incorrect—there is an increased risk of bleeding. Option 2 is incorrect because garlic does indeed affect blood coagulation. Even though garlic does help to support immune function (option 3), this fact does not directly relate to anticoagulation therapy.

Cognitive Level: Application **Client Need:** Physiological Integrity: Pharmacological and Parenteral Therapies **Integrated Process:** Nursing Process: Analysis **Content Area:** Foundational Sciences: Nutrition **Strategy:** Critical words are *garlic* and *anticoagulants.* Recall garlic's effect on clotting function to direct you to option 4. **Reference:** Rolfes, S., Pinna, K., & Whitney, E. (2006). *Understanding normal and clinical nutrition* (7th ed.). Belmont, CA: Wadsworth & Thomson Learning, p. 632.

7 **Answers: 2, 5** Isoflavones and phytoestrogens are deemed beneficial in protecting female clients from developing osteoporosis due to their estrogen-like enhanced effects. Option 1 is incorrect—phenolic acids are effective against cancers because they act as pro-oxidants. Option 3 is incorrect as indoles make estrogen less effective. Option 4 is incorrect—carotenoids are considered to be in the classification of phenolic acids and helps to decrease cancer risks.

Cognitive Level: Application **Client Need:** Health Promotion and Maintenance **Integrated Process:** Nursing Process: Analysis **Content Area:** Foundational Sciences: Nutrition **Strategy:** Critical words are *phytochemicals* and *osteoporosis.* Recall isoflavones and estrogen have a beneficial effect on bones to direct you to options 2 and 5. **Reference:** Nix, S. (2005). *Williams' basic nutrition and diet therapy* (12th ed.). St. Louis, MO: Mosby, p. 118.

8 **Answer: 3** It is important the client demonstrate an understanding of the basics of the treatment program, fo-

cusing on a multifaceted approach of intake, physical activity, and weight control. Each one of these is an interrelated variable that affects the client's ability to achieve and maintain weight control. Option 1 is incorrect because this may not be prudent (physical activity is usually increased). Option 2 is incorrect—it is not wise to utilize this feeding pattern because it may contribute to weight gain. Option 4 is incorrect—the total calories may be somewhat low, but the percentage of calories from fat is too high to effect substantial weight loss.

Cognitive Level: Application **Client Need:** Health Promotion and Maintenance **Integrated Process:** Nursing Process: Planning **Content Area:** Foundational Sciences: Nutrition **Strategy:** Recognize the need to reduce caloric intake as well as increase activity level to eliminate option 1. Eliminate option 2 since it does not provide specific suggestions, and eliminate option 4 since this caloric restriction is unsafe. **Reference:** Nix, S. (2005). *Williams' basic nutrition and diet therapy* (12th ed.). St. Louis, MO: Mosby, pp. 269–272.

9 **Answer: 2** Anesthesiologists recommend that all herbal and botanical preparations be stopped 2 to 3 weeks prior to scheduled surgery in order to minimize possible interactions between anesthesia induction and blood pressure response. Options 1 and 3 are incorrect for the reason just stated. Even though it may be good to discuss herbal therapies with a dietitian (option 4), it is more important to acknowledge that herbal therapies should be stopped prior to scheduled surgeries to minimize anesthesia risks.

Cognitive Level: Application **Client Need:** Physiological Integrity: Reduction of Risk Potential **Integrated Process:** Nursing Process: Implementation **Content Area:** Foundational Sciences: Nutrition **Strategy:** The core concept is preparation for outpatient surgery. Recall many drugs and herbs may take several days to be eliminated from the body to direct you to option 2. **Reference:** Rolfes, S., Pinna, K., & Whitney, E. (2006). *Understanding normal and clinical nutrition* (7th ed.). Belmont, CA: Wadsworth & Thomson Learning, p. 636–638.

10 **Answer: 500** An extra 3,500 kilocalories per week is needed for a 1 pound weight gain (500 kilocalories per day). Weight gain strategies revolve around consuming foods that provide many kilocalories in small volume along with building muscle.

Cognitive Level: Analysis **Client Need:** Health Promotion and Maintenance **Integrated Process:** Nursing Process: Implementation **Content Area:** Foundational Sciences: Nutrition **Strategy:** Focus on critical information of 3,500 kilocalorie = 1 lb of fat. **Reference:** Rolfes, S., Pinna, K., & Whitney, E. (2006). *Understanding normal and clinical nutrition* (7th ed.). Belmont, CA: Wadsworth & Thomson Learning, pp. 302–304.

References

Adams, M., Josephson, D., & Holland, L. (2005). *Pharmacology for nurses: A pathophysiologic approach.* Upper Saddle River, NJ: Pearson/Prentice Hall, p. 543.

Astrup, A., Lawsenton, E. & Harper, A. (2004). Atkins and other low-carbohydrate diets: Hoax or an effective tool for weight loss? Lancet *364,* 897–899.

Cataldo, C., DeBruyne, L. K., & Whitney, E. (2006). *Nutrition for health and health care* (7th ed.). Belmont, CA: Wadsworth, pp. 387–388, 426, 437-410.

Criston, N. V. (2004). Surgery decreases long-term mortality, morbidity, and health care use in morbidly obese patients. *Annals of Surgery, 240,* 416–423.

Dudek, S. G. (2006). *Nutrition essentials for nursing practice* (5th ed.). Philadelphia: Lippincott, pp. 206–240, 371–412.

Foster, G. D., Makris, A. P., & Boiler, B. A. (2005). Behavioral treatment of obesity. *American Journal of Clinical Nutrition, 82* (1 suppl), 2301–2355.

Greenway, F. (2005). Another type of intervention: Treating obesity with medication. *Journal of American Dietetic Association, 105,* 895–897.

Grodner, M., Anderson, S. L., & DeYoung, S. (2004). *Foundations and clinical applications of nutrition: A nursing approach* (3rd ed.). St. Louis, MO: Mosby, pp. 271–303, 396–436, 460–496, 632–652.

LeMone, P., & Burke, K. (2004). *Medical-surgical nursing: Critical thinking in client care* (3rd ed.). Upper Saddle River, NJ: Prentice Hall, p. 525.

Lutz, C., & Przytulski, K. (2006). *Nutrition and diet therapy* (3rd ed.). Philadelphia: F. A. Davis, p. 98.

Nix, S. (2005). *Williams basic nutrition and diet therapy* (12th ed.). St. Louis, MO: Elsevier Mosby, pp. 267–301.

Rolfes, S., Pinna, K. Whitney, E. (2006). *Understanding normal and clinical nutrition* (7th ed.). Belmont, CA: Wadsworth, pp. 626–649.

Super, R. B., Eisenberg, D. M., & Phillips, R. S. (2004). Common dietary supplements forweight loss. *American Family Physician, 70,* pp. 1731–1738.

10 Nutritional Management of the Client with Multisystem Disorders

Chapter Outline

Objectives

- Explain the importance of collaborative management of the client with multisystem disorders.
- Identify common concerns for the nutritional status of the client with multisystem disorders.
- Identify acute and chronic concerns for the client with nutritional multisystem disorders.
- Describe the impact of malnutrition and obesity on clients with multisystem disorders.

NCLEX-RN® Test Prep

Use the CD-ROM enclosed with this book to access additional practice opportunities.

Review at a Glance

acute illness disease process or traumatic event that has a rapid onset, requiring prompt medical attention to restore balance

acute respiratory failure (ARF) clearly defined metabolic parameters ($CO_2 > 50$ mm Hg and/or $O_2 < 60$ mm Hg) whereby immediate intervention is required to sustain ventilation and perfusion

anemia of chronic disease (ACD) anemia associated with the progression of chronic disease processes as a result of decreased erythropoietin production

anticoagulation therapy medical therapy whereby clients receive anticoagulants (blood thinners) to treat or prevent the risk of thromboembolic events

APACHE criteria systematic method that examines physiologic status, age, and presence of chronic disease to monitor the high-acuity client and provide prognostic indicators relative to treatment and outcome

chronic illness disease process that has no defined time limit and is characterized by periods of remission and exacerbations with resultant complications

graft versus host disease (GVHD) disease process that occurs in response to a transplanted organ that leads to acute and chronic changes culminating in possible organ rejection

immunosuppressive therapy utilization of azathioprine, cyclosporine, and prednisone therapy to prevent organ rejection in a client who has received an organ transplant

international normalized ratio (INR) diagnostic standardized laboratory test used to measure the effects of oral anticoagulation therapy

multiple organ dysfunction syndrome (MODS) a continuum disease process that can occur in high-acuity clients that affects multiple organ systems in the body and often leads to vascular collapse and death

polypharmacy use of multiple drug profiles in clients that leads to increased likelihood of drug reactions (DRAPE—drug-related adverse pharmacological events) and hospitalizations

prothrombin time (PT) diagnostic laboratory test that measures activity of the extrinsic clotting pathway, denoting the effects of oral anticoagulant therapy

systemic inflammatory response syndrome (SIRS) inflammatory process that can progress to the development of MODS; occurs through the stimulation of chemical mediators to an initial event

PRETEST

PRETEST

1 A client is admitted to the hospital with an acute painful attack of pancreatitis. The nurse anticipates that which of the following changes will impact nutritional status during treatment of this acute episode?

1. Altered taste perception due to increased pain
2. Inability to eat due to increased pain
3. Potential for gastroparesis to develop due to disease process
4. Weight loss of greater than 10% during management of the acute phase

2 A client with anemia of chronic disease (ACD) is referred for nutritional counseling regarding dietary intake. Which of the following methods would be the most helpful for the nurse to implement in order to meet nutritional goals?

1. Have the client continue to take epoetin alfa (Procrit) as prescribed because that will help to maintain adequate nutritional stores.
2. Have the client consume more calories in order to meet increased nutritional demands.
3. Evaluate client's dietary pattern for nutritional adequacy.
4. Instruct the client on adequate sources of iron in the diet.

3 An unlicensed caregiver asks the critical care nurse why it is so important to assess the nutritional status of a critically ill client on ventilator support, who has just been started on enteral nutritional support. Which of the following items would the nurse consider when formulating a response?

1. Parenteral feeding is associated with a decreased rate of sepsis and mortality.
2. Gastric emptying can be decreased in response to medication and acid-base and fluid/electrolyte imbalances.
3. The use of enteral feeding methods is associated with a decrease in liver function.
4. Enteral feedings lead to a decrease in mucosal blood flow.

PRETEST

4 The nurse would place highest priority on assessing which of the following critically ill clients for complications associated with enteral feedings?

1. A client who is receiving an elemental formula
2. A client receiving full-strength formula feeding in small volumes
3. A client receiving hypertonic enteral nutrition solutions
4. A client who is hemodynamically stable

5 The nurse should plan to monitor which of the following indicators as the most reliable method of assessing the nutritional status of a critically client on a mechanical ventilator who is receiving nutritional support via parenteral therapy?

1. Serum albumin levels
2. Intake and output
3. Daily weight
4. Skin turgor

6 A client with a longstanding history of diabetes, hypertension, and heart failure has been referred for dietary counseling. Which of the following should the nurse do initially?

1. Have the client provide a 3-day food diary at the next scheduled appointment.
2. Obtain a list of all medications currently taken, both prescription and OTC.
3. Obtain vital signs (blood pressure, pulse, and respirations) in order to calculate body mass index (BMI).
4. Ask if the client is satisfied with ease of maintaining current therapies.

7 The nurse would instruct the client taking sodium warfarin (Coumadin) for a deep vein thrombosis (DVT) of the left leg that it is acceptable to continue eating which of the following foods that the client prefers?

1. Broccoli
2. Spinach
3. Corn
4. Tomatoes

8 When caring for a client who has undergone a liver transplant, the nurse should consider which factor when assessing the nutritional status of the client?

1. Use of immunosuppressant drugs, which decreases nutrient needs
2. Nutritional status pre-transplant, which has little influence on post-transplant nutrition.
3. Increased weight, which may not correlate with adequate nutrition.
4. Awareness that no dietary restrictions are needed post-transplant.

9 Which of the following nutritional complications would the nurse assess for in a client with longstanding congestive heart failure (CHF)?

1. Weight gain due to fluid retention
2. Cardiac cachexia
3. An increase in activity tolerance
4. Increased airway clearance

10 Which of the following would be most helpful for the nurse to do when planning for the nutritional management of an obese client with multisystem disorders?

1. Refer to a psychiatrist for counseling.
2. Refer to a physician who specializes in weight disorders.
3. Make sure that the client continues to take all medications ordered to treat disease processes.
4. Discuss dietary meal planning activities with client.

See pages 306–308 for Answers and Rationales.

I. NUTRITIONAL IMPACT ON ACUTE AND CHRONIC DISORDERS

A. Refer to Table 10-1 for comparison of general characteristics of acute and chronic disorders

Table 10-1

Comparison of Characteristics of Acute and Chronic Disorders

Acute Disorders	Chronic Disorders
Behaviors associated with acute disorders • Rapid onset of symptoms that may require intervention. • Assumption of the "sick role" in that the client recognizes the need for therapeutic intervention and/or assistance from others. • Client becomes "dependent" on others and relies on healthcare professionals to treat the acute disorder. • Resolution of clinical condition leads to recovery as a consequence of intervention or because of the self-limiting nature of the disorder.	Behaviors associated with chronic disorders • A chronic disorder becomes a permanent state in which symptoms occur, leading to disability and compensation. • Adaptation to the "sick role" becomes a way of life for the client and family members on a daily basis. • The client becomes "interdependent" on others as they become a part of a collaborative health team approach to treat and manage symptoms and complications of the chronic disorder. • Eventually chronic disorders lead to increased mortality as they affect the client's physiological integrity.
Depending on their nature and severity, acute disorders can lead to long-term consequences such as surgical interventions, psychosocial adaptations, and financial impact of event.	Chronic disorders can become acute in nature due to the cyclic nature of illness and disease leading to exacerbations and remissions. These repeated events can lead to profound changes in the client's and family's ability to adapt, leading to significant physical, psychosocial and financial changes.

B. Acute illness concerns

! **1.** The primary approach used to manage acutely ill clients is the "ABCs"—airway, breathing, and circulation

a. Utilize the approach used by EMTs when dealing with acute (and/or traumatic) illnesses—establish airway, maintain hemodynamic stability, and treat clinical presentations

b. Adequate oxygenation is needed to establish circulation and maintain adequate tissue perfusion

c. Baseline monitoring and trending of client's vital signs are critical

d. Surgical management may be required to treat medical emergencies arising from acute illness

e. Pain management will take priority over nutritional interventions in acutely ill clients

f. Acute disease processes lead to alterations in activities of daily living, increased stress, and financial burdens on the client and family support systems

2. Fluid replacement is needed to stabilize hemodynamic values and maintain fluid and electrolyte balance

! **a.** Height, weight, and body frame parameters are critical parameters needed to establish fluid replacement

! **b.** Monitoring intake and output is critical in determining client's renal status and response to treatment

! **c.** NPO status may be required during the assessment and treatment phase in order to prepare client for surgical intervention or to institute bowel rest for emergent conditions to minimize gastric secretions

! d. Determination of appropriate IV therapy is required based on defined lab results (serum electrolytes and plasma osmolality) and renal function

3. Structural damage can occur as a result of acute trauma or a metabolic event leading to altered vascular integrity and end organ damage
   a. Stress of the disease process leads to catabolism
   b. Hypermetabolic body response leads to increased protein turnover, negative nitrogen balance, and decreased growth hormone, antioxidant, and selenium levels
   c. Final effects of the stress of catabolism lead to breakdown of skeletal muscle cells and loss of lean body mass
4. Preexisting baseline nutritional status affects acute illness
   ! a. A malnourished client with loss of visceral protein stores has increased medical risks due to inability to handle stress as a result of poor immune response, healing ability, and anemia of chronic disease
   ! b. A client with overnutrition is also at increased medical risk due to metabolic effects of increased fat stores and alterations in insulin resistance (increased) and sensitivity (decreased)

C. Chronic illness concerns

1. Primary approaches to care
   a. It is necessary to deal with compensatory changes of the disease process that have resulted in physiologic adaptations
   b. Recognize that established "norms" for client may be inconsistent with normal adaptable responses
   c. Use primary approach of airway, breathing, and circulation to determine priorties
   d. Evaluate the client's dietary pattern for nutritional adequacy
   e. Chronic disease leads to financial burdens, long-term stressors, and alterations and adaptations to recognized illness patterns
2. Fluid replacement
   a. Stabilization of fluid balance depends on individual client status, progression of disease process, and affected body systems
   ! b. Clients with fluid volume excess (FVE) as a result of the disease process may require fluid restriction or diuretic therapy in order to maintain normal fluid balance
   c. NPO status may be required depending on clinical presentation and/or medical-surgical management
3. Structural damage
   a. Chronic disease can affect baseline organ function, resulting in altered ability to perform metabolic functions
   ! b. End organ disease will affect the client's ability to handle physiologic stressors
   c. Vascular damage can lead to significant alterations in capillary permeability, causing fluid and electrolyte imbalances
   d. Deteriorating nature of chronic disease leads to inability to compensate effectively and increased likelihood of hospital admissions
4. Preexisting baseline nutritional status
   a. Length and duration of chronic disease process affects client's nutritional status

Box 10-1

Anemia of Chronic Disease (ACD)

- Hemoglobin and hematocrit are decreased.
- Serum iron and total iron binding capacity (TIBC) levels are decreased.
- Serum ferritin levels are increased.
- Low or low normal RBC count and normal red cell distribution width (RDW) are present.
- Mean corpuscular volume (MCV) can be normal or decreased.
- Morphology may indicate hypochromic or normochromic presentation.
- Clients who have contributory diseases may have more pronounced symptoms because of anemia in affected systems or organs (e.g., exaggerated edema and dyspnea in clients with heart failure).
- Anemia may be seen in clients who have chronic renal failure, any chronic inflammatory disease process, malignancy, or in those who receive chemotherapy/immunosuppressive treatment regimens.
- Presenting clinical symptoms may be mild or may not be evident due to long-standing condition and ability of the client to compensate.
- Usual symptoms seen are fatigue, weakness, decreased activity tolerance, palpitations, dyspnea on exertion (DOE), and orthostatic lightheadedness.
- Medication such as erythropoietin (Epogen or Procrit) is used to treat ACD and dose is titrated by evaluation of hematocrit. Refer to pharmacology textbook for specifics of drug therapy.

b. Anorexia and loss of visceral protein stores, leading to muscle wasting and immobility, can occur in response to disease progression

c. **Anemia of chronic disease (ACD)** requires medication therapy to improve RBC production but does not correct the underlying disease process and therefore becomes a chronic concern (refer to Box 10-1)

! **d.** It is important to determine nutritional adequacy of client's dietary selections in order to support metabolic functions of the body

! **e.** Alternate feeding methods (tube feedings) may already be in use for the client as a result of chronic illness that can contribute to the development of other problems (altered skin integrity and potential for infection)

5. Exacerbation of a chronic illness can lead to an acute presentation

! **a.** Clients with a chronic disease process often enter a cyclical pattern with exacerbations and remissions

b. Frequency of events can lead to progression of disease and inability to handle stressors

c. Financial considerations, altered body image, and poor coping mechanisms can contribute to both psychological as well as physiological stress

II. NUTRITIONAL CONCERNS FOR THE CLIENT ON A VENTILATOR

A. ABCs affecting care

1. Respiratory therapists (RT) monitor the ventilatory function of clients in acute care settings

2. Airway management is established for clients with specific criteria arising from diagnosis of **acute respiratory failure (ARF)**—(arterial $CO_2 > 50$ mmHg and arterial $O_2 < 60$ mmHg)
3. Clients in respiratory failure are prone to hyperventilation due to excessive work of breathing required to ventilate the airway; they usually suffer from underlying malnutrition

B. Course of therapy

1. Therapy is aimed at resolving the underlying cause of respiratory problems and depends on the client's ability to maintain respiratory effort
2. Acute care management of disease processes may require short-term intubation
3. Strict sterile technique is required in order to decrease the risk of infection in a client who is already undergoing profound stress
4. Arterial blood gas (ABG) results are trended in order to document client's baseline and monitor response to therapy
5. Medications used during the course of therapy (such as dopamine, opioid analgesic and diuretics) can lead to decreased gastric emptying and fluid/electrolyte and acid-base imbalances

C. Fluid replacement

1. Clients receiving mechanical ventilation are initially started on parenteral fluids as part of the initial acute care management based on individualized requirements; they are then given tube feedings and possibly receive free water boluses by tube; enteral vs. parenteral support considers risk of fluid overload
2. Long-term ventilatory support will require that the client receive nutritional support via an alternate feeding route when enteral feeding is indicated
3. Effects of medication therapy aimed at treating underlying disease processes can affect fluid requirements
4. Accurate intake and output must be recorded with results trended over the course of therapy to evaluate the client's response to therapy

D. Stabilization of the client and progression to being weaned off the ventilator

1. Goals for successful weaning from mechanical ventilation include correction of the underlying cause of respiratory failure, improvement of muscle strength, adequate nutritional intake, and psychological readiness
2. Criteria for weaning depend on the client's clinical condition and ability to tolerate extubation (presence of cough and gag reflex and adequate level of consciousness)
3. Effects of malnutrition have a profound impact on weaning a client from a ventilator due to compromised ventilatory muscle function, central ventilatory drive effort, and decreased defenses against lung infection
4. Clients on mechanical ventilation often have multisystem disorders (heart disease, infections, altered nutrition, oversedation, and fluid overload) that can affect ability to wean from the ventilator

Practice to Pass

How do the effects of malnutrition compromise a client on ventilator therapy?

E. Nutrient calculations

1. Caloric needs are based on the metabolic stress of both disease processes and mechanical ventilation itself
2. Determination of client's metabolic rate and energy requirements using a predictive equation or indirect calorimetry is critical in setting nutritional goals (see Chapter 1)

! 3. Collaboration with dietitian is necessary to manage the client's nutritional status during this hypermetabolic period

! 4. Obtain daily weights and document pertinent labs (chemistry panels and nitrogen balance) to monitor client's response to treatment

5. Enteral feeding route is the preferred feeding method as it maintains intestinal mucosal integrity and stimulates gut associated lymph tissue (GALT)

6. The use of parenteral feeding (TPN) is suggested for clients who have a nonfunctioning gut or if access become a problem

III. NUTRITIONAL CONCERNS FOR THE TRAUMA CLIENT

A. **ABCs affecting care**—the priority principles used to treat the trauma client are the ABCs and EMT approach

! B. **The course of therapy** depends on the nature of the traumatic event, age of the client, and baseline status of the individual client

1. Surgical intervention may be necessary in order to correct hemodynamic problems and stop internal bleeding
2. Multiple trauma victims may have the predominant trauma attended to in the acute care period
3. Elderly and young clients are at greatest risk to suffer from traumatic injuries due to fluid loss potential
4. Clients with contributory disease processes are at increased risk to develop complications during trauma events
5. The stress response occurs in three phases: ebb, flow, and anabolic (refer to Table 10-2); clients who have adequate nutritional stores are better able to respond to stress as they proceed through the different phases of the stress response

Table 10-2 Stress Response Phases

Ebb Phase	Flow Phase	Anabolic Phase
Initial stress to 24 hours Reduced body requirements are seen (BP, CO, temperature, and O_2 consumption) Requires 1.5 grams of protein/kg/day Hypothermia, hyperglycemia, and increased lactate levels seen in response to alterations in carbohydrate and lipid metabolism	Increased CO, urinary protein losses, and catabolism are seen as the body tries to compensate Hormonal changes occur in response to body stress Increased epinephrine, glucagon, ADH, and aldosterone secretion Decreased insulin Breakdown of body protein to provide fuel (glucose) Increased protein needs to 2 grams of protein/kg/day Decreased blood flow to GI tract and decreased mucus secretion Gastric acid secretion increases Symptom complaints of diarrhea and bloating	Different hormonal changes continue to occur in response to stress Increases in insulin and growth hormone now occur Increased protein needs are seen—2 grams of protein/kg/day

C. Fluid replacement

1. The trauma client is at risk to develop shock due to fluid losses (hypovolemic/hemorrhagic) and should be monitored closely for changes in level of consciousness and vital signs
2. If fluid/blood loss is significant, blood component therapy may have to be utilized in order to restore hemodynamic balance

D. Triage and stabilization of the client

1. Prioritization of care in emergent/nonemergent settings
   a. Use of a tagging system indicating the acuity of the client assists the health-care team in delivering care to clients who have a higher acuity status
   ! b. Evidence of internal bleeding and blunt penetrating trauma take priority over other less severe injuries
2. Stabilization
   ! a. Improvement of hemodynamic function is critical to maintain adequate blood volume and promote medication effects
   ! b. Restoration of vascular integrity leading to fluid and electrolyte balance is critical in managing the trauma client

E. Nutrient calculations

1. Depending on the nature of the trauma and intervention required, nutrient calculations can be managed using a variety of methods
   a. A dietitian will calculate specific nutrient requirements using predictive equations or indirect calorimetry in high-acuity clients (see Chapter 1)
   b. Increased stress demands may lead to an increased need for calories depending on the nature of the event
   ! c. Calculation of kilocaloric needs of a hypermetabolic client using the Harris-Benedict equation is with the following formula—Resting Energy Expenditure (REE) × Stress Factor = Estimated Energy Need
   d. Stress Factor relates to the amount of physical stress placed by specific disease/trauma that ranges from 1.2–2.0
   e. Initial fluid replacement will take priority over nutritional management of the client in the short-term period
   f. Hypermetabolic conditions may require an increase in caloric intake as well as an increase in protein sources
2. Adequate amounts of micronutrients will help to support immune function and restore healing in the trauma client; a multivitamin with minerals is indicated; evidence for specific doses of individual micronutrients is currently lacking

Practice to Pass

What is the nutritional priority in the trauma client?

IV. NUTRITIONAL CONCERNS FOR THE CLIENT WITH MODS

! **A. Stabilization of the client** is achieved by maintaining hemodynamic and vascular integrity in the presence of multiple organ dysfunction syndrome (MODS), in which more than one organ system fails

1. The clinical goal is to prevent infection and treat aggressively all clients who present with this continuum disorder
2. It is vital to maintain oxygenation and prevent effects caused by hypoperfusion leading to hypoxemia

3. Therapeutic management is aimed at decreasing emerging oxygen demands and increasing oxygen delivery to the tissues
4. Complications related to the development of SIRS and MODS (see section below) should be treated aggressively and may require the use of mechanical ventilation and/or dialysis therapy to support affected organs and maintain hemodynamic stability

B. Clinical course and impact of disease process

1. Physiological response of body systems leads to organ failure as a result of chemical mediators (refer to Box 10-2)
   a. **SIRS (systemic inflammatory response syndrome)** is characterized by an inflammatory response in organs as a result of chemical mediators from a localized event
   b. **MODS (multiple organ dysfunction syndrome)** is characterized by the progression of SIRS, leading to multiple organ failure

Box 10-2

Clinical Presentations Associated with Organ Dysfunction

- Temperature variations (> 38°C or < 36°C)
- Tachycardia > 90 bpm
- Respiratory rate > 20 min or $PaCO_2$ < 32 mm Hg
- WBC > 12,000/mm^3 or < 4,000/mm^3 or increase in bands > 10%
- Changes in capillary permeability as a result of chemical mediators leading to vast and dramatic changes in organ function and ability of the client to compensate
- Acute lung injury usually seen as the first organ system involved with progression to acute respiratory distress syndrome (ARDS)
- Cardiac changes leading to decreased systemic vascular resistance (SVR) and increased O_2 consumption
- Gastrointestinal changes leading to decreased tissue perfusion, translocation of normal flora bacteria, and colonization with pathogens
- Liver changes as a result of inability to detoxify bacteria from translocation, decreased production of proteins to control inflammatory response, and increased bilirubin levels
- Renal changes leading to renal failure due to decreased perfusion and ischemia; the use of potent nephrotoxic drugs during therapy may further play a role in the development of renal failure
- Coagulation pathway alterations resulting in the development of disseminated intravascular coagulation (DIC) and hemorrhage as a result of consumption of clotting factors, platelets, and production of excessive fibrinogen degradation products
- Neurological changes resulting in altered mental status due to capillary leakage, tissue damage, and resulting cerebral edema
- Hypermetabolism occurs in response to body's efforts to maintain balance; initial depletion of glycogen stores to fuel the body occurs during high stress state; once stores are depleted, then catabolism of protein begins resulting in loss of lean body mass as body switches to fat metabolism as primary fuel source
- Fluid and electrolyte imbalances as the body attempts to balance metabolic shifts caused by vascular insults, release of chemical mediators, and in response to secretion of catecholamines and glucocorticoids; these dramatic fluid and electrolyte shifts can cause the development of metabolic acidosis that can further compound the body's ability to maintain balance and lead to increased deterioration
- Losses in potassium, sodium, calcium, magnesium, and phosphate in response to hormone release of antidiuretic hormone (ADH) and aldosterone

c. Primary MODS is the result of direct organ dysfunction, whereas secondary MODS occurs in organs not directly affected by the initial event

! d. The gastrointestinal (GI) tract is critical to clients with SIRS or MODS because it is the largest source of immune tissue in the body (GALT—gastrointestinal associated lymphoid tissue)

2. The **APACHE criteria** are a set of parameters that are used to monitor the high-acuity client, establish and monitor response to treatments, and serve as a prognostic indicator
   a. Components of APACHE II criteria are acute physiologic state, age, and presence of chronic disease (refer to Table 10-3)
   b. Points range from 0 to 71 with higher scores denoting an increased relationship between client status and death

C. Fluid replacement

1. Fluid replacement is 30–40 mL/kg/day or 1 mL H_2O per calorie in the adult; however, in critical illness, fluid measurement is very complex and involves pulmonary and renal issues
2. Fluid replacement is based on replacement of sensible and insensible losses, although fluid replacement equations may or may not be appropriate to use
3. Parenteral administration of fluids is required to correct fluid and electrolyte imbalances that commonly occur during this disease process

Practice to Pass

What are the implications of micronutrient deficiencies in a client who has multiple organ dysfunction syndrome (MODS)?

D. Nutrient calculations

1. Caloric requirements are calculated using a predictive equation such as Harris-Benedict or by indirect calorimetry
2. ! Micronutrients (Na, K, Mg, Fe, Cu, Zn, PO_4, and Se) are critical in promoting an immune response because clinical deficiencies can occur in response to cellular death, hypermetabolic conditions, and progression of stress response
3. ! Meeting the nutrient demands of the hypermetabolic client helps prevent development of associated protein-calorie malnutrition that is often associated with clients who have MODS
   a. Energy expenditure ranges from 1.5 to 2.0 times the normal metabolic rate
   b. It is important to minimize weight loss and cachexia by providing client with necessary nutrients during the hypermetabolic phase

Table 10-3
APACHE II Criteria

Physiologic Parameters	Age Parameters	Chronic Disease Parameters
Temperature Mean arterial pressure Heart rate Respiratory rate A-aPO_2(FiO_2 > 50%) or PaO_2(FiO_2 < 50%) Arterial pH or HCO_3 Serum Na Serum K Serum creatinine Hematocrit WBC count Glasgow Coma Score	Extremes in aging (young and old) can cause increased risk for adverse health consequences	Biopsy-proved liver cirrhosis NY Heart Association Class IV Severe COPD Chronic dialysis Immunocompromised Surgical vs. nonsurgical

4. Monitoring nitrogen balance is helpful in determining the adequacy of nutrient provision

V. NUTRITIONAL CONCERNS FOR CLIENTS WITH DRUG AND ALCOHOL DEPENDENCIES

A. Effects of drug use

1. Drug use can lead to impaired metabolism and altered behavioral responses
2. ! Physiological addiction and dependency can lead to alterations in lifestyle dynamics, impaired coping mechanisms, and financial devastation
3. Withdrawal effects can be just as prominent as "medication" effects, and the client should be closely monitored during withdrawal therapy
4. Correlation of smoking with development of cancers has been clinically proven; evidence is also emerging about effects of secondhand smoke

B. Effects of alcohol use

1. Alcohol ingestion can lead to impaired metabolism (MEOS system activation) with resultant liver damage
2. ! Alcohol as a source of empty calories can contribute to poor nutritional intake and unhealthy dietary patterns
3. Addiction/dependency can result in physiological as well as psychological effects
4. ! Treatment of clinical nutrient deficiencies (B complex vitamins) associated with alcoholism should be instituted as soon as possible
5. Referral of client and family members to support systems such as Alcoholics Anonymous can be an important part of any alcohol withdrawal program
6. Identification of client behaviors using the CAGE questionnaire (a 4-question format to detect alcohol abuse) may help identify clients at risk for alcohol dependency

VI. NUTRITIONAL CONCERNS FOR THE CLIENT WITH CONTRIBUTORY DISEASES

A. Existing diseases in the same body—how can you treat them all?

1. Clients often experience multiple disease processes such as diabetes, heart disease, and respiratory diseases that progress over time as the client ages
2. ! Clients are often on multiple medication profiles (polypharmacy) and may have adverse outcomes related to therapies
3. Treating the symptoms rather than the disease progression is a consequence of multiple disease profiles
4. Table 10-4 outlines nutritional effects of common disorders grouped by body system

B. Concerns over drug to food and herb interactions

1. ! **Polypharmacy** approach increases the risk for potential interactions
   a. It is critical to have a complete listing of all the medications and herbs that the client is currently taking, both OTC and prescription
   b. The client's medication profile should be reviewed during each hospitalization and/or physician visit in order to verify medication status
2. ! The greater the number of medications, the greater is the likelihood of concerns about bioavailability

Table 10-4

Contributory Diseases and Their Effects on Nutritional Profile

System	Nutritional Profile
Cardiac	Cardiac cachexia and PEM Anorexia, dyspnea, and associated fatigue Restrictive diets (salt and fluids) Potential for weight gain Nutrient deficiencies related to thiamine as a consequence of high output failure Potential electrolyte imbalances related to medication therapy
Gastrointestinal	Bacterial translocation leading to sepsis Malabsorption related to disease processes Alterations in gastric emptying affected by disease process and/or medications Symptom management of elimination problems
Hematological	Fatigue issues related to clinical deficiencies Nutritional anemias requiring treatment Cyclic nature of disease may require frequent blood transfusions and medical management
Immune	Protein depletion affects immune status Immunosuppression leads to increased likelihood of infection and poor healing response
Infectious	Hypermetabolic response to septic process Increased stress leading to inflammatory response and release of chemical mediators
Musculoskeletal	Bone loss and demineralization occur over time with aging Adequate calcium, protein, vitamin D, sunlight, and exercise are needed to support bone status Mobility issues can be affected by other contributory disease processes, leading to poor outcomes as evidenced by increased likelihood of falls
Neurological	Nature and extent of injury leading to hypermetabolic response and release of chemical mediators Alterations in fluid and electrolyte status with compensatory acid base changes due to increased cerebral O_2 consumption can result in anaerobic metabolism Medication therapy can affect vascular dynamics
Renal	Acute and chronic insults require aggressive medical therapy due to hypermetabolism, dramatic fluid and electrolyte changes, acid-base disturbances, and protein limitation
Respiratory	Restrictive and obstructive changes cause fatigue due to increased respiratory effort to maintain compensation Frequently occurring malnutrition associated with chronic lung disease and low protein levels Excessive administration of carbohydrates or total calories can further increase respiratory effort, as client is unable to blow off built-up CO_2 levels

Medical treatment of disease processes can in themselves affect multiple body systems resulting in complex management issues.

a. Depending on the medication profile, it is important to note when client is taking medications (morning, night, on an empty stomach, or with meals) in order to note factors affecting bioavailability

b. The use of alcohol is contraindicated in conjunction with medication therapy because it can lead to increased effects (sedative or changes in blood pressure), altered metabolism of drug therapy, and potential for liver damage

c. Clients taking antibiotics, MAO inhibitors, HMG-CoA reductase inhibitors, antifungals, and diuretics should receive individualized dietary instruction regarding foods that can affect absorption and drug therapy

d. It is important to note effects and reactions that the client is experiencing from medication therapy in order to access drug efficacy and to identify potential untoward reactions

! 3. Knowledge deficit can affect client compliance

a. It is important to instruct the client in proper administration of medications and potential interactions

b. It is important that the client have an understanding of why the medication is being ordered and the desired effects of medication therapy

c. Medication therapy should only be taken as directed by the healthcare provider; the client should inform the healthcare provider immediately of any reactions or changes in therapy

Practice to Pass

How does polypharmacy contribute to increased likelihood of hospitalizations? What methods could be used to decrease the risk of increased hospitalizations due to polypharmacy?

C. Progression of disease and the aging process

1. Disease progression creating lifestyle changes and physiological adaptations, coupled with aging, leads to an overall decline in function
2. Effects of systemic disease can cause profound changes in many organ systems, leading to increased likelihood of complications, increased medication therapy, and frequent hospitalizations
3. Life expectancy has increased, leading to a greater number of disease processes

VII. NUTRITIONAL CONCERNS FOR THE CLIENT TAKING SODIUM WARFARIN (COUMADIN)

A. Types of clients

1. Clients with heart valve replacements require long-term **anticoagulation therapy** in order to minimize clotting
2. Clients with deep vein thrombosis (DVT) require anticoagulation therapy in order to minimize risk of clotting
3. Initially, the client may be placed on heparin therapy and then switched over to warfarin (Coumadin) therapy for long-term maintenance
4. Dose is titrated in response to **prothrombin time (PT)** or **international normalized ratio (INR)** levels to achieve maximum desired effect

! **B. Lifelong treatment concerns** with numerous drug–drug and drug–food interactions

1. Sodium warfarin (Coumadin) is the prototype medication for possible drug–drug and drug–food interactions due to the large number of documented possible interactions
2. Referral to a dietitian and use of the Coumadin client teaching booklet is a critical element for in clients placed on Coumadin anticoagulation therapy
3. Client should wear a Medic Alert™ bracelet indicating that the client is on Coumadin therapy
4. The antidote for warfarin is vitamin K, which is administered in the presence of bleeding concurrently with fresh frozen plasma (FFP) or factor IX concentrate if there are underlying clinical conditions
5. A consult with a hematologist is appropriate if client is nonresponsive to Coumadin therapy or if client is experiencing side effects
6. Multiple drug interactions can occur when a client is taking Coumadin therapy (refer to Box 10-3)

Box 10-3

Listing of Potential Drug Interactions with a Client on Warfarin Therapy

- Plasma protein drugs potentiate effects of sodium warfarin
- Sodium warfarin potentiates effects of anticonvulsants and hypoglycemics
- Herbal medicines may either increase or decrease effects of warfarin
- High doses of vitamin E ($\geq$ 400 IU) can increase the risk of bleeding by prolonging clotting time
- Vitamin K supplementation can reduce the effectiveness of warfarin

7. Drug interactions can occur through multiple pathways: synergistic (reduced or impaired clotting synthesis), competitive (vitamin K activity), or hereditary resistance (altered vitamin K metabolism)

C. Dietary teaching principles

1. Clients should receive instructions about vitamin K activity in foods (refer to Box 10-4)
2. Dietary planning is an essential part of evaluating the client's knowledge base and monitoring compliance with treatment regimen
3. Maintain a consistent well-balanced diet that is adequate and constant in vitamin K but not excessive

D. Monitoring client's response

1. ! Pertinent lab work specific to warfarin therapy should be regularly evaluated, specifically PT/INR ratio
2. PT (prothrombin time) is the testing used to determine the clotting ability of the extrinsic pathway
3. INR (international normalized ratio) is the standardized method used to evaluate the PT level
4. Followup labs should be done at appropriate intervals noting INR between 2.0 and 3.0 or higher, or between 2.5 and 3.5 if the client has a mechanical heart valve
5. An increased PT/INR indicates that there is increased potential for bleeding and the dose should be decreased to minimize this effect
6. A decreased PT/INR indicates that treatment is not effective and the dose should be increased to maintain adequate anticoagulation
7. ! The client should receive adequate instructions about potential side effects of medication therapy and when to notify the healthcare provider (refer to Box 10-5)

Box 10-4

Food Sources High in Vitamin K

- Green leafy vegetables (broccoli, brussel sprouts, cabbage, collard greens, endive, green scallions, kale, lettuce, mustard greens, parsley, spinach, turnip greens, swiss chard, and watercress)
- Liver (beef and chicken)
- Mayonnaise and oils (salad, canola, and soybean)
- Green tea leaves
- Garbanzo beans (chick peas)

Box 10-5

Anticoagulant Instructions

- Take the medication exactly as ordered by your healthcare provider.
- Wear a medical alert bracelet and know your prescribed dosage.
- Do not use any new medications or OTC preparations without notifying your healthcare provider, as there can be potential interactions.
- Maintain a balanced diet making note of vitamin K activity in food choices.
- Be careful when shaving and use electric razors to minimize chance of irritation or bleeding.
- The use of alcohol in conjunction with anticoagulant therapy can cause potential problems.
- Notify your healthcare provider if you experience any of the following:
  - Any bleeding episodes (nose, gums, urine, or bowel)
  - Headaches or abdominal pain
  - Increase in menstrual flow
  - Persistent bruising
  - Rash
  - Fatigue or unexplained weakness

VIII. NUTRITIONAL CONCERNS FOR THE CLIENT WITH A TRANSPLANT

A. Treatment protocol to prevent rejection

1. **Immunosuppressive therapy** is used to prevent rejection of transplanted organ and often consists of azathioprine (Imuran), cyclosporine (Neoral), and prednisone
2. High-dose radiation is used to irradiate the client's existing bone marrow defenses and allow for replacement of new bone marrow
3. Prevention of **graft versus host disease** (organ or tissue rejection that leads to systemic manifestations) is critical in terms of establishing a favorable prognosis for the transplant client

B. Baseline nutritional status prior to transplant

1. A pretransplant evaluation is performed on every client in order to ascertain overall health status and nutritional baseline
2. Improvement of nutritional status is an established goal in most transplant clients because they are likely to have depletion of nutrient stores and suffer from preexisting malnutrition due to organ/system failure
3. ! Reaction to treatment therapies can cause significant nutritional complications ranging from nausea, vomiting, and diarrhea to anorexia, alterations in taste, and weight loss

C. Dietary teaching principles

1. Neutropenic/low-bacteria diet is utilized when the client is at risk for infection due to profound immunosuppression either as a result of treatment therapies or as a consequence of disease processes
2. ! Monitoring of absolute neutrophil count (ANC) is critical in determining client's response to treatment and progression of diet status

! 3. Immunosuppressive therapy with cyclosporine (Neoral) can lead to increased risk of hyperkalemia and hyperuricemia as well as elevations of cholesterol and triglycerides levels

! 4. Immunosuppressive therapy with corticosteroids (prednisone) can lead to weight gain, fluid and electrolyte imbalances, and GI upset

! 5. Immunosuppressive therapy with azathioprine (Imuran) can lead to diarrhea, vomiting, esophageal sores, and anemia

! 6. The nurse must be aware of potential drug effects as a result of therapy, client's food preferences, altered taste perception, and client's overall activity level when planning dietary selections

D. Monitoring client's response

! 1. Short-term goals include adequate intake and output, correction of fluid/electrolyte imbalances, and limited weight loss

   a. Symptom management (nausea, vomiting, diarrhea, taste alterations, and anorexia) is done utilizing medication therapy

   b. Appropriate dietary selections that offer the client nutrient-dense calories and satisfy the client's preferences are very important

   c. Referral to dietitian may be needed to individualized nutritional client goals

! 2. Long-term goals include stable weight, adequate caloric intake, and adequate nutritional stores

   a. Continued followup with dietitian is needed to monitor client's response to therapy and determine whether goals have been met or require modification based on the individual client's response

   b. In response to immunosuppressive therapy, restriction of sodium and fluids may be advised to minimize the potential for edema formation and development of hypertension

   c. Caloric intake and protein, fat, and carbohydrate intake should be adjusted to meet adequate weight goals

   d. The diet should be adequate in calcium in order to prevent problems with bone mineral density and development of osteoporosis (estrogen and vitamin D supplements may be considered to support bone mineral density)

   e. The initiation of immunosuppressive therapy can lead to restrictions and monitoring of potassium (increased levels are seen), and of magnesium and phosphorus (decreased levels are seen)

   f. The use of a multivitamin supplement is recommended for transplant clients

   g. Evaluation of the functional status of the transplanted organ is done on an ongoing basis

! 3. It is important to use medical nutrition therapy to prevent or treat common comorbidities of transplant procedures such as diabetes mellitus, hyperlipidemia, hypertension, obesity, and osteoporosis

   a. Diabetes mellitus can occur in response to treatment by immunosuppressive therapy

   b. Hyperlipidemia can already be established in a majority of clients receiving transplants but maybe further stimulated by immunosuppressive therapy

   c. Hypertension may be a prior existing problem in many transplant clients; organ replacement does not change the client's general vascular status

Practice to Pass

Why is a transplant client at greater risk for nutritional problems during the post-transplant period?

d. Clients are prone to develop obesity in response to immunosuppressive therapy

e. The presence of osteoporosis may be further evident in clients receiving immunosuppressive therapy posttransplant

IX. NUTRITIONAL CONCERNS FOR THE MALNOURISHED CLIENT WITH MULTISYSTEM DISORDERS

A. Impact of baseline status on long term outcomes

1. Depleted visceral stores and impaired immune function with subsequent wasting syndrome are commonly occurring health problems in the malnourished client
2. Dynamic effects of malnutrition superimposed on disease processes lead to poor outcomes and increased likelihood of mortality

B. Therapeutic management concerns

1. ! Malnutrition increases the metabolic demands and places the client at increased risk for mortality
2. Inability to restore adequate nutritional status due to imposed effects of chronic malnutrition is an important concern
3. Refeeding syndrome can occur in response to the introduction of nutritional support in the malnourished client who has contributory disease processes
   a. Response to introduction of carbohydrates leads to an increase in insulin secretion with accompanying sodium and fluid retention
   b. Increases in metabolic rate, oxygen consumption, and production of carbon dioxide occur
   c. ! Increased shifting of electrolytes into cells is seen, especially phosphorus, potassium, and magnesium, which can severely reduce intravascular levels
   d. It is critical to evaluate and correct hemodynamic status and fluid and electrolyte balance and to start feedings at a prescribed stepwise rate in order to avoid further metabolic stress, and to replace electrolytes separately

X. NUTRITIONAL CONCERNS FOR THE OBESE CLIENT WITH MULTISYSTEM DISORDERS

A. Impact of baseline status on long-term outcomes

1. Clinical syndromes resulting in altered respiratory status (Pickwickian syndrome—obesity hyperventilation syndrome—or obstructive sleep apnea syndrome—OSAS) can lead to significant changes in a client's ability to compensate
2. ! Excess weight on heart and lungs leads to impaired vascular status and increased workload
3. ! If obese clients experience sleep disturbances, they are likely to be even more fatigued, leading to decreased physical activity and sedentary lifestyle, which can lead to further weight gain

B. Therapeutic management concerns

1. ! Life expectancy is decreased because of effects of obesity coupled with multisystem disorders

! 2. Weight reduction may become a secondary priority as emerging physiological needs of various systems (heart and lung) may require immediate attention

! 3. Evaluation of the client's nutritional status by looking at meal patterns, types of food eaten, amount of alcohol consumed (source of empty calories), exercise habits, stress level, and contributory health problems is critical in determining realistic individualized goals

Case Study

A 38-year-old male client is admitted to the hospital with a diagnosis of deep vein thrombosis (DVT) of the left leg. He has been receiving anticoagulation therapy with heparin and has now been switched to sodium warfarin (Coumadin). Anticipated discharge is in 2 days, pending the client's documented response to therapy. Client's vital signs are BP 150/70, pulse 72, and respirations 22. His height is 5 feet 8 inches and weight is 200 pounds. Past medical history indicates no specific abnormalities; however, the client states he has a family history of diabetes.

1. What pertinent diagnostic/laboratory testing is critical to evaluate client's overall response to treatment?
2. What dietary information should be reviewed with the client prior to discharge?
3. What type of followup schedule should the client adhere to in order to determine effectiveness of therapy?
4. What nutritional factors could help to decrease the risk of thrombolic events?
5. The client is unhappy that he will be taking this medication for several months and wants to know why this is so important. How would you respond to the client's concerns?

For suggested responses, see pages 320–321.

POSTTEST

POSTTEST

1 A client taking warfarin (Coumadin) has had difficulty regulating prothrombin times. Which of the following questions should the nurse ask to identify dietary factors that could influence the drug levels?

1. "Do you use a lot of mayonnaise and salad oils?"
2. "How many times a day do you eat?"
3. "Do you eat a diet high in carbohydrates (CHOs)?"
4. "Are you drinking a lot of fruit juices?"

2 A 68-year-old male client who has longstanding diabetes with resultant complications has been hospitalized with recurring frequency over the years and is extremely upset over this most current admission. The client does not want to eat and repeatedly pushes away the food tray at each meal. How should the nurse best respond to the client's actions?

1. Tell the client that you can get him something else that would be more to his liking.
2. Take the tray away and try again with the next meal to get the client to eat.
3. Consult with the dietitian to improve client compliance.
4. Ask the client to share with you why he doesn't feel like eating.

3 The nurse is caring for a 32-year-old female client with multiple trauma. The nurse identifies which of the following as a priority intervention for nutritional support?

1. Determine if the client is hungry and what her favorite foods are.
2. Provide IV access and increase fluid rate to maintain nutritional status.
3. Offer sips of water and ice chips as tolerated.
4. Assess skin turgor, vital signs, and diagnostic test results before seeking a diet order.

4 When caring for a client diagnosed with multiple organ dysfunction syndrome (MODS), the nurse would utilize which of the following parameters to determine overall nutritional status?

1. Plasma osmolality and presence of chronic disease process
2. Age of client, presence of chronic health conditions, and physiologic parameters
3. Rectal temperature and respiratory rate
4. CBC with differential, electrolyte panel, and liver function tests

5 A 42-year-old male client states, "I am an alcoholic. I heard that drinking is good for you in terms of preventing heart disease, so why should I stop?" What is the best response of the nurse to the client's statement?

1. "Alcohol is only beneficial if used in moderate amounts; so this fact does not apply to your situation."
2. "Alcohol is a risk factor in many disease processes and the type and amount of alcohol consumed do have significant health consequences."
3. "Are you interested in seeing a counselor for help with alcohol dependency?"
4. "Will you complete a CAGE questionnaire so we can accurately determine if you really are an alcoholic?"

6 The nurse determines which of the following clients would be at the greatest risk for nutritional problems?

1. A 42-year-old male admitted with a fracture of the femur as a result of a fall
2. A 36-year-old obese female client admitted for pyelonephritis
3. A 20-year-old female client admitted with exacerbation of asthma
4. A 48-year-old female client who has a history of hypertension (HTN) and diabetes admitted for abdominal pain

7 The nurse determines that a client taking sodium warfarin (Coumadin) is being compliant with treatment if the client:

1. Doubles the dose when he misses a pill.
2. Is taking OTC cold medication in addition to warfarin therapy.
3. Takes the pill at the same time every day but is not aware of the dosage.
4. Maintains a balanced diet and eats a constant amount of green leafy vegetables.

8 When caring for a client who has had a liver transplant, the nurse would consider which of the following when planning for the client's post-transplant nutritional needs?

1. There is a decrease in protein catabolism.
2. Urinary nitrogen losses stabilize in the acute post-transplant period.
3. Early tube feeding is favored over parenteral feeding.
4. Branched chain amino acids are found in adequate amounts in the post-transplant period.

9 The nurse will include dietary teaching on what micronutrient to help support the client's immune function and restore healing?

1. Vitamin C
2. Vitamin D
3. Niacin
4. Magnesium

10 The nurse plans to monitor for which of the following consequences of refeeding syndrome in a critically ill client receiving total parenteral nutrition (TPN)?

1. Increase in serum phosphorus and sodium levels
2. Hypoglycemia
3. Decreased fasting blood sugar levels
4. Decreased serum potassium, magnesium, and phosphorus levels

See pages 308–310 for Answers and Rationales.

POSTTEST

ANSWERS & RATIONALES

Pretest

1 **Answer: 2** The client is usually kept NPO in order to minimize secretion of digestive enzymes that can contribute to the condition, and the client in acute pain is unlikely to want to eat until the pain is adequately controlled. IV therapy may be instituted to maintain hydration levels, and the client may also require administration of total parenteral nutrition (TPN) if the case is severe. The client with a mild case may receive enteral nutrition for support. The client will not have altered taste perception, and gastroparesis is not part of the clinical picture. The client should not lose more than 10% body weight if enteral or parenteral nutritional support is adequate.

Cognitive Level: Application **Client Need:** Physiological Integrity: Physiological Adaptation **Integrated Process:** Nursing Process: Analysis **Content Area:** Foundational Sciences: Nutrition **Strategy:** Critical words are *acute pancreatitis* and *pain.* Recall impact of severe pain on appetite and need to be NPO until acute inflammatory stage is over to direct you to option 2. **Reference:** Lemone, P., & Burke, K. (2004). *Medical surgical nursing: Critical thinking in client care* (3rd ed.). Upper Saddle River, NJ: Pearson/Prentice Hall, pp. 601–602.

2 **Answer: 3** To make valid recommendations to meet nutritional goals with regard to ACD, it is vital to evaluate the client's present dietary pattern for nutritional adequacy. This helps to establish a nutritional baseline and determine food preferences and other related factors that influence the client's intake pattern. Option 1 is incorrect—even though medication therapy is aimed at increasing RBC production, it does not specifically address nutritional adequacy in terms of maintaining nutritional stores. Option 2 is incorrect—merely increasing caloric intake without regard to adequacy or balance may place the client at an increased risk of nutritional imbalance. Consuming an adequate diet with all essential nutrients is as important as increasing caloric intake in clients with chronic disease processes. Although it is important to instruct the client about good sources of iron, this option is limited, since it will not provide the most comprehensive approach in dietary evaluation.

Cognitive Level: Application **Client Need:** Health Promotion and Maintenance **Integrated Process:** Nursing Process: Assessment **Content Area:** Foundational Sciences: Nutrition **Strategy:** The critical words are *most helpful.* Recognize importance of assessing baseline data in a client. Eliminate option 2 since it does not address the anemia or nutritional status. Eliminate options 1 and 4 since they are specific to only one aspect of the problem.

Reference: Rolfes, S., Pinna, K., & Whitney, E. (2006). *Understanding normal and clinical nutrition* (7th ed.). Belmont, CA: Wadsworth & Thomson Learning, pp. 586–588.

3 **Answer: 2** Critically ill clients on ventilator support must be provided nutritional support in order to maintain nutritional adequacy, prevent depletion of nutrient stores, and respond to increasing hypermetabolic demands of illness and therapies. Clients receiving medications such as dopamine and narcotics (opiates) are at risk to develop delayed gastric emptying, which can lead to further problems. In addition, changes in acid-base and fluid/electrolyte balance can lead to decreased gastric emptying.

Cognitive Level: Analysis **Client Need:** Physiological Integrity: Physiological Adaptation **Integrated Process:** Nursing Process: Analysis **Content Area:** Foundational Sciences: Nutrition **Strategy:** Option 1 is a factually incorrect statement. Options 3 and 4 are incorrect because enteral feeding is associated with a stimulation of blood flow in the gut and improved mucosal integrity and liver function. **Reference:** Rolfes, S., Pinna, K., & Whitney, E. (2006). *Understanding normal and clinical nutrition* (7th ed.). Belmont, CA: Wadsworth & Thomson Learning, p. 710.

4 **Answer: 3** The use of hypertonic enteral nutrition can lead to bowel necrosis and therefore should not be used for a critically ill client. All of the other choices would not lead to feeding complications in the critically ill client. Elemental formulas require minimal digestion and are readily absorbed. The use of full-strength formula feedings in small volumes with appropriate monitoring according to individual tolerance is an accepted practice. A client should be hemodynamically stable prior to the initiation of enteral feeding.

Cognitive Level: Analysis **Client Need:** Physiological Integrity: Physiological Adaptation **Integrated Process:** Nursing Process: Analysis **Content Area:** Foundational Sciences: Nutrition **Strategy:** Read each option and determine if a risk factor is present. Note the word "stable" in option 4 and eliminate it. Recall knowledge of osmolarity and physiology to choose option 3. **Reference:** Rolfes, S., Pinna, K., & Whitney, E. (2006). *Understanding normal and clinical nutrition* (7th ed.). Belmont, CA: Wadsworth & Thomson Learning, Appendix J-3.

5 **Answer: 3** A client who is critically ill on a ventilator and receiving parenteral nutrition should have daily weight measured as a reliable indicator of nutritional status. Serum albumin levels are not reliable indicators of effectiveness of nutritional therapy, although prealbumin levels reflect nutritional status over the last few days. Intake and output are excellent measures of fluid volume status, but not overall nutritional status. Skin turgor is a measure of fluid volume, but can be affected by other factors, such as age, and is not a reliable indicator of overall nutritional status.
Cognitive Level: Application **Client Need:** Health Promotion and Maintenance **Integrated Process:** Nursing Process: Assessment **Content Area:** Foundational Sciences: Nutrition
Strategy: Focus on the critical words *most reliable.* Eliminate vague options such as option 4 first. Eliminate next the two options that reflect fluid volume status only.
Reference: Lemone, P., & Burke, K. (2004). *Medical surgical nursing: Critical thinking in client care* (3rd ed.). Upper Saddle River, NJ: Pearson/Prentice Hall, p. 1166.

6 **Answer: 2** A client with a multiple disease profile is at great risk both medically and nutritionally because of multiple organ system problems that could alter metabolism and absorption of nutrients. Since the client is likely to have a multiple medication profile, it would be prudent to obtain a listing of all medication (both prescription and OTC) in order to evaluate potential drug–drug and drug–food interactions. Option 1 is incorrect—a 3-day food diary will only provide information relative to intake. Option 3 is incorrect—vital signs will not enable the nurse to calculate a BMI, since height and weight are needed. Even though it is important to ask if the client is satisfied with current management of disease processes, option 4 is stated as a closed-ended question, which will provide no further information, and the client may not be able to provide an accurate assessment of his or her own treatment.
Cognitive Level: Application **Client Need:** Health Promotion and Maintenance **Integrated Process:** Nursing Process: Assessment **Content Area:** Foundational Sciences: Nutrition
Strategy: Note that the client has history of three different chronic conditions. Recall that multiple food and drug interactions that are possible. Eliminate option 3 since the BMI is not calculated with those parameters. Options 1 and 4 can be eliminated as they may provide some valuable information after baseline information is gathered.
Reference: Rolfes, S., Pinna, K., & Whitney, E. (2006). *Understanding normal and clinical nutrition* (7th ed.). Belmont, CA: Wadsworth & Thomson Learning, p. 707.

7 **Answer: 3** A client on Coumadin (sodium warfarin) needs to avoid foods that are high in vitamin K, which acts as an antidote to the drug. Foods high in vitamin K include green leafy vegetables (options 1 and 2), and tomatoes (option 4), as well as wheat grains and liver. Corn is not high in vitamin K.
Cognitive Level: Application **Client Need:** Health Promotion and Maintenance **Integrated Process:** Teaching and Learning **Content Area:** Foundational Sciences: Nutrition
Strategy: Recall that green leafy vegetables are high in vitamin K to eliminate the first two options. It is then necessary to understand that tomatoes are a rich source of vitamin K to choose correctly between this option and the one containing corn. **Reference:** Nix, S. (2005). *Williams' basic nutrition and diet therapy* (12th ed.). St. Louis, MO: Mosby, p. 98.

8 **Answer: 3** Increased weight gain can be attributed to fluid retention due to medical treatment therapies post-transplant and as such does not reflect accurate information about nutritional status. Option 1 is incorrect—the use of immunosuppressant drugs can lead to increased nutrient needs due to side effects (nausea, vomiting, mouth lesions, and diarrhea). Option 2 is incorrect because the client's pre-transplant nutritional baseline status has a very profound impact on post-transplant nutritional status. The organ is being replaced, not the vascular system, and clients with liver failure often have longstanding nutritional deficits as a result of altered liver metabolism. Option 4 is incorrect—a post-transplant client still has to follow dietary restrictions due to existing medical treatment regimens and is followed closely by a dietitian.
Cognitive Level: Application **Client Need:** Health Promotion and Maintenance **Integrated Process:** Nursing Process: Analysis **Content Area:** Foundational Sciences: Nutrition
Strategy: Read each option, checking for accuracy of content and relevance to the question. Eliminate options 1, 2, and 4 since they are incorrect. **Reference:** Rolfes, S., Pinna, K., & Whitney, E. (2006). *Understanding normal and clinical nutrition* (7th ed.). Belmont, CA: Wadsworth & Thomson Learning, p. 778.

9 **Answer: 2** A client with a longstanding history of congestive heart failure is likely to develop chronic protein energy malnutrition resulting in cardiac cachexia. Option 1 is incorrect because clients with chronic CHF often have weight loss with superimposed edema that goes unnoticed, thereby masking poor nutritional status. Options 3 and 4 are incorrect—clients with chronic CHF have decreased activity tolerance and airway clearance due to disease pathology.
Cognitive Level: Application **Client Need:** Health Promotion and Maintenance **Integrated Process:** Nursing Process: Assessment **Content Area:** Foundational Sciences: Nutrition
Strategy: Critical words are *nutritional complications.* Eliminate options 3 and 4 since they are complications

related to airway and oxygenation. Note the word *cachexia* to direct you to option 2. **Reference:** Rolfes, S., Pinna, K., & Whitney, E. (2006). *Understanding normal and clinical nutrition* (7th ed.). Belmont, CA: Wadsworth & Thomson Learning, p. 838.

10 **Answer: 4** Discussing dietary meal planning activities with an obese client who has multisystem disorders would be the most helpful in terms of prospective therapeutic management. This option would allow the client to provide information relative to meal planning and demonstrate both application and compliance with medical/nursing treatments. Option 1 is incorrect—there is no indication that the client requires intervention by a psychiatrist. This option reflects a judgment by the nurse with no other defining information to suggest that the client is having a psychological problem. Option 2 is incorrect because there is no information to suggest that the client needs or is ready to accept medical treatment for obesity. Although it is important to ascertain that the client is being compliant with medication therapy, option 3 does not answer the question with regard to the nutritional management of the client. **Cognitive Level:** Application **Client Need:** Health Promotion and Maintenance **Integrated Process:** Nursing Process: Implementation **Content Area:** Foundational Sciences: Nutrition **Strategy:** Note the question addresses the nutritional needs of an obese client. First, eliminate option 3 since neither of the topics is addressed. Eliminate option 1 since there is no mention of a mental health problem. Eliminate option 2 once this defers the problem and does not involve the nurse. **Reference:** Rolfes, S., Pinna, K., & Whitney, E. (2006). *Understanding normal and clinical nutrition* (7th ed.). Belmont, CA: Wadsworth & Thomson Learning, pp. 587–588.

Posttest

1 **Answer: 1** Mayonnaise and salad oils are high in vitamin K, which will prolong the anticoagulation effects of warfarin. CHOs and fruit juice are not high in vitamin K. Option 2 does not directly affect coagulation. **Cognitive Level:** Application **Client Need:** Physiological Integrity: Pharmacological and Parenteral Therapies **Integrated Process:** Communication and Documentation **Content Area:** Foundational Sciences: Nutrition **Strategy:** Critical words are *warfarin* and *dietary factors.* Recall type of drug warfarin is and recognize dietary factors that would impact this drug. Eliminate option 2 since it would affect coagulation. Recall foods with vitamin K content to direct you to option 1. **Reference:** Rolfes, S., Pinna, K., & Whitney, E. (2006). *Understanding normal and clinical nutrition* (7th ed.). Belmont, CA: Wadsworth & Thomson Learning, p. 778.

2 **Answer: 4** A client who has frequent hospitalizations due to chronic disease is likely to exhibit signs of sadness, depression, and loss of control regarding the disease process. The nurse should allow the client to vent his feelings in the hopes of sharing concerns and offering emotional support. Option 1 is incorrect—although it is important to ascertain a client's food preference, the information provided states that the client is repeatedly pushing away the food tray at several meals. Option 2 is incorrect—this client behavior presents as a continued pattern and not an isolated incident. Therefore, the nurse should do more than try again with the next meal to get the client to eat. Option 3 is incorrect because although it might be important to consult with the dietitian regarding food selections, this option does not address the immediate problem of the client pushing away the foods trays.
Cognitive Level: Application **Client Need:** Health Promotion and Maintenance **Integrated Process:** Communication and Documentation **Content Area:** Foundational Sciences: Nutrition **Strategy:** Note the nature of the question is psychosocial. Review options for the one which best addresses clients refusal to eat to choose option 4. **Reference:** Nix, S. (2005). *Williams' basic nutrition & diet therapy* (12th ed.). St. Louis, MO: Elsevier Mosby, p. 11.

3 **Answer: 4** The first priority with any trauma client is to establish baseline information by assessing skin turgor, vital signs, and review of pertinent diagnostic tests in order to stabilize the client and determine the extent of injuries. Looking at the client's physical and diagnostic presentations will help to determine the client's fluid balance and pertinent stressors. Option 1 is incorrect—even if the client is hungry, the existing trauma condition may preclude any feeding attempts at this time. Although it is important to establish IV access for a trauma client, the nurse cannot increase the rate without a physician's order, therefore option 2 is incorrect. More importantly, increasing the IV rate will not help to maintain nutritional status but rather will help to restore fluid balance. Option 3 is incorrect because the client's underlying trauma may require surgical intervention and therefore the client should be kept NPO until the exact extent of injuries is known.
Cognitive Level: Analysis **Client Need:** Health Promotion and Maintenance **Integrated Process:** Nursing Process: Planning **Content Area:** Foundational Sciences: Nutrition **Strategy:** Critical words are *multiple trauma* and *priority.* Recognize need to obtain baseline data to determine specific needs of clients to direct you to option 4. **Reference:** Rolfes, S., Pinna, K., & Whitney, E. (2006). *Understanding normal and clinical nutrition* (7th ed.). Belmont, CA: Wadsworth & Thomson Learning, p. 584.

4 **Answer: 2** A client who is diagnosed with MODS in an ICU setting is critically ill. Determination of overall health status is usually reviewed using the APACHE scoring, which provides relative information regarding risk of mortality. APACHE scoring looks at acute physiological indicators, age, and presence of chronic health conditions to evaluate a client's response and prognosis. Option 1 is incorrect—plasma osmolality does not serve as an indicator for acute physiology scoring. Option 3 is incorrect—these choices only reveal information about the client's age and possibly chronic respiratory health problems. Option 4 is incorrect because a CBC with differential does not provide comprehensive information about the client's overall health status.
Cognitive Level: Application **Client Need:** Health Promotion and Maintenance **Integrated Process:** Nursing Process: Assessment **Content Area:** Foundational Sciences: Nutrition **Strategy:** The core concept is *MODS.* Eliminate options 1, 3, and 4 since they focus on one type of parameter, which would be insufficient to identify nutritional needs. **Reference:** Rolfes, S., Pinna, K., & Whitney, E. (2006). *Understanding normal and clinical nutrition* (7th ed.). Belmont, CA: Wadsworth & Thomson Learning, p. 711.

5 **Answer: 2** It is important to provide a client with the most comprehensive information available to answer questions and clarify concerns. The consumption pattern (type and amount) of alcohol has been shown to be a risk factor in many disease processes—this should be clearly stated to the client. Option 1 is incorrect because even though moderate alcohol consumption has been documented to provide some cardiovascular benefits, the last portion of the statement indicates bias relative to the client's alcoholism. Option 3 is incorrect because it does not address the client's concern at this time. Option 4 is incorrect because it implies that the nurse does not believe the client's statement that he is an alcoholic. It is important for the nurse to respond to the question asked before delving further into confirming a diagnosis of alcoholism.
Cognitive Level: Application **Client Need:** Physiological Integrity: Physiological Adaptation **Integrated Process:** Communication and Documentation **Content Area:** Foundational Sciences: Nutrition **Strategy:** Note the psychological nature of the question as well as need to clarify misinformation. Option 1 makes an assumption, so eliminate it. Eliminate options 3 and 4 as they do not address the client's question. **Reference:** Rolfes, S., Pinna, K., & Whitney, E. (2006). *Understanding normal and clinical nutrition* (7th ed.). Belmont, CA: Wadsworth & Thomson Learning, p. 245–249.

6 **Answer: 4** A 48-year-old female client with the contributory diseases of hypertension (HTN) and diabetes is at a greater risk for nutritional problems than any of the other clients. HTN and diabetes both have dramatic effects on vascular status and lipid physiology. Option 1 is incorrect because there is no information to suggest that the client has any underlying health problems. Even though the client is obese in option 2, this represents only a single risk factor for nutritional status. Similarly, the client in option 3 has only a single risk factor, that of asthma.
Cognitive Level: Analysis **Client Need:** Physiological Integrity: Physiological Adaptation **Integrated Process:** Nursing Process: Analysis **Content Area:** Foundational Sciences: Nutrition **Strategy:** Read each option, identifying risk factors that would contribute to nutritional problems. Eliminate options 1 and 3 since each contains only one risk factor. Choose option 4 since this client has two chronic conditions. **Reference:** Rolfes, S., Pinna, K., & Whitney, E. (2006). *Understanding normal and clinical nutrition* (7th ed.). Belmont, CA: Wadsworth & Thomson Learning, p. 711.

7 **Answer: 4** A client taking warfarin should be aware of pertinent medication facts prior to initiation of therapy to avoid possible interactions and to maintain an adequate anticoagulation response. The client should eat a well-balanced diet and consume a constant amount of vitamin K that can interfere with the action of the medication. Green leafy vegetables are high in vitamin K. Option 1 is incorrect—the client should not double the dose because this can lead to severe consequences and altered coagulation. Option 2 is incorrect because a client taking warfarin should not take other medications unless the physician prescribes them. Option 3 is incorrect—even though it is important for the client to take the medication at the same time every day, it is also critical that the client be aware of the dosage. This information should be related as part of the client's pertinent medical history and can influence medical treatment by other healthcare providers.
Cognitive Level: Analysis **Client Need:** Physiological Integrity: Reduction of Risk Potential **Integrated Process:** Nursing Process: Evaluation **Content Area:** Foundational Sciences: Nutrition **Strategy:** Critical words are *complications* and *warfarin.* Recall this drug is an anticoagulant that requires maintenance of consistent blood levels and eliminate options 1 and 2 since they would alter steady blood levels. Choose option 4 since it addresses the most significant dietary information regarding warfarin. **Reference:** Rolfes, S., Pinna, K., & Whitney, E. (2006). *Understanding normal and clinical nutrition* (7th ed.). Belmont, CA: Wadsworth & Thomson Learning, pp. 382–384

8 **Answer: 3** Early tube feeding leads to fewer complications than parenteral feedings in the acute post-transplant period and is the preferred method if the client

has a functioning GI tract. Options 1 and 2 are incorrect because there is increased protein catabolism in the acute post-transplant period as well as an increase in the amount of urinary nitrogen. Option 4 is incorrect because the presence of end-stage liver disease is associated with a decrease in the amounts of branched chain amino acids, leading to an alteration in aromatic amino acids, which may further contribute to the presentation of hepatic encephalopathy.
Cognitive Level: Application **Client Need:** Health Promotion and Maintenance **Integrated Process:** Nursing Process: Planning **Content Area:** Foundational Sciences: Nutrition **Strategy:** The critical words are *post-transplant needs* and *liver.* Recall protein needs in catabolic and acute stress conditions to eliminate options 1 and 2. Eliminate option 4 since these acids are decreased in the post-operative state. If you had difficulty with this question, review content on the post-transplant client. **Reference:** Rolfes, S., Pinna, K., & Whitney, E. (2006). *Understanding normal and clinical nutrition* (7th ed.). Belmont, CA: Wadsworth & Thomson Learning, p. 778.

9 **Answer: 1** Adequate amounts of micronutrients (vitamins A and C, calcium, and zinc) will help support immune function and restore healing in the trauma client.
Cognitive Level: Application **Client Need:** Health Promotion and Maintenance **Integrated Process:** Nursing Process: Planning **Content Area:** Foundational Sciences: Nutrition **Strategy:** The core issue of the question is knowledge of which micronutrients play a key role in immune function and healing. Use this information and the process of elimination to make a selection. **Reference:** Rolfes, S., Pinna, K., & Whitney, E. (2006). *Understanding normal and clinical nutrition* (7th ed.). Belmont, CA: Wadsworth & Thomson Learning, pp. 350, 370–371.

10 **Answer: 4** Refeeding syndrome can occur in the critically ill client in response to feeding attempts whereby glucose and electrolytes (phosphorus, potassium, and magnesium) rapidly enter into body cells. These electrolytes are involved in enzyme reactions and ATP physiology that is part of metabolizing the TPN. Option 1 is incorrect because serum phosphorus levels are decreased dramatically in response to increased glucose needs. Options 2 and 3 are incorrect because hyperglycemia is present along with increased insulin resistance.
Cognitive Level: Application **Client Need:** Physiological Integrity: Physiological Adaptation **Integrated Process:** Nursing Process: Assessment **Content Area:** Foundational Sciences: Nutrition **Strategy:** Recall that refeeding syndrome occurs secondary to utilization of electrolytes involved in energy metabolic pathways to direct you to option 4. **Reference:** Rolfes, S., Pinna, K., & Whitney, E. (2006). *Understanding normal and clinical nutrition* (7th ed.). Belmont, CA: Wadsworth & Thomson Learning, p. 683.

References

Cataldo, C., DeBruyne, L.K., & Whitney, E. (2005). *Nutrition and diet therapy* (3rd ed.). Belmont, CA: Wadsworth & Thomson Learning, pp. 701–704.

Dudek, S. (2006). *Nutrition essentials for nursing practice* (5th ed.). Philadelphia: Lippincott, pp. 634–692.

Grodner, M., Anderson, S. L., & DeYoung, S. (2005). *Foundations and clinical applications of nursing: A nursing approach* (3rd ed.). St. Louis, MO: Mosby, pp. 519–526, 593–595, 621-631.

LeMone, P., & Burke, K. (2004). *Medical-surgical nursing: Critical thinking in client care* (3rd ed.). Upper Saddle River, NJ: Prentice Hall, pp. 601–602, 1166.

Lutz, C., & Przytulski, K. (2006). *Nutrition and diet therapy* (4th ed.). Philadelphia: F. A. Davis, pp. 529–544.

Rolfes, S., Pinna, K., & Whitney, E. (2006). *Understanding normal and clinical nutrition* (7th ed.). Belmont, CA: Wadsworth & Thomson, Learning, pp. 634–641.

Appendix

➤ Practice to Pass Suggested Answers

Chapter 1

Page 6: *Suggested Answer*—The Healthy People 2010 initiative from the federal government (Department of Health and Human Services) has two goals: to achieve an increase in the span of healthy life for Americans and to reduce health disparities among Americans. In order to attain these nutritional goals, the federal government has established these objectives: to establish and promote healthy behaviors and healthy food communities, to provide access to preventive healthcare for all Americans, and to prevent disease and clinical disorders.

Page 8: *Suggested Answer*—Important information includes:

- What is her definition of vegetarianism? What type of vegetarian diet is she following? Ask if she is eating eggs, dairy products, and/or fish.
- Does she understand and make an effort to use complementary proteins? If not, she will need teaching on matching food sources to ensure intake of complete proteins.
- Is her calcium intake adequate? If she is not eating dairy products, she will need information on other calcium sources.
- Is she taking any vitamin or mineral supplements?
- Is her family also following a vegetarian diet? What meal planning options does she have in the school setting or on a daily basis to meet vegetarian diet goals?

Page 9: *Suggested Answer*—The terms *free, low, very low, reduced, less, light* (or *lite*), *good source, high, rich in, excellent source, more, lean,* and *extra lean* are the only terms that can be used in making a health claim on a food product label. The food product must meet strict criteria in order to have the health claim on the label. Each term has a specific meaning:

- *Free:* Contains virtually none of the nutrient; can refer to calories, sugar, sodium, salt, fat, saturated fat, and cholesterol.
- *Low:* Contains a small enough amount of a nutrient that the product can be used without concern for exceeding dietary recommendations; can refer to sodium, calories, fat, saturated fat, and cholesterol.
- *Very Low:* Refers to sodium only; ≤ 35 mg.
- *Reduced or Less:* At least a 25% reduction in a nutrient from a comparable regular product.
- *Light or Lite:* 1/3 fewer calories or 50% less fat than a comparable regular product.
- *Good Source:* Provides 10–19% of the Daily Value for a nutrient.
- *High, Rich in, or Excellent Source:* Provides ≥ 20% of the Daily Value for a nutrient.
- *More:* Provides ≥ 10% of a desirable nutrient compared to a comparable product.
- *Lean:* Meat or poultry product containing < 10 grams fat, < 4 grams saturated fat, and < 95 mg cholesterol per 100 grams and standard-sized serving.
- *Extra Lean:* Meat or poultry product containing < 5 grams fat, < 2 grams saturated fat, and < 95 mg cholesterol per 100 grams and standard-sized serving.

Page 12: *Suggested Answer*—Height and weight are obtained and compared to tables such as the Metropolitan Life Insurance Table. The Body Mass Index is also computed. In addition, the use of BMI silhouettes can be used to have clients identify body image perceptions. The use of growth charts can be used to correlate height and weight patterns for newborn and pediatric clients. Determination of waist/hip ratio and skin fold thickness (TSF, MAC, and MAMC) can also be used to assess physical status.

This data provides information relative to whether the client is experiencing malnutrition (overnutrition or undernutrition) because anthropometric data are based on standardized measurements that have proven reliability and validity. If the data represents an abnormal weight pattern, then the client can be referred for more diagnostic testing looking for underlying contributory disease processes and other risk factors that may have caused these abnormal findings. An appropriate referral to a healthcare provider with follow up is needed in cases with abnormal findings.

Page 12: *Suggested Answer*—The BMI is calculated by first converting the height into meters and the weight into kilograms.

6 feet = 72 inches × 2.54 cm/inch ÷ 100 cm/meter
= 1.83 meters
275 lbs × .454 kilograms/pound = 124.8 kg

The formula for determining BMI is:

$$\text{Weight} \div (\text{Height})^2 = \text{BMI}$$
$$124.8 \div (1.83 \times 1.83) = 37.2$$

A BMI ≥ 30.0 indicates obesity.

Page 13: *Suggested Answer*—An albumin less than 3.5 grams/dL indicates protein deficiency malnutrition. It is important to ascertain more information relative to the client's medical status to see if there is any contributory disease that may be affecting the client's protein status. Usually, low albumin levels are evidence of poor nutritional status, although they can be influenced by other metabolic conditions resulting in loss (GI or renal), increased catabolism (fever, burns, or malignancy) and dilutional factors (dilutional hyponatremia or excess IV fluid administration). Looking at prealbumin and transferrin levels in conjunction with a full history and physical examination on this client would provide more definitive information.

Chapter 2

Page 25: *Suggested Answer*—One of the functions of protein is to participate in chemical reactions that influence acid-base and fluid/electrolyte balance. Low protein levels are associated with decreased colloid osmotic pressure and cause fluid shifting, leading to edema formation. High protein levels are associated with increased colloid osmotic pressure and capillary membrane integrity. Albumin (major protein of the plasma) participates in the interaction between colloid osmotic pressure and hydrostatic pressure of the capillaries to maintain vascular integrity.

Page 25: *Suggested Answer*—BCAA formulations are used in certain TPN solutions to replace essential amino acids (valine, leucine, and isoleucine) that may be needed in clients who have sustained losses due to extensive trauma or liver or renal failure. The provision of these essential nutrients helps to replace losses and restore balance.

Page 26: *Suggested Answer*—First, it would be important to establish the client's baseline weight, frame, and current health status in order to recommend instructions for adequate protein levels in the diet. A healthy adult client needs 0.8 gram/kg/day of protein in the diet. Next, it would be important to discuss the concepts of protein quality so that the client will realize which sources of protein will provide adequate value in his diet. It will also be important to include food preferences, potential allergies, and diet preferences in order to make reasonable choices with which the client can comply.

Page 28: *Suggested Answer*—Cholesterol is a necessary substance produced in the body that functions in lipid transport. HDL cholesterol has cardioprotective effects and clinical evidence has supported that it is as important to have a minimum level of HDL as it is to have reduced levels of LDL in the body. Cholesterol is needed for the synthesis of certain hormones; it is a component of bile salts; and it is normally found in the brain, nerve tissue, and throughout the blood.

Page 30: *Suggested Answer*—Hydrogenated food products reflect additional sources of saturated fats in the diet. Clients who increase their use of hydrogenated food products in the diet are at risk for developing associated cardiac and vascular manifestations that are attributable to a high saturated fat diet. These can include hypertension, coronary artery disease, and vascular changes that can result in serious health consequences.

Page 33: *Suggested Answer*—Adequate sources of fiber in the diet contribute to regulation of elimination patterns, blood glucose levels, decrease in cholesterol levels, and decrease in risk of certain cancers and diverticular disease. Fiber in the diet can also contribute to satiety.

Chapter 3

Page 45: *Suggested Answer*—Bioavailability relates to the amount of a substance that can be utilized by the body to perform metabolic functions. If there is a high bioavailability, then the absorption of the micronutrient will be increased. If there is a low bioavailability, then there is the potential for clinical deficiencies to occur because the micronutrient, even if supplied to the body, may not be in a form that can participate in metabolic reactions.

Page 56: *Suggested Answer*—Clients with alcoholism are likely to present with clinical evidence of malnutrition, altered metabolism, and impaired absorption leading to deficiencies of B complex vitamins (thiamin, folate, and B_{12}).

Page 61: *Suggested Answer*—Clients who are receiving antibiotic therapy may be at risk for developing vitamin K deficiency as the body is depleted of its normal protective flora. Intestinal bacteria are needed for vitamin K synthesis.

Page 63: *Suggested Answer*—Increased water requirements would be needed in response to increased physical activity; diets that are already high in protein, sodium, caffeine, and/or sodium; high environmental temperatures that lead to insensible fluid losses; and in metabolic conditions that lead to fluid loss.

Page 69: *Suggested Answer*—Magnesium functions as a coenzyme in multiple metabolic reactions involving neuromuscular transmission and leads to the relaxation of skeletal muscles.

Page 77: *Suggested Answer*—Trace elements are needed by the body to perform essential metabolic reactions and to prevent clinical deficiencies. While only small amounts are necessary, they should not be overlooked—clinical deficiencies can result in significant metabolic abnormalities of macronutrients and compromise the immune function of the individual.

Chapter 4

Page 86: *Suggested Answer*—Digestion of nutrients in the body is facilitated by muscular actions (peristalsis, segmentation, and sphincter contractions), chemical actions (digestive enzymes), mechanical actions (chewing in combination with enzyme support), and emulsification of fat. Factors that assist the body in the absorption of nutrients include the increased surface area of the microvilli found on the brush border. Factors that assist the body in the transport of nutrients include the vascular and lymphatic channels.

Page 88: *Suggested Answer*—Different pH environments of the body facilitate the process of digestion because they either promote or deter specific enzymatic activity. These differences in the chemical environment encourage the enzymatic action on specific substrates and assist the body to derive the most benefit from ingested nutrients.

Page 92: *Suggested Answer*—The clinical state of malabsorption affects the absorption and utilization of nutrients leading to poor nutritional status; altered fluid, electrolyte, and acid-base balance; and specific clinical deficiencies if not identified and treated. Malnutrition can arise from clinical states of malabsorption and depletion of body stores can occur, which can increase a client's risk for infection and ability to tolerate and withstand stress.

Page 94: *Suggested Answer*—Anabolism refers to chemical reactions in the body that require energy in the form of ATP and involve the building-up of body tissues. Catabolism refers to chemical reactions in the body that release energy in the form of ATP and involve the breaking-down of body tissues.

Page 95: *Suggested Answer*—Ketone bodies are formed as a response to the incomplete breakdown of fats due to decreased carbohydrate (CHO) levels. This acidotic state is due to impairment of CHO metabolism and can be seen in the diabetic client. Diabetic clients have altered CHO metabolism because they either do not produce insulin (Type 1—formerly known as IDDM) or they have increased resistance, decreased sensitivity at the peripheral tissues, and/or alterations in hepatic uptake (Type 2—formerly known as NIDDM). In addition, diabetic clients have altered lipid metabolism and usually present with some form of dyslipidemia.

Page 96: *Suggested Answer*—Fats are not considered to be a primary energy source in the body because multiple chemical reactions are required to generate energy release. Since the process requires so many steps to achieve energy release, it is not considered an efficient method to provide energy. Lipids are broken down into their constituent parts of glycerol and fatty acids and it is these very long fatty acid chains that require multiple degradation steps. In addition, only a small portion of fats can participate in conversion to glucose. CHOs are more energy efficient and the catabolic process takes place over a shorter period of time.

Page 98: *Suggested Answer*—Proteins are unique in the aspect of metabolism because they can enter the catabolic process via three pathways: glucogenic, ketogenic, or direct. The glucogenic pathway reflects amino acids that can be used to synthesize glucose. The ketogenic pathway reflects amino acids that can be directly converted to acetyl-coenzyme A (acetyl-coA). The direct pathway reflects amino acids that can enter the TCA cycle directly without undergoing chemical restructuring. Fats and carbohydrates do not have the ability to enter the catabolic pathway in this manner.

Chapter 5

Page 110: *Suggested Answer*—Preconceptual nutrition is a critical factor in providing a nutritional baseline for both the mother and fetus. It provides an accurate assessment of nutrient stores, identifies potential deficits, and allows the healthcare provider to assist in maintaining nutritional goals and outcomes for the soon-to-be pregnant client. In addition, it is possible to ascertain food preferences, dietary habits, and patterns of intake and incorporate them into an adequate plan to meet increased nutritional requirements during the time of pregnancy. Merely starting at the time of conception does not allow for the development of adequate nutritional stores and can lead to starting off the pregnancy in a nutritionally deficient state.

Page 123: *Suggested Answer*—Many working women are able to continue breastfeeding, if they are committed, even with periodic absences from their infants. The easiest solution is to pump breasts and freeze the milk for later use by the infant. If this technique is used, it is necessary to get the infant used to drinking from a bottle.

Page 135: *Suggested Answer*—Measures that may help avert feeding resistance include holding the infant during the enteral feedings, interacting face-to-face with the infant during enteral feedings, providing a pacifier, and gradually stroking the oral area from cheeks to lips.

Page 137: *Suggested Answer*—It is not uncommon for toddlers to demonstrate erratic patterns of eating. Provide a variety of foods for the child to select from. Other measures to increase intake include providing finger foods, increasing caloric density by adding powdered milk to regular milk, and trying one new food with a favorite food.

Page 137: *Suggested Answer*—The nurse must first inquire what the parent considers "excessive weight." It is not uncommon in later school age for children to appear heavier because they are laying down stores for the puberty growth spurt. If the child is truly gaining too much weight, information must be collected about dietary patterns and activity levels. If inactive, the child should be encouraged to increase activity levels slowly. If dietary patterns are inappropriate, suggest keeping high-calorie and high-fat foods to a minimum at home and offering healthy alternatives such as fruit and raw vegetables.

Page 141: *Suggested Answer*—The nurse should first determine what weight management techniques have been used in the past to screen for possible eating disorder (bulimia in particular) and to determine if past measures to manage weight could be adapted to college life. If the client does not seem to have a history of eating disorder, the nurse and client could collaboratively develop an exercise and eating plan to fit the changes in college—for instance, making time for exercise each day, finding a "buddy" at school to exercise with, utilizing campus fitness facilities, avoiding high-fat choices in the dining hall, and watching portion sizes in the dining hall. Even though the client has not had a past history of an eating disorder, the nurse should discuss the prevalence of this activity among college students and caution the client against using purging as a weight control method.

Page 145: *Suggested Answer*—As a normal consequence of aging, one's body undergoes metabolic rate changes that are consistent with level of activity and changes in eating patterns associated with lifestyle and occupational requirements. One normally expects to gain a few pounds as one ages. This is not related to any pathological concern, but rather is generally attributed to a decrease in activity and higher stress demands of family and job. It would be important to consider both dietary intake pattern, physical activity level, and overall physiologic function (adequate sleep and rest) in order to ascertain that caloric intake is sufficient to meet energy needs and not be excessive so as to cause weight gain.

Page 149: *Suggested Answer*—The nurse can assist the elderly client in meeting nutritional goals by performing an adequate nutritional assessment that focuses on dietary intake, available resources (both personal and financial), and determining whether there are any underlying/contributory medical conditions that may impact nutritional status. Many elderly clients are on limited financial budgets and as such may be at risk to develop nutritional deficiencies merely due to income factors rather than preference. It is important to perform a community assessment, looking at available resources—both community- and culturally based—that may assist the client in meeting nutritional goals.

Chapter 6

Page 161: *Suggested Answer*—Relevant assessment data includes fear of rejection by significant others, negative feelings verbalized about the body, feelings of helplessness or powerlessness, preoccupation with body change, client's family role, client's family support systems.

Page 163: *Suggested Answer*—

- Parkland formula: 4 mL Lactated Ringers solution × 84 kg × 45% = 15,120 mL; 7,560 mL over first 8 hours; 3,780 mL over second 8 hours; and 3,780 mL over third 8 hours
- Curreri formula: (25 kcal × 84 kg) + (40 kcal × 45%) = 3,900 kcal/24 hours

Page 168: *Suggested Answer*—Relevant admission data would include compliance with diet: three-day recall, sodium intake, food preparation techniques; compliance with medications; daily weights; use of over-the-counter drugs; daily exercise.

Page 173: *Suggested Answer*—Relevant subjective data would include usual weight; three-day diet recall; diet prescription; when diagnosed; diabetic and other medications; daily exercise pattern; blood glucose records; family history; symptoms (intermittent claudication, visual changes, skin dryness, itching, bloating, diarrhea, fatigue), wound healing; self-concept; job; support systems.

Page 181: *Suggested Answer*—Nursing interventions include monitor fluid I&O; daily weight; monitor vital signs; monitor serum electrolytes and hematocrit; monitor skin turgor, thirst, dry mucous membranes; provide good oral care; maintain IV fluids as ordered; promote skin integrity for client on bedrest.

Chapter 7

Page 196: *Suggested Answer*—Early intervention strategies for clients with HIV/AIDS should include a high kcal intake to help maintain body weight and body protein stores. Kilocalorie intake should be as high as 3,500 kcal/day. Liquid nutritional supplements may be necessary to supply extra energy. Several small meals throughout the day may be necessary to meet these requirements. A multivitamin or liquid supplements containing RDA level of vitamin and minerals in addition to meals/supplements is recommended. Clients should be referred to a dietitian to determine nutritional baseline status and develop individualized goals. Specific symptoms such as nausea and diarrhea should be aggressively managed in order to prevent dehydration and resulting fluid and electrolyte imbalances.

Page 199: *Suggested Answer*—Clients should:

- Eat frequent small meals using calorie-dense foods and liquid supplements fortified with vitamins and minerals.
- Limit liquids at meal times to ensure intake of foods.
- Serve foods at room temperature.
- Limit highly seasoned or greasy foods.
- Exercise regularly.
- Eat in a pleasant setting with companions.

Page 203: *Suggested Answer*—Hepatitis A (HAV) is a reversible liver disorder spread through a virus via contaminated food or water. Quite often, HAV is contracted in developing areas of the world with poor sanitation. Due to vomiting, adequate fluids must be given to prevent dehydration. In addition, a diet high in kcals and protein (2,000–4,000 kcals and 1.5–2.0 g protein/kg) is recommended. Hepatitis B (HBV) and Hepatitis C (HCV) in contrast, are irreversible liver diseases also spread by virus. Modes of transmission are primarily through blood, blood products, and, to a lesser extent, body fluids. These clients should be given a diet adequate in calories, protein, and most micronutrients. Iron is required by the virus for reproduction and may interfere with treatment using Interferon and thus should be limited. Goals should be maintenance of optimum body weight and maintenance of lean body mass.

Page 205: *Suggested Answer*—Painful swelling of the joints and limitation of mobility characterize osteoarthritis (OA). Most individuals will experience some effect of OA during their lifetime because it is a degenerative joint disease characterized by wear and tear. In order to optimize function, maintenance of optimal body weight is essential. Since pain is a predominant feature in the disease process, clients often are on prolonged pain medication that can cause GI side effects. Limitation of mobility can occur in response to arthritic pain and further affect weight status, as the client is unable to exercise or maintain activity level. Eventual progression of disease and pain symptoms can lead to surgical intervention and joint replacement, which can affect the client's nutritional status and reserves during the operative and postoperative periods. Rehabilitation can be a long-term process leading to increased nutrient needs during the healing period.

Page 218: *Suggested Answer*—A reduced protein, sodium, and potassium diet, along with reduced fluid intake, is recommended for the predialysis client. Adequate kcals must be provided to maintain body weight and provide energy. Fats and oils, simple carbohydrates, and low-protein starches should provide the nonprotein calories.

Chapter 8

Page 234: *Suggested Answer*—MNT utilizes a comprehensive nutritional assessment in the treatment of clients with defined healthcare needs. By including a baseline nutritional assessment, MNT provides a critical element in client care. Too often, the nutritional aspect of a client's case has been overlooked or minimized, leading to acute exacerbations with chronic implications. By recognizing a client's nutritional status and using it to establish comprehensive treatment goals, a client with defined healthcare needs will have better clinical outcomes.

Page 237: *Suggested Answer*—Ideal body weight (IBW), actual body weight, BEE, and pertinent labs such as electrolytes, serum chemistries, albumin, prealbumin, transferrin, and hemoglobin/hematocrit are necessary to establish overall nutritional requirements for the clients on nutritional support therapy. It is also important to recognize potential allergies/sensitivities (to foods and drugs) and the underlying clinical condition that initially places the client in need for this type of therapy.

Page 243: *Suggested Answer*—Clinical gout is due to an increase in uric acid either from excessive production or impaired excretion. Uric acid is the end product of purine catabolism, and increased ingestion of purine sources in the diet can lead to exacerbation of clinical symptoms if there is defective protein metabolism as in gout. It is important for the client to be educated about foods that are high in purines (such as organ meats, alcohol, anchovies, and seafood) and to limit intake in order to avoid clinical symptoms.

Page 245: *Suggested Answer*—This amount would indicate that the client is not adequately digesting the tube feeding. The feeding should be held and the residual evaluated again in 1 hour to determine client status. Adjustment of rate and/or method of feeding may be required in order to help the client manage the feeding. If the feeding continues and the client is unable to process the feeding, this can lead to metabolic complications and place the client at risk for fluid and electrolyte imbalances.

Page 251: *Suggested Answer*—TPN solutions are extremely concentrated hypertonic solutions with large amounts of dextrose and as such they are excellent mediums for bacterial overgrowth. The changing of TPN solutions every 24 hours helps to minimize this potential.

Page 252: *Suggested Answer*—It is necessary to follow a test diet in the clinical setting in order to obtain results that are consistent and reliable. Certain foods may be restricted or provided in order to assess how the body handles their absorption and/or metabolism. If the test diet is not followed correctly, then the results may be inconclusive or the diagnostic test may have to be repeated, leading to client and financial stress and possibly increasing the hospitalization or treatment time.

Page 254: *Suggested Answer*—Progressive diets (clear, full, soft, to regular) are used for postoperative surgical clients based on the resumption of gag reflex, gastrointestinal motility, and food tolerance without nausea or vomiting. The postoperative period is one in which clients recover from anesthesia and regain function of their GI tract and other body systems (musculoskeletal and neurological). If food or liquids are administered orally before a client is able to function, aspiration could occur. The client must be adequately assessed for clinical findings that demonstrate progression and resumption of "normal" body functioning.

Chapter 9

Page 264: *Suggested Answer*—Phytochemicals represent non-nutrient chemical substances that are found naturally in plants. Functional foods represent nutrient substances found in food items. Nutraceuticals represent a more comprehensive group that bridges the gap between phytochemicals and functional foods. Nutraceuticals include naturally made products such as botanicals and phytochemicals. All of the above classifications are being viewed as having potential health benefits, ranging from antioxidant function to cancer prevention. These categories represent a new field of therapeutic treatment that is being actively pursued for its beneficial effects on the human body.

Page 266: *Suggested Answer*—Client teaching should include (1) A review of the client's present health status, pertinent PMH, and medications (both prescription and OTC)—this will allow the nurse to adequately assess the client for potential interactions and contraindications relative to the herbal product. It will also allow the nurse to assess if the client's practitioner is aware of the client's starting a new therapy. It is important that all members of the healthcare team are aware of herbal therapy use. (2) Ascertain what health benefit the client thinks will be gained from taking this herbal product—this will establish the factual nature of the herbal product as there may be some confusion about what health benefit is available and/or if the product is clinically indicated. (3) Discuss which form of the herbal preparation the client will take—this information will affect the dosage and application of the herbal product. (4) Discuss the time frame of herbal therapy—many herbal products require several weeks of use before any health benefits are realized. The client needs to understand this fact because he or she might think that the benefits will be more immediate; this could lead to discontinuation of the therapy. (5) Discuss the importance of reported side effects—it is important for the client to understand what effects can be realized from the use of these types of products (beneficial, side effects, and toxicity symptoms).

Page 270: *Suggested Answer*—A diabetic client already has an underlying problem with carbohydrate metabolism, thus, the addition of chromium as a nutritional supplement may cause potential problems for this type of client. It is important to ascertain what type and dosage of chromium the client is planning to take along with the frequency of administration. If the client has existing problems with glycemic control and is prone to hypoglycemia, the use of chromium supplements might exacerbate this clinical condition. It would also be important to find out why the client wants to use this supplementation and what health benefit he thinks will be achieved.

Page 271: *Suggested Answer*—It is critical that nurses (and all members of the healthcare team) be aware of nutritional supplements that a client may be taking. Clients with defined health problems (and even those who are considered to be healthy) may be affected by the use of nutritional supplements. It is important to assess and evaluate the client for potential interactions and adverse effects on the client's overall metabolic state. If the client has a defined health problem, the use of certain nutritional supplements could be contraindicated. Once the information is received, it is up to the nurse performing the assessment to notify members of the healthcare team about the use of nutritional supplements.

Page 279: *Suggested Answer*—The nurse can assist the client in meeting defined weight goals by helping the client to set realistic goals based on individualized client needs. The nurse, using available subjective (behaviors, beliefs, and culture) and objective (BMI, pertinent labs, and evaluation of client baseline health) data, can help the client to achieve outcomes. Incorporating interventions that are based on scientific principles and yet realize individual preferences and financial and cultural resources will facilitate compliance. Continued follow-up, client education, and monitoring with possible revision will lead to goal achievement.

Chapter 10

Page 292: *Suggested Answer*—A client who has preexisting malnutrition and is on ventilator therapy already has compromised muscle function, central ventilatory drive effort, and inability to mount a suitable defense against possible lung infection. Decreased visceral protein stores lead to increased likelihood of fatigue and an ineffective immune response in a client who is further experiencing stress and hypermetabolism.

Page 294: *Suggested Answer*—The nutritional priority in a trauma client is restoration of adequate fluid volume and maintenance of hemodynamic status. Dietary interventions are not needed during the acute phase management of the trauma client. Critical dietary information that could be helpful in the management of the trauma client would relate to prior dietary intake if surgical intervention is necessary. This information would relate to choice of anesthesia and likelihood of aspiration.

Page 296: *Suggested Answer*—High-acuity clients are prone to micronutrient deficiencies that can have substantial impact on a client's ability to mount an immune response. Clinical research has demonstrated that selenium deficiencies occur during periods of critical illness and that the use of selenium therapy improves APACHE scoring. Low phosphorus levels correlate with increased likelihood of refeeding syndrome, seen in clients experiencing starvation. Potassium losses can occur in response to cell death. As the acuity of the client increases, so does the metabolic response, leading to increased deficiency states as a result of cellular death. Low iron levels are associated with anemia, and examination of transferrin levels will reveal accurate information relative to the body's iron stores. A clinical deficiency of zinc and copper has been correlated with a poor immune response. Deficits of sodium and magnesium affect fluid balance and neuromuscular transmission of impulses.

Page 299: *Suggested Answer*—The more medications that a client is taking, the greater the chance of drug interactions leading to multiple systemic effects. It is critical to have an accurate history of what medications a client takes, the prescribed dosage, and how the client is taking medication therapy. Too often, clients continue to take medication even though it may no longer be required. In addition, clients may store medications and self-medicate when they experience similar problems without going to a healthcare provider for diagnosis and therapeutic management. Periodically, all medication therapy should be reviewed and evaluated with the client, making note of both OTC and prescription drugs. In addition, the increased effects of herbal supplements can cause potential drug interactions and so should be included in a medication review.

Page 302: *Suggested Answer*—A client who has had a transplant already has documented end organ damage and alterations in vascular integrity. Poor nutritional status is a common presentation in any transplant client due to the effects of the disease process, treatment methods used, and medication therapy instituted. In addition, transplant clients often have altered intake patterns related to side effects of treatment protocols and adverse effects of the disease process that has led to the need for organ transplant. During the post-transplant phase, the client undergoes a hypermetabolic response and is at increased nutritional risk due to immunosuppressive protocols used to prevent clinical signs of organ rejection. The use of immunosuppressive therapy places the client at increased risk for weight gain, hypertension, hyperlipidemia, diabetes mellitus, and osteoporosis.

➤ Case Study Suggested Answers

Chapter 1

1. Important information to include would be (a) how the goals were developed by the federal government (Office of Disease Prevention and Health Promotion of the U.S. Department of Health and Human Services), (b) what the goals are and how they apply to this community group, and (c) how this group can achieve the goals.
2. Not just an increase in the amount of time Americans live, but that all Americans, especially the elderly, will be healthy while they are alive.
3. Currently, middle- and upper-class Caucasians live longer, have healthier pregnancies, and have better survival rates of MI (heart attack), CVA (stroke), and all forms of cancer. This goal seeks to improve health outcomes for poor Americans and Americans of color regardless of income.
4. The nutritional target areas addressed in Healthy People 2010 relate to weight control issues (obesity, overweight, and underweight), dietary intake issues (fats, fruits and vegetables, grains, sodium, and iron), school nutrition issues (meals and snacks and anemia in pregnancy) and nutrition education issues (assessment, planning, and security).
5. MyPyramid seeks to increase dietary consumption of vegetables and complex carbohydrates and decrease intake of animal protein (meat) and all fats in order to decrease the risk of cardiovascular disease and obesity (and subsequent sequelae). Explaining the benefits of more healthful eating to this community group may help decrease the risk factors associated with poor nutrition.

Chapter 2

1. The lipid profile reveals a somewhat decreased HDL level (normal range for HDL is 35–70 mg/dL based on client's age). LDL level is slightly elevated (normal range for LDL is 60–180 mg/dL based on client's age). Triglyceride level is within normal range (51–197 mg/dL). Results imply that the HDL level is not sufficient to exert cardioprotective effects; increased LDL level is contributing to hypercholesterolemia; and triglycerides are WNL at this time.
2. Elevated serum cholesterol places the client at an increased risk for cardiovascular events. The client already has an established diagnosis of coronary artery disease and hypertension, which suggests the client's overall vascular status has already been altered by fat and plaque deposition leading to vascular changes. The client requires aggressive clinical management in order to prevent end organ damage and increased risk of cardiac events that could lead to increased mortality.
3. Dietary instructions that can be given to the client to reduce dietary fat intake and lower serum cholesterol levels include (a) read food labels to look for hidden sources of fat in the diet and limit foods accordingly that may contribute to this type of hidden intake, (b) trim excess fat from foods and do not use additional fat sources during the cooking process, (c) select food items that have a lower fat content or use fat alternatives/substitutes in the diet, (d) include adequate fiber in the diet, and (e) eat a well-balanced diet that consists of fruits and vegetables and adequate fluid intake.
4. Serum protein levels, albumin, prealbumin, transferrin, serum chemistry profile, CBC with differential, and UA may provide information about protein stores, glucose balance, and renal/liver status. Clients who have been diagnosed with coronary artery disease, hypertension, and hypercholesterolemia are at risk to develop other disease states such as diabetes and renal problems and should be assessed for normal function. If any of the specific tests reveal abnormalities, additional testing may be required to further determine the etiology.
5. Although not specifically mentioned, the client's medication status has not been listed in the above clinical scenario, and it is possible that the client may be taking a diuretic and/or antihypertensive agent to control hypertension. In addition, if dietary interventions fail to reduce cholesterol levels, the use of antilipidemic agents may be indicated to decrease serum cholesterol levels. Closer follow-up monitoring of the client's condition and response to treatment may be indicated for better compliance. Referral to a dietitian should be included in order to educate client and evaluate compliance in meeting individualized dietary goals.

Chapter 3

1. It would be important to ascertain food preferences (likes and dislikes) in order to make reasonable recommendations that will increase compliance. In addition, it would be important to note what type of diet pattern the client follows and whether she uses any type of supplement or OTC preparations that might affect dietary intake. A review of elimination patterns may lead to discovery of potential GI disturbances that might affect the client's nutritional status. A baseline review of lab work (CBC and serum chemistries) will help to identify potential deficiencies that may influence dietary recommendations. Finally, a review of the client's physical activity status (time frame schedule), cooking/dining lifestyle, and financial status will impact dietary recommendations.
2. In order to maximize the absorption of vitamins and minerals, it is important not to overcook vegetables, which leads to vitamin and mineral loss in cooking fluids. Steaming of fresh vegetables is suggested to prevent loss of nutrients. Fruits and vegetables can be eaten in their raw state after a thorough rinsing. Vegetables can be sautéed in a small amount of water or oil; if fluid remains in the cooking pan, it would be wise to use that fluid as part of a sauce base in order to retain the nutrients lost during cooking. Microwave cooking can lead to inactivation of

certain B vitamins and should not be utilized as a primary preparation method.

3. A referral to a dietitian would be helpful to coordinate resources and to provide more extensive dietary teaching and instruction.
4. While dietary supplements may be helpful for certain clients, this particular client expressed a desire to achieve goals through dietary intake. The use of a multivitamin supplement may be indicated to support the client in meeting identified needs, but it is important to follow the RDA recommendations so that intake remains within an acceptable range.
5. The use of megavitamin therapy is not without problems because excessive intake levels of vitamins and minerals can lead to the development of toxicity symptoms. It is important to have the client look at scientific clinical evidence that will support the use of additional therapies. Client education to facilitate accurate reading of labels and knowledge of nutrients will help the client to make realistic decisions.

Chapter 4

1. It would be important to determine the type, amount, and frequency of alcohol ingestion, as well as the time frame pattern during which the client has consumed alcohol. Information about the client's perception of whether alcohol use is a problem would also be pertinent. The use of the CAGE questionnaire would help in determining whether the client has a problem with alcohol consumption and may bring the issue to the forefront of discussion. Note whether the client has experienced any physical or emotional changes relative to alcohol ingestion. Obtain a complete nutritional assessment on this client, focusing on dietary patterns and usual food consumption. This is critical to determine nutritional status and will help ascertain what role alcohol plays in the diet structure.
2. Consuming alcohol can lead to the development of metabolic acidosis in the body. NAD becomes oxidized to NADH + H, which interferes with acetyl-coA's entering the TCA cycle. This in itself leads to the development of fatty acids and ketone bodies. This acidotic state increases the amount of fatty acids present and changed into triglycerides. The resulting effect is that the liver experiences fatty liver changes, which becomes clinically significant and leads to liver failure.
3. Alcohol provides empty calories (7 kcal/g), as it contributes calories but no proteins, vitamins, or mineral content. Usually alcohol consumption is accompanied by a decrease in appetite because of these "empty" calories. The presence of alcohol can lead to alterations in gastric activity because it reduces the absorption of certain nutrients (vitamins and minerals) as well as alters the gastric mucosa leading to other GI complaints. Decreased intake of B vitamins can lead to increases in homocysteine levels; this can correlate with an increased incidence of cardiac disease. The prolongation of nutritional deficiencies can lead to the development of nutritional anemia (vitamin B_{12} and folate deficiencies) with resultant clinical effects.
4. One would expect to see multiple deficiencies of the B vitamins, notably thiamin, folate, and vitamin B_{12}. The presence of alcohol in the diet leads to decreased absorption, decreased intake, and increased urinary excretion of vitamins and other nutrients. Multiple electrolyte deficiencies may also be seen, notably magnesium, calcium, and potassium.
5. Supplementation with vitamins may be indicated for this client to correct deficiencies. However, it is important to alter the pattern of consumption by obtaining appropriate referrals and having the client involved in a therapeutic program to stop alcohol intake. Depending on the nature and amount of alcohol consumed, the client may not feel that he even has a problem and therefore, unless the client is experiencing physical/mental changes or lifestyle alterations, it may be hard to start a treatment program. Continued monitoring and follow-up of the client with regularly established visits with a healthcare provider may foster compliance and prevent complications from occurring. Client education about the effects of continued alcohol consumption must be clearly provided without prejudice and continued support must be offered to the client and family members. It is important to keep the lines of communication open and acknowledge emerging client concerns.

Chapter 5

1. Minimum information required would include weight, height, BMI, activity level at work and home, vital signs, complete physical exam looking for signs of chronic illness (hypertension, diabetes, etc.), usual dietary patterns, and personal health goals. A more comprehensive assessment would include past history, family history, and laboratory studies (CBC, renal panel, serum protein, and urinalysis).
2. Follow these 4 steps to calculate the client's caloric needs:

   Step one—Calculate BMR (11 × ideal weight = BMR)
   Step two—Calculate energy for physical activity (0.20 × BMR = calories for physical activity or CPA)
   Step three—Calculate thermic effect (BMR + CPA × 0.10 = thermic effect)
   Step four—Add answers from first three steps (BMR + CPA + thermic effect) = total caloric expenditure

3. It is important to ascertain the type of eating patterns, food preferences (likes and dislikes), preferred preparation methods, restricted food items, and what value the client places on food and eating behaviors. Ethnic, cultural, and religious factors can have considerable impact on choice, preparation, and importance of food in the diet. Many foods can have symbolic meanings and affect dietary selections.

4. The client needs to engage in aerobic exercise, strength training, and stretching. Aerobic exercise should be a minimum of 30 minutes of low to moderate physical activity most days. Examples of moderate activity include walking at 3–4 mph, swimming, canoeing, and ice skating. The activity duration, intensity, and frequency should increase over time; more vigorous activities include brisker walking, cycling, and running. Strength training exercises should be performed two times per week and stretching exercises a minimum of three times per week. Perform 8–10 strength training exercises that work the major muscle groups, 8–12 repetitions of each exercise. Increase the weight over time; maintain proper form and breathing throughout weight lifts. Select stretching exercises that maintain posture; hold stretch for 30 seconds and repeat 3–5 times. To ensure safe exercising, obtain the resting heart rate, the target heart rate zone, and the maximum heart rate. Most beginning exercisers should exercise at 50–75% of maximum heart rate.

Chapter 6

1. Increasing age leads to reduced elasticity in arteries; atherosclerosis; family history; HTN is more prevalent in men; postmenopausal women lose the protective qualities of estrogen and are at greater risk for development of coronary artery disease (CAD).
2. Smoking, sedentary lifestyle, high sodium intake, weight gain, stress (loss of spouse).
3. Teach client to read labels for sodium content; increase intake of potassium-rich foods; decrease fat intake to < 30% of total calories; decrease cholesterol intake to < 200 mg/day; decrease use of canned foods; increase use of fresh fruits and vegetables; reduce caloric intake to reduce weight.
4. Regular daily exercise; stop smoking (offer cessation classes or support groups); stress management techniques.
5. Nursing diagnoses could include the following:
   - Altered health maintenance related to lack of knowledge about hypertension, effects of smoking, and sedentary lifestyle
   - Altered nutrition: more than body requirements related to high sodium intake, weight gain, and high fat and cholesterol intake
   - Ineffective coping related to loss of husband and possible use of food as coping mechanism
   - Social isolation related to loss of husband and withdrawal from friends and family

Chapter 7

1. Using the client's height and weight, the BMI can be calculated as 23 (23.16 to be exact), which indicates that the client is of normal weight at the present time. A BP of 138/98 indicates hypertension because the diastolic is > 90. Respirations and pulse are within normal limits. At the present time, other than the noted hypertension, the client appears to be stable.
2. On inspection of CBC results, one would expect to see anemia due to decreased erythropoietin production and possible hemoconcentration. The differential may reveal a normocytic normochromic anemia. Chemistry profile would reveal increased creatinine and BUN levels, elevated BUN/creatinine ratio, hyperkalemia, hyperphosphatemia, decreased bicarbonate level, and hypocalcemia secondary to renal failure. Because the client also has Type 1 diabetes, labs may reveal an elevated glucose level. Urinalysis might reveal presence of blood, protein, or casts dependent on etiology of renal failure or whether the client's diabetes is under good control.
3. Since the client is already being treated for diabetes and hypertension, it would be important to determine the client's current diet pattern and what medications the client is taking because medications can impact nutritional status. We know that the client is taking insulin therapy, but there is no information regarding treatment for hypertension. In addition, it would be important to learn results of Hemoglobin A_{1c} levels in order to assess client compliance with diabetes regimen and provide information as to client's nutritional status. It would also be helpful to have the client complete a 24-hour diet recall in order to determine how he is eating on a daily basis. It would also be important to determine if the client eats out a lot, smokes, or drinks because these behaviors can influence nutritional intake and disease processes.
4. Even though dialysis may ultimately be a necessary treatment option, at the present time, it is important for the client to understand that a collaborative approach between him and the healthcare team members (physician, practitioner, nurse, and dietitian) will help to establish treatment goals and help the client achieve the optimal function. Frank discussion of the client's risk factors—diabetes and hypertension—should occur, but the underlying cause of the renal failure should be determined because this will provide necessary information relative to prognosis and treatment. Offer emotional support to the client by being available to talk to both the client and family members. Answer questions honestly and openly and assist client as needed.
5. Clients with renal failure will have dietary restrictions in potassium, protein, and phosphorus. The dietitian will calculate specific energy requirements, calcium, and fluid levels on an individualized basis. The client will be placed on a renal diet that will reflect these restrictions, and intake and output will be monitored closely along with daily weights. Depending on the stage of renal failure the client is experiencing, alterations in specific nutrient values will occur based on lab values and current kidney function. Since food and fluid intake are critical at this point in time, it is important that all food and fluid intake be counted in the client's daily intake. Dietary counseling with the dietitian and initiation of medical nutrition therapy will help to maintain an optimal nutritional intake. Evaluation of the client's diabetic status will help to determine if the diabetes is adequately controlled or if the stress of this new disease process is causing

fluctuations in the client's ability to maintain glycemic control. The use of medication therapy and treatment regimens can affect both the client's nutritional status and intake ability; therefore, the healthcare team must collaborate in effective management goals for this client.

Chapter 8

1. The initial baseline monitoring parameters include height/weight (IBW, actual body weight, and BSA), individualized energy needs based on specific nutrients (macronutrients, micronutrients, and fluids), serum electrolytes (glucose, creatinine, BUN, Mg, Ca, and PO_4), protein stores (albumin, prealbumin, and transferrin), fat stores (triglycerides and cholesterol), and determination of liver and renal function.
2. The client should be weighed every 24 hours using the same scale, clothing, and at the same time in order to trend results and assess for possible fluid imbalances during the course of therapy.
3. A client receiving TPN often experiences elevated glucose levels because this hypertonic solution has dextrose as a major component. Orders for insulin by a sliding scale are part of the protocol and regular insulin is administered to normalize serum glucose levels. If the client's blood glucose continues to be elevated, then insulin can also be included as an additive in the TPN solution.
4. A suitable response would include the information that TPN is indicated for clients who do not have a functioning GI tract. At the present time, this treatment regimen is being prescribed to meet his nutritional and metabolic needs. This doesn't mean that the therapy will be permanent, but at the present time it will provide the best form of nutritional support.
5. In order to evaluate the client's response to treatment, it is important to monitor and trend pertinent lab results, weight gain patterns, and assess for return of "normal" GI functioning as evidenced by bowel sounds and elimination patterns.

Chapter 9

1. Two medications have currently been approved by the FDA for weight loss in the obese client: sibutramine HCl monohydrate (Meridia) and orlistat (Xenical).
2. It would be necessary to perform a complete history and physical with pertinent laboratory and diagnostic studies so that the client's health status and baseline are established prior to starting any drug therapy. It would also be important to note if the client has any past history of weight loss treatments (exercise, medications, or OTC preparations), normal dietary pattern/behaviors, and exercise pattern. It is important to note that merely taking a pill does not ensure that weight loss will be effective or be maintained. Lifestyle modifications including behavior, exercise, and approach to food are all required to establish healthy eating patterns and establish weight control.
3. Depending on the medication that the physician chooses for this client, the client will need instructions about expected side effects, and the client must be alerted to potential complications for any medication therapy. In addition, follow-up appointments focusing on pertinent labs and diagnostics with monitoring of weight patterns will help the client to realize that the healthcare team is supportive. Lifestyle modifications that are instituted can be evaluated periodically as the client sees what works and what doesn't. The client may also require supportive counseling so as to be able to share feelings and foster compliance.
4. It would be important to note behaviors related to eating, exercise pattern, and lifestyle behaviors that influence dietary selections and how the client perceives her body image. In order to set realistic goals, it is critical that the client be closely involved in identifying and selecting dietary measures to achieve weight control. The client must understand what medication can and can't do and that medication therapy is only one part of the comprehensive therapy that will work toward achieving a realistic goal. It is important to determine what the client thinks is a realistic goal, because the client's goal might not be realistic based on the physical characteristics of the individual, and this would need further discussion.
5. Clients who have weight control issues (obesity or underweight) often have altered perception of body image and psychological sensitivities about to their weight status. It is important to recognize the client's needs and worries and offer emotional support. Depending on the nature of the client's stated "depression," referral to psychological counseling may be indicated. It is very hard to assure the client that weight loss (or gain) will be permanent, but, rather, it is essential to talk about the total picture of lifestyle modifications, as this will provide the greatest chance of meeting and maintaining goals.

Chapter 10

1. It is critical to have documented baseline results of coagulation studies, specifically looking at aPPT, PT, and INR levels. A client who is being discharged on warfarin therapy will have scheduled follow-up lab work that evaluates PT and INR levels to determine response to therapy. Follow-up vascular studies may be indicated if the client presents with symptom complaints based on swelling or pain. If the client's PT and INR levels do not indicate adequate response to treatment, referral to a hematologist may be indicated for further diagnostic workup related to clotting abnormalities and possibility of antiphospolipid syndrome.
2. Referral to a dietitian is a critical component for any client who will be discharged on anticoagulant therapy. Dietary information is given after obtaining an accurate dietary history, noting diet selections and client's prefer-

ences, and establishing IBW (ideal body weight) and caloric intake. Dietary instruction should be given regarding food choices that are high in vitamin K. The client and family members should receive an instruction booklet noting clearly identified food choices and how anticoagulation therapy has significant potential food and drug interactions. It is important that this dietary information be given in several recurring sessions and that understanding of information is evaluated prior to discharge. The client should be allowed to ask questions and information should be given both verbally and in written form in order to maintain accuracy and prevent errors in assumption or translation.

3. The client taking warfarin therapy should have regularly scheduled blood work as ordered by his healthcare provider and continue to receive dietary counseling from the dietician. It is important for the client to keep all regularly scheduled appointments with the healthcare provider and to report any signs or symptoms of potential interactions/side effects immediately. The client must understand that the prescribing healthcare provider should evaluate all medication, both OTC and prescription, to avoid potential interactions. Adequate communication among all members of the healthcare team should be stressed.
4. The client should maintain a diet that is balanced in terms of vitamin K activity. In addition, the client should not alter his diet drastically (as this may affect levels of vitamin K) or eat foods that are high in vitamin K on a daily basis. Given the client's height and weight, the client should be advised to lose weight as this will help to decrease the risk of thrombolic events.
5. It would be important to acknowledge the client's concerns regarding the length of medication therapy, but it is also important to tell the client that long-term anticoagulation therapy (as prescribed by his physician) is warranted to prevent further episodes of blood clots. The nature of the therapy is not defined by a week or even a 10-day period as with certain types of medication therapy (antibiotics). The client should be educated about the importance of maintaining a therapeutic regimen to reduce the risk of blood clot formation leading to further hospitalizations in the future. It is important to offer support to the client and apprise him that his care will be both supportive and ongoing and that a collaborative effort by members of his healthcare team is in place.

Index

Page numbers followed by f indicate figure; those followed by b indicate box; those followed by t indicate table.

O

P

Q

R

U

V

Pearson Education, Inc.

YOU SHOULD CAREFULLY READ THE TERMS AND CONDITIONS BEFORE USING THE CD-ROM PACKAGE. USING THIS CD-ROM PACKAGE INDICATES YOUR ACCEPTANCE OF THESE TERMS AND CONDITIONS.

Pearson Education, Inc. provides this program and licenses its use. You assume responsibility for the selection of the program to achieve your intended results, and for the installation, use, and results obtained from the program. This license extends only to use of the program in the United States or countries in which the program is marketed by authorized distributors.

LICENSE GRANT

You hereby accept a nonexclusive, nontransferable, permanent license to install and use the program ON A SINGLE COMPUTER at any given time. You may copy the program solely for backup or archival purposes in support of your use of the program on the single computer. You may not modify, translate, disassemble, decompile, or reverse engineer the program, in whole or in part.

TERM

The License is effective until terminated. Pearson Education, Inc. reserves the right to terminate this License automatically if any provision of the License is violated. You may terminate the License at any time. To terminate this License, you must return the program, including documentation, along with a written warranty stating that all copies in your possession have been returned or destroyed.

LIMITED WARRANTY

THE PROGRAM IS PROVIDED "AS IS" WITHOUT WARRANTY OF ANY KIND, EITHER EXPRESSED OR IMPLIED, INCLUDING, BUT NOT LIMITED TO, THE IMPLIED WARRANTIES OR MERCHANTABILITY AND FITNESS FOR A PARTICULAR PURPOSE. THE ENTIRE RISK AS TO THE QUALITY AND PERFORMANCE OF THE PROGRAM IS WITH YOU. SHOULD THE PROGRAM PROVE DEFECTIVE, YOU (AND NOT PRENTICE-HALL, INC. OR ANY AUTHORIZED DEALER) ASSUME THE ENTIRE COST OF ALL NECESSARY SERVICING, REPAIR, OR CORRECTION. NO ORAL OR WRITTEN INFORMATION OR ADVICE GIVEN BY PRENTICE-HALL, INC., ITS DEALERS, DISTRIBUTORS, OR AGENTS SHALL CREATE A WARRANTY OR INCREASE THE SCOPE OF THIS WARRANTY.

SOME STATES DO NOT ALLOW THE EXCLUSION OF IMPLIED WARRANTIES, SO THE ABOVE EXCLUSION MAY NOT APPLY TO YOU. THIS WARRANTY GIVES YOU SPECIFIC LEGAL RIGHTS AND YOU MAY ALSO HAVE OTHER LEGAL RIGHTS THAT VARY FROM STATE TO STATE.

Pearson Education, Inc. does not warrant that the functions contained in the program will meet your requirements or that the operation of the program will be uninterrupted or error-free.

However, Pearson Education, Inc. warrants the diskette(s) or CD-ROM(s) on which the program is furnished to be free from defects in material and workmanship under normal use for a period of ninety (90) days from the date of delivery to you as evidenced by a copy of your receipt.

The program should not be relied on as the sole basis to solve a problem whose incorrect solution could result in injury to person or property. If the program is employed in such a manner, it is at the user's own risk and Pearson Education, Inc. explicitly disclaims all liability for such misuse.

LIMITATION OF REMEDIES

Pearson Education, Inc.'s entire liability and your exclusive remedy shall be:

1. the replacement of any diskette(s) or CD-ROM(s) not meeting Pearson Education, Inc.'s "LIMITED WARRANTY" and that is returned to Pearson Education, or

2. if Pearson Education is unable to deliver a replacement diskette(s) or CD-ROM(s) that is free of defects in materials or workmanship, you may terminate this agreement by returning the program.

IN NO EVENT WILL PRENTICE-HALL, INC. BE LIABLE TO YOU FOR ANY DAMAGES, INCLUDING ANY LOST PROFITS, LOST SAVINGS, OR OTHER INCIDENTAL OR CONSEQUENTIAL DAMAGES ARISING OUT OF THE USE OR INABILITY TO USE SUCH PROGRAM EVEN IF PRENTICE-HALL, INC. OR AN AUTHORIZED DISTRIBUTOR HAS BEEN ADVISED OF THE POSSIBILITY OF SUCH DAMAGES, OR FOR ANY CLAIM BY ANY OTHER PARTY.

SOME STATES DO NOT ALLOW FOR THE LIMITATION OR EXCLUSION OF LIABILITY FOR INCIDENTAL OR CONSEQUENTIAL DAMAGES, SO THE ABOVE LIMITATION OR EXCLUSION MAY NOT APPLY TO YOU.

GENERAL

You may not sublicense, assign, or transfer the license of the program. Any attempt to sublicense, assign or transfer any of the rights, duties, or obligations hereunder is void.

This Agreement will be governed by the laws of the State of New York.

Should you have any questions concerning this Agreement, you may contact Pearson Education, Inc. by writing to:

Director of New Media
Higher Education Division
Pearson Education, Inc.
One Lake Street
Upper Saddle River, NJ 07458

Should you have any questions concerning technical support, you may contact:

Product Support Department: Monday–Friday 8:00 A.M. –8:00 P.M. and Sunday 5:00 P.M.-12:00 A.M. (All times listed are Eastern). 1-800-677-6337

You can also get support by filling out the web form located at http://247.prenhall.com

YOU ACKNOWLEDGE THAT YOU HAVE READ THIS AGREEMENT, UNDERSTAND IT, AND AGREE TO BE BOUND BY ITS TERMS AND CONDITIONS. YOU FURTHER AGREE THAT IT IS THE COMPLETE AND EXCLUSIVE STATEMENT OF THE AGREEMENT BETWEEN US THAT SUPERSEDES ANY PROPOSAL OR PRIOR AGREEMENT, ORAL OR WRITTEN, AND ANY OTHER COMMUNICATIONS BETWEEN US RELATING TO THE SUBJECT MATTER OF THIS AGREEMENT.